Essentials of Biostatistics

Essentials of Biostatistics

DR. NISHI AGGARWAL
PhD (Statistics)

New Delhi Tuberculosis Centre
State TB Training and Demonstration Centre
Jawaharlal Nehru Marg
New Delhi - 110002

PEEPEE

PUBLISHERS AND DISTRIBUTORS (P) LTD

Essentials of Biostatistics

Published by
Pawaninder P. Vij

Peepee Publishers and Distributors (P) Ltd.
Head Office: 160, Shakti Vihar, Pitam Pura, Delhi-110 034 (India)

Correspondence Address:
7/31, First Floor, Ansari Road, Daryaganj, Post Box-7243
New Delhi-110 002 (India)

Ph: 65195868, 9811156083, 23246245

e-mail: peepee160@yahoo.co.in

e-mail: peepee160@rediffmail.com

e-mail: peepee160@gmail.com

www.peepeepub.com

First Edition: **2010**

ISBN: 81-8445-080-X

Printed at
Lordson, C-5/19, Rana Pratap Bagh, Delhi-110 007

This book is the result of encouragement of my loving parents
Dr. P.K. Aggarwal and Mrs. Prem Aggarwal

Gifted to my beloved
Husband ***Dr. K.K. Aggarwal***
Sons: ***Shashwat and Suchet***

To
Friends and Colleagues

Foreward

One of the most important aspects of research in medical practice is analysis of results of any study. Interpretation of results of any study or project requires understanding of the basic principles of Biostatistics and their applications to assess the results and present the same as required for the study or the project in a more comprehensive as well as eye catching manner. The medical students both undergraduates as well as postgraduates usually find themselves at a disadvantage when planning a protocol and their research study, ascertain about the sample size, designing a project, applying suitable tests for the estimates and interpreting the results as per the study requirement.

This book written by Dr. Nishi Aggarwal, Statistician, New Delhi Tuberculosis Centre fills the gap for the medical students and researchers in this field and will be an asset for them in understanding statistics and its application for the data management and its analysis for their research work.

I wish her good luck.

Dr. V.K. Dhingra
MBBS, MD (TB and Chest Diseases), MCAI, MNCCP (I)
Director
New Delhi Tuberculosis Centre
State TB and Training Demonstration Centre
Jawaharlal Nehru Marg
New Delhi - 110002

Preface

The book will provide students with an overview of qualitative and quantitative methods useful for collation, display and analysis of data. An applied statistical focus is integrated and is concentrating on evaluation of general issues like in operational studies as well as health related statistics and emphasizing when and how a statistical procedure should be performed. The book will provide a broad framework for understanding and applying commonly used data analysis techniques in research. Basic concepts necessary to the interpretation and application of statistics will be included, such as types of distribution, concept of significance of testing and discussion of basic descriptive statistics. The students are also introduced to common parametric and non-parametric statistical tests of association and trend analysis, including examples and illustrations which provide experience with various methods to handle a data set. With this book the students will gain experience in common data analysis techniques and in reading and interpretation of computer printouts. Students are often not in use of practical approach of statistics applications. This book will guide them how vastly we can use statistics in various fields of sciences.

Dr. Nishi Aggarwal

Contents

CHAPTER 1

GENERAL STATISTICS

1.1 INTRODUCTION OF STATISTICS

Broadly speaking, statistics are merely numerical statements about certain subject for example; medical matters, how many people die from a certain cause each year, how many hospital beds are available in a certain hospital, how much money is spend on certain medical services. Such facts are clearly of administrative importance. Numerical facts also supply the basis for a great deal of medical research, operational research; examples are given throughout this book. Such facts may be found in official publication of national and international health departments, in the published report of research investigations and even in the textbooks and monographs on various subjects.

What is Statistics?

Statistics is mathematical sciences which involve collection, selection, presentation, tabulation and interpretation of any form of data. The details about the data we will discuss in the later part of this chapter.

The word 'Statistics' is derived from the Latin word 'Statis' which means a **"political state".** Clearly, statistics is closely linked with the administrative affairs of a state such as facts and figures regarding defense force, population, housing, food, financial resources etc. What is true about a government is also true about industrial administration units, and even one's personal life.

The word statistics has several meanings. In the first place, it is a **plural noun** which describes a collection of numerical data such as employment statistics, accident statistics, population statistics, birth and death, income and expenditure, of exports and imports etc. It is in this sense that the word 'statistics' is used by a layman or a newspaper.

Secondly; the word statistics as a **singular noun**, is used to describe a branch of applied mathematics, whose purpose is to provide methods of dealing with collections of data and extracting information from them in compact form by tabulating, summarizing and analyzing the numerical data or a set of observations.

The various methods used are termed as **statistical methods** and the person using them is known as a statistician. A statistician is concerned with the analysis and interpretation of the data and drawing valid worthwhile conclusions from the same. It is in the second sense that we are writing this guide on statistics.

The word 'statistics' in the first sense is defined by Professor Secrit as follows:

"By statistics we mean aggregate of facts affected to a marked extent by multiplicity of causes, numerically expressed, enumerated or estimated according to reasonable standard of accuracy, collected in a systematic manner for a predetermined purpose and placed in relation to each other."

This definition gives all the **characteristics** of statistics which are: (1) Aggregate of facts (2) Affected by multiplicity of causes (3) Numerically expressed (4) Estimated according to reasonable standards of accuracy (5) Collected in a systematic manner (6) Collected for a pre-determined purpose (7) Placed in relation to each other.

The word 'statistics' in the second sense is defined by Croxton and Cowden as follows: "The collection, presentation, analysis and interpretation of the numerical data."

This definition clearly points out four stages in a statistical investigation, namely:

(1) Collection of data
(2) Presentation of data
(3) Analysis of data
(4) Interpretation of data

In addition to this, one more stage i.e. organization of data is suggested.

Uses of Statistics

To present the data in a concise and definite form: Statistics helps in classifying and tabulating raw data for processing and further tabulation for end users.

1. To make it easy to understand complex and large data: This is done by

presenting the data in the form of tables, graphs, diagrams etc., or by condensing the data with the help of means, dispersion etc.

2. For comparison: Tables, measures of means and dispersion can help in comparing different sets of data.
3. In forming policies: It helps in forming policies like a production schedule, based on the relevant sales figures. It is used in forecasting future demands.
4. Enlarging individual experiences: Complex problems can be well understood by statistics, as the conclusions drawn by an individual are more definite and precise than mere statements on facts.
5. In measuring the magnitude of a phenomenon: Statistics has made it possible to count the population of a country, the industrial growth, the agricultural growth, the educational level (of course in numbers).

Limitations

1. Statistics does not deal with individual measurements. Since statistics deals with aggregates of facts, it cannot be used to study the changes that have taken place in individual cases. For example, the wages earned by a single industry worker at any time, taken by itself is not a statistical datum. But the wages of workers of that industry can be used statistically. Similarly the marks obtained by John of your class or the height of Beena (also of your class) are not the subject matter of statistical study. But the average marks or the average height of your class has statistical relevance.
2. Statistics cannot be used to study qualitative phenomenon like morality, intelligence, beauty etc. as these cannot be quantified. However, it may be possible to analyze such problems statistically by expressing them numerically. For example we may study the intelligence of boys on the basis of the marks obtained by them in an examination.
3. Statistical results are true only on an average: The conclusions obtained statistically are not universal truths. They are true only under certain conditions. This is because statistics as a science is less exact as compared to the natural science.
4. Statistical data, being approximations, are mathematically incorrect. Therefore, they can be used only if **mathematical** accuracy is not needed.

5. Statistics, being dependent on figures, can be manipulated and therefore can be used only when the authenticity of the figures has been proved beyond doubt.

Distrust of Statistics

It is often said by people that, "statistics can prove anything". There are three types of lies-lies, demand lies and statistics-wicked in the order of their naming. A Paris banker said, "Statistics is like a miniskirt, it covers up essentials but gives you the ideas."

Thus by "distrust of statistics" we mean lack of confidence in statistical statements and methods. The following reasons account for such views about statistics:

1. Figures are convincing and, therefore people easily believe them.
2. They can be manipulated in such a manner as to establish foregone conclusions.
3. The wrong representation of even correct figures can mislead a reader. For example, John earned Rs. 4000 in 1990-1991 and Jem earned Rs. 5000. Reading this one would form the opinion that Jem is decidedly a better worker than John. However, if we carefully examine the statement, we might reach a different conclusion as Jem's earning period is unknown to us. Thus while working with statistics one should not only avoid outright falsehoods but be alert to detect possible distortion of the truth.

Statistics Can Be Misused

In one factory, which I know, workers were accusing the management for not providing them with proper working conditions. In support they quoted the number of accidents. When I considered the matter more seriously, I found that most of the staff was inexperienced and thus responsible for those accidents. Moreover many of the accidents were either minor or fake. I compared the working conditions of this factory to other factories and I found the conditions far better in this factory. Thus by merely noting the number of accidents and complaints of the workers, I would not dare to say that the working conditions were worse. On the other hand due to the proper statistical knowledge and careful observations I came to conclusion that the management was right.

Thus the usefulness of the statistics depends to a great extent upon its user. If used properly, by an efficient and unbiased statistician, it will prove to be an efficient tool.

Collection of facts and figures and deriving meaningful information from them is an important program.

As an example, suppose "Jerry Greval" has a drug company. His company wants to establish their business in India, particularly in Mumbai. Let us see a few ways in which statistics will be useful to him.

1. Leaflets among people: For this he needs to know the mother-tongues of various groups of people in Mumbai. This information is the most important factor of his business. In order to get this information, his company will have to appoint personnel who will go from door to door and find out the necessary information about the drug market. Jerry would like to know which pain reliever are more in demand and which are in less demand. Knowing this they can devise the manufacturing strategy.
2. Now the company wants to advertise the 'Brand name' and thus their product in the market. To make the product popular the brand name must be attractive: Jerry selects the name 'Pain Relieved'. The 'Pain Relieved' and its qualities have to be made to look appealing to the people in Mumbai and this requires publicity. Nothing is more appealing than what has been said in one's own mother tongue. So Jerry wants to print and distribute choice, their mother tongue etc. This process is known as taking a survey. The objects under study are known as Individuals or Units and the collection of individuals is known as the population.

   Often it is not possible or practical to record observations of all the individuals of the groups from different areas, which comprise the population. In such a case observations are recorded of only some of the individuals of the population, selected at random. This selection of some individuals which will be a subset of the individuals in the original group, is called a Sample, i.e., instead of an entire population survey which would be time-consuming, the company will manage with a 'Sample survey' which can be completed in a shorter time.

   Note that if a sample is representative of the whole population, any conclusion drawn from a statistical treatment of the sample would hold reasonably good for the population. This will of course, depend on the proper selection of the sample. One of the aims of statistics is to draw inferences about the population by a statistical treatment of samples.

Thus, choosing a random sample is a critical part of the statistical process and we will discuss this in more details in the chapter "Sampling".

Types of Statistics

As mentioned earlier, for a layman or people in general, statistics means numbers numerical facts, figures or information. The branch of statistics wherein we record and analyze observations for all the individuals of a group or population and draw inferences about the same is called "Descriptive statistics" or "Deductive statistics". On the other hand, if we choose a sample and by statistical treatment of this, draw inferences about the population, then this branch of statistics is known as Statistical Inference or Inductive Statistics.

In our discussion, we are mainly concerned with two ways of representing descriptive statistics: Numerical and Pictorial.

1. Numerical statistics are numbers. But some numbers are more meaningful such as mean, standard deviation etc.
2. When the numerical data is presented in the form of pictures (diagrams) and graphs, it is called the Pictorial statistics. This statistics makes confusing and complex data or information, easy, simple and straightforward, so that even the layman can understand it without much difficulty.

Common Mistakes Committed in Interpretation of Statistics

1. Bias: Bias means prejudice or preference of the investigator, which creeps in consciously and unconsciously in proving a particular point.
2. Generalization: Sometimes on the basis of little data available one could jump to a conclusion, which leads to erroneous results.
3. Wrong conclusion: The characteristics of a group if attached to an individual member of that group, may lead us to draw absurd conclusions.
4. Incomplete classification:- If we fail to give a complete classification, the influence of various factors may not be properly understood.
5. There may be a wrong use of percentages.
6. Technical mistakes may also occur.

7. An inconsistency in definition can even exist.
8. Wrong causal inferences may sometimes be drawn.
9. There may also be a misuse of correlation.

Example

Individual	Characteristic		Type of Characteristic
1. A person	Height in cm	→	Continuous variate
	Color of eyes	→	Attribute
	Age	→	Continuous variate
	Weight in lbs	→	Continuous variate
	Sex	→	Attribute
	Mother tongue	→	Attribute
	Marks in biology	→	Discrete variate
2. Mr. Brown's family	Number of members	→	Discrete variate
	Monthly income in Rupees	→	Discrete variate
3. A washer	Diameter and thickness in cm	→	Continuous variate
	Defective or non-defective	→	Attribute

In brief, statistics may be broadly divide as shown in figure given below:

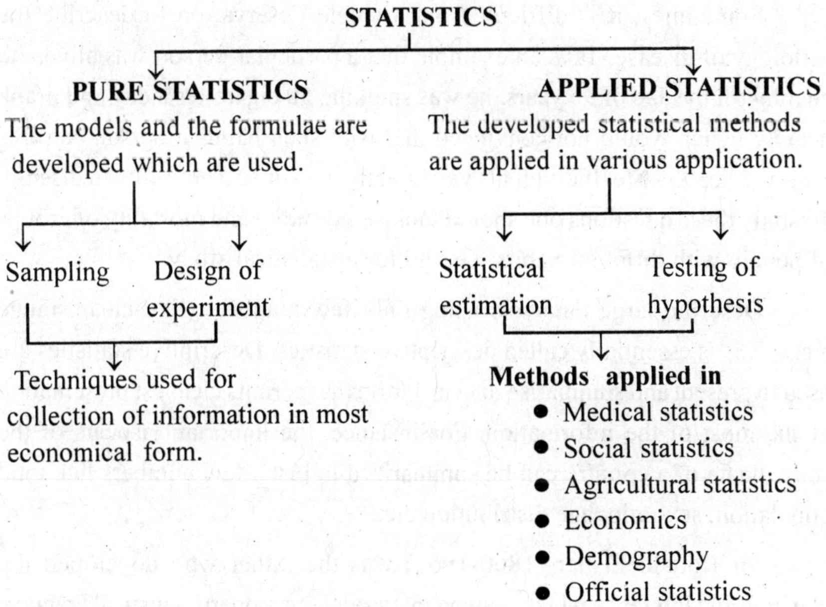

Figure 1.1

Many occasions, it is assumed that statistical information does not yield much to the progress of medicine as the physicians are concerned at any one time with the treatment of a single patient and every patient differs in important aspect from the other patient. Take an example, the physicians assumes that the normal human body temperature is 98.4 °C . What is the basis of this statement? This basic concept of temperature which even a lay person is aware, is based on simple logical calculations of statistics. Many more examples can be seen for the uses of statistics. Now the argument is that whether such information should be stored in rather informal ways in the clinicians' mind or whether it should be collected and reported in a systematic way. Very few professionals acquire, by personal experience, factual information over the whole range of medium, it is partly by the collection, analysis and reporting of statistical information that a common body of knowledge is built and solidified.

Why Should We Go For Statistics?

Sometimes, it is difficult from a single observation to describe the aetiology of disease. Take an example that a particular person was alive and healthy till the age of 90 years, he was smoking 50 cigarettes a day and drank heavily which would not convinced that with such habits a person can live long and healthy life. Individuals vary greatly in their susceptibility to disease. To study these questions one should look at morbidity and mortality of groups of people with different habits; i.e.; go for a statistical study.

Describe large data sets using only few numbers (like mean, range etc.). This is essentially called descriptive statistics. Descriptive statistics are used to present and summarise data in a form that permits cleanest presentation of the most of the information. For instance, the important aspects of the census data of a country can be summarized in just a few numbers like total population, sex ratio, age distribution etc.

Sir Ronald Fisher (1860-1962) was the father who developed the planning and inference which is apparent throughout modern statistical practice.

Statistics in Clinical Medicine

The statistical methods are required in the analysis and interpretation of figures which are at the mercy of numerous influences. Its object is to determine whether these individuals influences can be isolated and their effects measured. The essence of the method lies in the determination that we are really comparing like, and we have not overlooked a relevant factor which is present in Group A and absent from Group B. The variability of human beings in their illness and in their reactions to them and to their treatment is a fundamental reason for the planned clinical trial and not against it. Large numbers are not invariably required and it is clear that in particular circumstances even one or two cases well observed may give information of vital importance. Vital statistics and their analysis are essential features of public health work, to determine its problems, to determine, as far as possible, cause and effect, and to measure the success or failure of the steps taken to deal with such problems.

Descriptive and Inferential Statistics

Statistics can be divided into two major areas. **Descriptive statistics** comprises the statistical methods dealing with the collection, tabulation and summarization of data, so as to present meaningful information. **Statistical inference**, on the other hand, consists of the methods involved with the analysis and interpretation of data that will enable the statistician to develop meaningful inferences about the data. Both subfields are interrelated; while descriptive statistics organize the collected data in a systematic manner, statistical inference analyzes the data and enables one to produce significant inferences about it.

1.2 PRESENTATION OF STATISTICS

CLASSIFICATION AND TABULATION

In any statistical investigation, the collection of the numerical data is the first and the most important matter to be attended. Often a person investigating, will have to collect the data from the actual field of inquiry. For this he may issue suitable questionnaires to get necessary information or he may take actual interviews; personal interviews are more effective than questionnaires, which may not evoke an adequate response. Another method of collecting data may be available in publications of Government bodies or other public or private organizations.

Such data, however, is often so numerous that one's mind can hardly comprehend its significance in the form that it is shown. Therefore it becomes, very necessary to tabulate and summarize the data to an easily manageable form. In doing so we may overlook its details. But this is not a serious loss because statistics is not interested in an individual but in the properties of aggregates. For a layman, presentation of the raw data in the form of tables or diagrams is always more effective.

Tabulation

It is the process of condensation of the data for convenience, in statistical processing, presentation and interpretation of the information. A good table is one which has the following requirements:

1. It should present the data clearly, highlighting important details.
2. It should save space but attractively designed.
3. The table number and title of the table should be given.
4. Row and column headings must explain the figures therein.
5. Averages or percentages should be close to the data.
6. Units of the measurement should be clearly stated along the titles or headings.
7. Abbreviations and symbols should be avoided as far as possible.
8. Sources of the data should be given at the bottom of the data.
9. In case irregularities creep in table or any feature is not sufficiently explained, references and foot notes must be given.
10. The rounding of figures should be unbiased.

Classification

"Classified and arranged facts speak of themselves, and narrated they are as dead as mutton." This quote is given by J.R. Hicks.

The process of dividing the data into different groups (viz. classes) which are homogeneous within but heterogeneous between themselves, is called a classification.

It helps in understanding the salient features of the data and also the comparison with similar data. For a final analysis it is the best friend of a statistician.

Methods of Classification

The data is classified in the following ways:

1. According to attributes or qualities this is divided into two parts:
   (A) Simple classification.
   (B) Multiple classification.
2. According to variable or quantity or classification according to class intervals.

Qualitative Classification

When facts are grouped according to the qualities (attributes) like religion, literacy, business etc., the classification is called as qualitative classification.

(A) Simple Classification:

It is also known as classification according to Dichotomy. When data (facts) are divided into groups according to their qualities, the classification is called as 'Simple Classification'. Qualities are denoted by capital letters (A, B, C, D ......) while the absence of these qualities are denoted by lower case letters (a, b, c, d, ... etc.) For example:

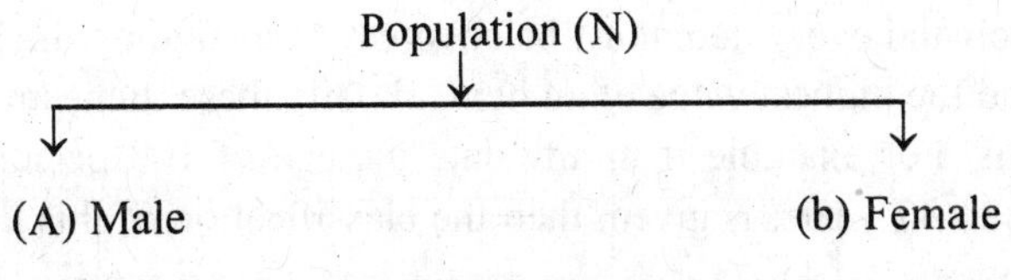

(B) Manifold or Multiple Classification:

In this method data is classified using one or more qualities. First, the data is divided into two groups (classes) using one of the qualities. Then using the remaining qualities, the data is divided into different subgroups. For example, the population of a country is classified using three attributes: sex, literacy and business as:

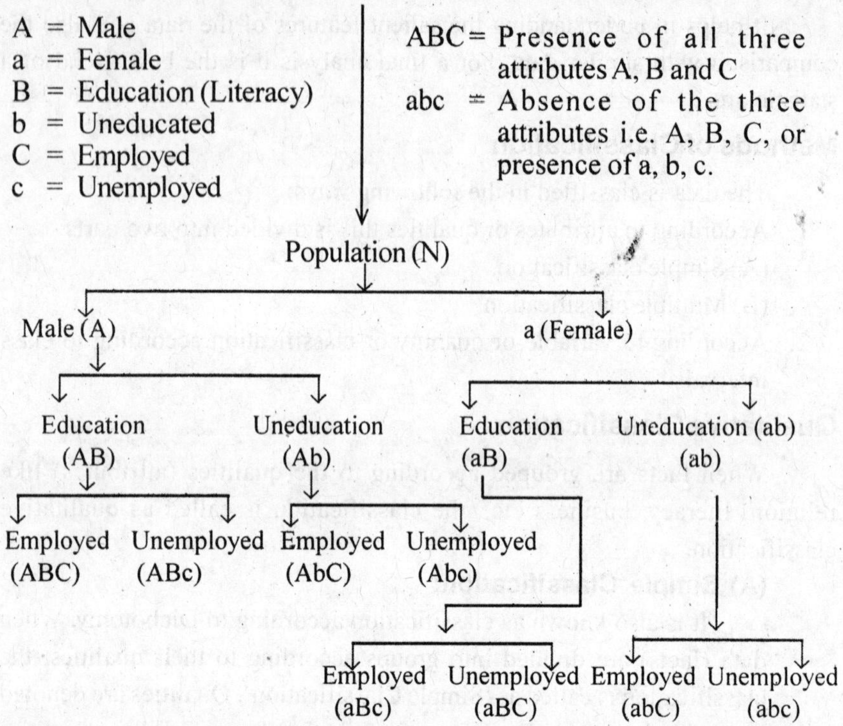

Classification According to Class Intervals or Variables

The data which is expressed in numbers (quantitative data), is classified according to class-intervals. While forming class-intervals one should bear in mind that each and every item must be covered. After finding the least value of an item and the highest value of an item, classify these items into different class-intervals. For example if in any data the age of 100 persons ranging from 2 years to 47 years, is given, then the classification of this data can be done in this way:

Table - 1.1

Age in year	No. of persons
0-10	5
10-20	9
20-30	32
30-40	34
40-50	20

In deciding on the grouping of the data into classes, for the purpose of reducing it to a manageable form, we observe that the number of classes should not be too large. If it were so then the object of summarization would be defeated. The number of classes should also not be too small because then we will miss a great deal of detail available and get a distorted picture. As a rule one should have between 10 and 25 classes, the actual number depending on the total frequency. Further, classes should be exhaustive; they should not be overlapping, so that no observed value falls in more than one class. Apart from exceptions, all classes should have the same length.

According to the Class-Intervals in Classification the Following Terms are Used

(i) Class-limits

A class is formed within the two values. These values are known as the class-limits of that class. The lower value is called the lower limit and is denoted by l_1 while the higher value is called the upper limit of the class and is denoted by l_2. In the example given above, the first class-interval has $l_1 = 0$ and $l_2 = 10$.

(ii) Magnitude of the Class-Intervals

The difference between the upper and lower limits of a class is called the magnitude or length or width of a class and is denoted by 'i' or 'c'. Thus 'i' = $(l_2 - l_1)$.

(iii) Mid-Value or Class-Mark

The arithmetical average of the two class limits (i.e. the lower limit and the upper limit) is called the mid-value or the class mark of that class-interval. For example, the mid-value of the class-interval (0 - 10) is

$$\frac{\lambda_1 + \lambda_2}{2} = \frac{0+10}{2} = 5, \text{ of } (10\text{-}20) \text{ it is } \frac{10+20}{2} = 15$$

and so on

(iv) Class Frequency

The units of the data belong to any one of the groups or classes. The total number of these units is known as the frequency of that class and is denoted by fi or simply f. In the above example, the frequencies of the classes in the given order are 5, 9, 32, 34 and 40 respectively.

Classification is of two types according to the class-intervals- (i) Exclusive Method (ii) Inclusive Method.

(i) Exclusive Method: In this method the upper limit of a class becomes the lower limit of the next class. It is called 'Exclusive' as we do not put any item that is equal to the upper limit of a class in the same class; we put it in the next class, i.e., the upper limits of classes are excluded from them. For example, a person of age 20 years will not be included in the class-interval (10-20) but taken in the next class (20-30), since in the class-interval (10-20) only units ranging from 10-19 are included. The exclusive types of class-intervals can also be expressed as:

0 and below 10 or 0 - 9.9
10 and below 20 or 10 - 19.9
20 and below 30 or 20 - 29.9 and so on.

(ii) Inclusive Method: In this method the upper limit of any class interval is kept in the same class-interval. In this method the upper limit of a previous class is less by 1 from the lower limit of the next class interval. In short this method allows a class-interval to include both its lower and upper limits within it. For example:

Table - 1.2

Inclusive Method		Inclusive Method	
Class	**Frequency**	**Class**	**Frequency**
0 - 4	5	0 - 4.9	5
5 - 9	7	5 - 9.9	7
10 - 14	9	10 - 14.9	9
15 - 19	12	15 - 19.9	12
20 - 24	11	20 - 24.9	11
25 - 29	14	25 - 29.9	14

Class Boundaries

Weights are recorded to the nearest Kg. The class-intervals 60 - 62 includes all measurements from 59.50000... to 62.50000 ... Kg; the variable being a continuous one. These numbers, indicated briefly by the exact numbers 59.5 and 62.5, are called class-boundaries or true class limits. The smaller number 59.5 is the lower class boundary and the larger one 62.5 is the upper class boundary.

In any problem if the class-intervals are given as the inclusive type, then they should first be converted into the exclusive type. For this we require a correction factor.

Correction factor = $\frac{1}{2}$ (the upper limit of a class—the lower limit of the next class) which is generally 0.5.

Now you subtract it from the lower limits and add it to the upper limits of the class-intervals given in the inclusive method. The class-intervals given above can be written after correction as:

Class-interval	Frequency
0 - 4.5	5
4.5 - 9.5	7
9.5 - 14.5	9
14.5 - 19.5	12
19.5 - 24.5	11
24.5 - 29.5	14

To obtain class-intervals when their mid-values are given, use the following formulae:

Lower limit (l_1) = $m - i/_2$ and upper limit (l_2) = $m + i/_2$

where m = mid-value and i = class-length.

For example, we are given some mid-values as 72, 77, 82, 87, ... Now, consider the first mid-value 72 and also the differences between successive mid-values.

We have 77 - 72 = 5, 82 - 77 = 5, 87 - 82 = 5 ....

which gives the class-length i = 5.

For the first class-interval, $l_1 = m - i/_2 = 72 - 5/_2 = 69.5$

and $l_2 = 72 + 5/_2 = 74.5$

Thus the first class-interval is 69.5 - 74.5

and other class-intervals then are 74.5 - 79.5, 79.5 - 84.5, 84.5 - 89.5

Open-end Class Intervals

In any question when the lower limit of the first class-inteval or the upper limit of the last class-interval, are not given then subtract the class length of the next immediate class-interval from the upper limit. This will give us the lower limit of the first class-interval. Similarly add the same class length to the lower limit of the last class-interval. But always notice that the lower limit of the first class (i.e. the lowest class) must not be negative or less than 0. For example:

Table - 1.3

With open ends	Completed Class	With open ends	Completed Class
Below 10	0 - 10	Below 10	0 - 10
10 - 20	10 - 20	10 - 25	10 - 25
20 - 30	20 - 30	25 - 40	25 - 40
30 - 40	30 - 40	40 - 70	40 - 70
40 - 50	40 - 50	above 70	70 - 100
above 50			

Relative Frequency Distribution

The relative frequency of a class is the frequency of the class divided by the total number of frequencies of the class and is generally expresse as a percentage.

Example

The weight of 100 persons were given as under:

Weight (in Kgs)	60 - 62	63 - 65	66 - 68	69 - 71	72 - 74
No. of Person (f_1)	5	18	42	27	8

Solution

Table - 1.4

Weight (in Kgs)	No. of Persons (f_i)	Relative Frequency
60 - 62	5	$\frac{5}{100}$ x 5% or 0.05

63 - 65	18	$\frac{18}{100}$ x 18% or 0.18
66 - 68	42	$\frac{42}{100}$ x 42% or 0.42
69 - 71	27	$\frac{27}{100}$ x 27% or 0.27
72 - 74	8	$\frac{8}{100}$ x 8% or 0.08
Total	$\Sigma f_1 = 100$	

Note

The word frequency of a class means, the number of times the class is repeated in the data or the total number of items or observations of the data belongs to that class.

Cumulative Frequency

Many a times the frequencies of different classes are not given. Only their cumulative frequencies are given. The total frequency of all values less than or equal to the upper class boundary of a given class-interval is called the cumulative frequency upto and including that class- interval. In this situation both the limits of a class-interval are not written; either lower or upper limit is written. These cumulative frequencies are called less than or more than cumulative frequencies. For example,

Table - 1.5

Class-interval	0-10	10-20	20-30	30-40	40-50
Frequency	4	9	5	12	15

Less than cumulative frequency		More than cumulative frequency	
(Upper limits)	**(Cum. freq.)**	**(Lower limits)**	**(Cum. freq.)**
Less than 10	4	More than 0	45 = 41 + 4
Less than 20	4+ 9 = 13	More than 10	41 = 32 + 9
Less than 30	18 + 12 = 20	More than 20	32 = 27 + 5
Less than 40	18 + 12 = 30	More than 30	27 = 15 + 12
Less than 50	30 + 15 = 45	More than 40	15

Preparation of Frequency Distribution

We shall now study how to classify the raw data in a tabular form. Consider the data collected by one of the surveyors, interviewing about 50 people. This is as follows:

Size of the liver: 2, 5, 6, 8, 2, 5, 6, 7, 6, 8, 7, 4, 3, .. This is called the raw data. Here some values repeat themselves. For instance the size 5 is repeated 10 times in 50 people. We say that the value of 5 of the variate has the frequency of 10. Frequency means the number of times a value of the variate or an attribute, as the case may be, is repeated in the data. A table which shows each value of the characteristic with its corresponding frequency, is known as a **Frequency Distribution**. The procedure of preparing such a table is explained as below:

Discrete Variate

Consider the raw data which gives the size of liver of 30 persons

2, 5, 6, 4, 5, 7, 4, 4, 6, 2
3, 5, 5, 4, 5, 6, 5, 4, 3, 2
4, 4, 5, 4, 5, 5, 3, 2, 4, 4

The least value is 2 and the highest is 7. All sizes are integers between 2 and 7 (both inclusive). We can prepare a frequency distribution table as follows:

Table – 1.6

Sizes of liver	Tally marks	Frequency
2	||||	4
3	|||	3
4	~~||||~~ ~~||||~~	10
5	~~||||~~ ~~||||~~	9
6	|||	3
7	|	1
Total		30

In this example the size difference from 2 to 7 is very small. If the range of a variate is very large, it is inconvenient to prepare a frequency distribution for each value of the variate. In such a case we divide the variate into convenient groups and prepare a table showing the groups and their corresponding frequencies. Such a table is called a **grouped frequency distribution**.

Consider the marks (out of 100) of 50 students as below:

40, 39, 43, 62, 30, 47, 33, 31, 17, 28

36, 29, 40, 32, 39, 24, 57, 42, 15, 30

50, 52, 47, 65, 31, 07, 37, 47, 17, 20

25, 53, 65, 85, 89, 56, 55, 41, 43, 10

44, 40, 69, 22, 40, 65, 39, 36, 71, 12

The range of the variate (marks) is very large. Also we are eager to know the performance of the students. The passing limit is 35 and above. Marks between 35 and 44 form the third class (or grade). Marks ranging between 45 - 59 are considered as second class and 60 - 100 form the first class. Thus we have a grouped frequency distribution as:

Table - 1.7

Sizes	Tally Marks	Frequency
0–34	𝍸 𝍸 𝍸 I	16
35–44	𝍸 𝍸 𝍸 III	18
45–59	𝍸 IIII	9
60–100	𝍸 II	7
Total		50

Bivariate Frequency Distribution

In Table 1.7, we have classified students according to their marks in one subject. Suppose we have marks of a number of students in two subjects, say anatomy and physiology and we want to consider the variation of marks in both the subjects simultaneously. Then we have to prepare a table (known as a bivariate table) for the following data:

No. of Students	1	2	3	4	5	6	7	8	9	10	11	12
Marks in Anatomy	60	56	42	33	40	13	27	12	19	50	23	16
Marks in physiology	50	45	53	54	49	23	50	24	31	41	47	20
No. of Students	13	14	15									
Marks in Anatomy	32	42	30									
Marks in physiology	38	21	45									

Table – 1.8

<table>
<tr><th rowspan="2">Marks in Anatomy</th><th colspan="6">Marks in physiology</th></tr>
<tr><th>10–20</th><th>20–30</th><th>30–40</th><th>40–50</th><th>50–60</th><th></th></tr>
<tr><td>10–20</td><td></td><td>|| = 2</td><td>| = 1</td><td>0</td><td>0</td><td>3</td></tr>
<tr><td>20–30</td><td></td><td>| = 1</td><td></td><td>| = 1</td><td>| = 1</td><td>3</td></tr>
<tr><td>30–40</td><td></td><td></td><td>| = 1</td><td>| = 1</td><td>| = 1</td><td>3</td></tr>
<tr><td>40–50</td><td></td><td>| = 1</td><td></td><td>| = 1</td><td>| = 1</td><td>3</td></tr>
<tr><td>50–60</td><td></td><td></td><td></td><td>| = 1</td><td>| = 2</td><td>3</td></tr>
<tr><td>Total</td><td></td><td>4</td><td>2</td><td>4</td><td>5</td><td>15</td></tr>
</table>

Example

Make a table showing the frequencies, cumulative frequencies (both less than and more than type) for the words having different numbers of letters in the following passage (ignore the punctuation marks).

"In Asia the complications are likely to be greater still. There will be four major powers in the Asian balance: Russia, China, Japan and the United States. To some extent, this increases the chance that the forces will emerge sufficient to contain China and it may lead to a real reapproachment between Russia and the West. But who knows, with so many factors, what the pattern will be like, ten years from now ?"

Solution

We find that the smallest word ' a ' has one letter; and the longest word "re-approachment" has 14 letters. We prepare a tally sheet by writing the number of letters in the first column from 1 to 14. The table is as follows :

Table – 1.9

Number of letters	Tally Marks	Total
1	|	1
2	~~||||~~ ~~||||~~ |	11
3	~~||||~~ ~~||||~~ ~~||||~~ |	16
4	~~||||~~ ~~||||~~ ~~||||~~ |	16
5	~~||||~~ ||||	9
6	~~||||~~ ~~||||~~	10
7	~~||||~~ |	6
8	-	0
9	|	1
10	|	1
11	-	0
12	-	0
13	|	1
14	|	1
Total		73

Thus, the table showing frequencies, cumulative frequencies is:

Table - 1.10

Number of Letter (Xi)	Frequency	Cumulative frequency (< or =, type)	Cumulative frequency (> or =, type)
1	1	1	73
2	11	12	72
3	16	28	71
4	16	44	71
5	9	53	71
6	10	63	70
7	6	69	69
8	0	69	69
9	1	70	63
10	1	71	53
11	0	71	44
12	0	71	28
13	1	72	12
14	1	73	1
Total	**73**		

Thus, statistical representation of data is the task of summarizing large amount of data in a compact format that yields meaningful information concerning the data. Without displaying the values for each observation taken for the population, it is possible to present the data concisely and meaningful using certain procedures. Such procedures often involve frequency distribution or graphs of the data. Graphically we can represent with bar chart, histogram, frequency polygon, frequency ogive, pie chart.

While describing the set of data graphically, students should keep the following rules for making a diagram:

1. As simple as possible and self-explanatory.
2. Mostly to show important points.
3. Tables followed by diagrams is not advisable.
4. Must specify: names of the variables, units, legends.
5. Like tables, graphs and text can be on the same page.
6. Golden rule is that it should speak by itself.

A bar chart/graph is the frequency distribution of the data on an xy co-ordinate system. The class-intervals are plotted on x-axis, the absolute frequencies on y-axis. Each interval is represented by a rectangle whose base corresponds to a class interval and whose height is equal to the frequency associated with the classinterval.

Population and Sample

A (statistical) population is the complete set of possible measurements or the record of some qualitative trait corresponding to the entire collection of units for which inferences are to be made. The population represents the target of an investigation, and the objective of the process of data collection is to draw conclusions about the population.

A sample from a statistical population is the set of measurements that are actually collected in the course of an investigation. e.g.:

Population = (Set of all even numbers between 1 & 20 inclusive)

= (2, 4, 6, 8, 10, 12, 14, 16, 18 and 20)

S1 = (set of all numbers between 1 & 20 who are multiple of 3)
= (6, 12, 18)

S2 = (Set of all numbers between 1 & 20 which are multiple of 5)

= (10, 20)

1.3 SUMMARIZING NUMERICAL DATA

Statistical Representation of Data

The statistician is often faced with the task of summarizing large amount of data in a compact format that yields meaningful information concerning the data. Without displaying the values for each observation taken from the population, it is possible to present the data concisely and meaningfully using certain procedures. Such procedures often involve frequency distributions or graphs of the data.

Frequency Distribution

A **frequency distribution** is a tabular arrangement of data whereby the data is grouped into different intervals, and then the number of observations that belong to each interval is determined. Data that is presented in this manner are known as **grouped data**.

The smallest value that can belong to a given interval is called the **lower class limit,** while the largest value that can belong to the interval is called the **upper class limit**. The difference between the upper class limit and the lower class limit is defined to be the **class width.** When designing the intervals to be used in a frequency distribution, it is preferable that the class widths of all intervals be the same. The main steps in this process are as follows:

Step 1 Find the range of data set, range = Max Value – Min Value.

Step 2 Choose a number of subintervals of equal length that cover the range without overlapping. These are called class-intervals and their end points are known as class boundaries.

Step 3 Count the number of observations in the data that belong to each classinterval. The count in each class is the class frequency.

GRAPHICAL REPRESENTATION

A graph is a visual representation of data by a continuous curve on a squared (graph) paper. Like diagrams, graphs are also attractive, and eye-catching, giving a bird's eye-view of data and revealing their inner pattern.

The methods used to represent a grouped data are:

1. Histogram
2. Frequency Polygon
3. Frequency Curve
4. Ogive or Cumulative Frequency Curve

These types of graphical representation of data summarizes data in comprehensive manner. While the method used to represent a grouped data in tabular form are (i) Frequency distribution table (ii) Relative frequency distribution table (iii) Cummulative frequency distribution table.

Comparison Between Tabular and Diagrammatic Presentation

1. Diagrams and graphs are meant for a layman.	1. Tables are meant for statisticians for the purpose of further analysis.
2. Diagrams give only an approximate idea.	2. Tables contain precise figures. Exact values can be read from tables.
3. Diagrams can be more easily compared, and can be interpreted by a layman.	3. Comparison and interpretations of tables can only be done by statisticians and it is a difficult task.
4. Diagrams and graphs cannot present much information.	4. Tables can present more information.
5. Diagrams are more attractive and have a visual appeal.	5. Tables are dry for a layman (may be attractive to a statistician).

William play fair - 1759 - 1823 said in his 'Commercial and political Atlas of 1801' that "Information take days through data presented in tables, but can be obtained in minutes through diagrams."

Cold figures are uninspiring to most people. Diagrams help us to see the pattern and shape of any complex idea, just as a map gives a bird's eye view of wide sketch of a country, so diagrams help us to visualize the whole meaning of a numerical complex at single glance. Diagrams register a meaningful impression almost before you think ...." (Moroney).

Difference Between Diagrams and Graphs

There is no clear-cut line of demarcation between a diagram and a graph yet:

1. A graph needs a graph paper but a diagram can be drawn on a plain paper. In the technical way we can say that a graph is a mathematical relation between two variables. This, however, is not the case of a diagram.

2. As diagrams are attractive to look at; they are used for publicity and propaganda. Graphs on the other hand are more useful to statisticians and research workers for the purpose of further analysis.

3. For representing frequency distribution, diagrams are rarely used when compared with graphs. For example, for the time series graphs are more appropriate than diagrams.

General Principles of Constructing Diagrams

1. The diagrams should be simple.
2. Each diagram must be given a clear, concise and suitable title without damaging clarity.
3. A proper proportion between height and width must be maintained in order to avoid an unpleasant look.
4. Select a proper scale; it should be in even numbers or in multiples of five or ten.

   e.g. 25, 50, 75 or 10, 20, 30, 40, ... etc. But no fixed rule.
5. In order to clear certain points, always put footnotes.
6. An index, explaining different lines, shades and colors should be given.
7. Diagrams should be absolutely neat and clean.

"The important point that must be borne in mind at all times that the pictorial representation chosen for any situation must depict the true relationship and point out the proper conclusion. Above all the chart must be honest." .... C. W. LOWE

Uses

A pie diagram is useful when we want to show relative positions (proportions) of the figures which make the total. It is also useful when the components are many in number.

Box and Whiskers

It is one step further to stem-and-leaf. It displays a number of statistics like, median, lower quartile (Q1), upper quartile (Q3), inter-quartile range (IQR). It tells us about the symmetry of the distribution and also gives us the idea about the highest and the lowest values.

Example

Verbal GMAT scores of 12 students 10, 22, 24, 27, 31, 33, 39, 40, 42, 43, 44, 45.

Solution

The scores is arranged in the ascending order

10, 22, 24, 27, 31, 33, 39, 40, 42, 43, 44, 45

1. Since n = 12 (total items)

   The two middle scores are $\frac{12+2}{2} = 6\text{th}$ and $\frac{12}{2} = 7\text{th}$.

   i.e. 33 and 39 respectively.

   Therefore the average of the two is the median

   i.e. Median $= \frac{1}{2}[33 + 99] = \frac{1}{2}[72] = 36$

2. The quartile (Q_1) is the median of the bottom half. i.e.

   25th percentile.

   Thus $Q_1 = N/4 = 12/4$ 3rd Score = 24

3. The upper quartile (Q_3) is the median of the top half. i.e.

   75th percentile.

   $Q_3 = 3N/4 = 3(12)/4 = 9\text{th}$ Score = 24

   Now the box-plot is constructed as follows:

   i. The line inside the box indicates the median.

   ii. The left side of this box indicates the lower quartile (Q_1).

   iii. The right side of this box indicates the upper quartile (Q_3)

   iv. A straight line is then drawn from the lowest value of this distribution through the box to the highest value of this distribution. This horizontal straight line is called the "Whiskers".

   Then the above GMAT score in box-plot will look like this:

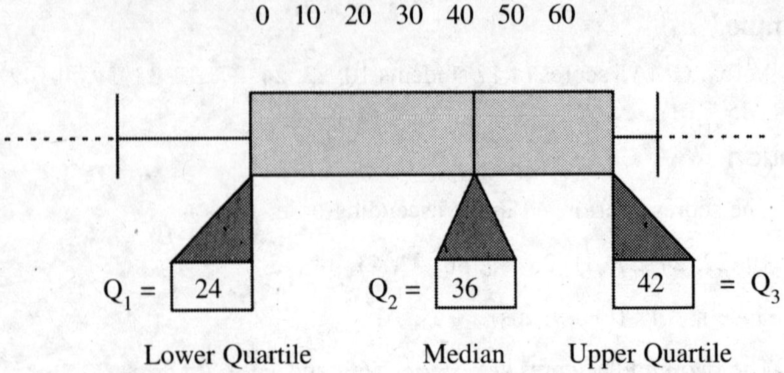

The information presented in a frequency distribution table can be more easily grasped if it is presented in a graphical format. Absolute, relative or cumulative frequencies can be represented in the graphs, depending on the particular objectives for creating the graph. There are various graphical means to visualize a frequency distribution; bar charts, histograms, pie charts and frequency polygons/ogives are among the most popular.

A **bar chart** graphs the frequency distribution of the data on an x-y coordinate system. The class-intervals are plotted on the x-axis, the absolute (or relative) frequencies on the y-axis. Each interval is represented by a rectangle whose base corresponds to a class-interval and whose height is equal to the frequency associated with the class-interval.

1. Simple 'Bar Diagram'

It represents only one variable. For example sales, production, population figures etc. for various years may be shown by simple bar charts. Since these are of the same width and vary only in heights (or lengths), it becomes very easy for readers to study the relationship. Simple bar diagrams are very popular in practice. A bar chart can be either vertical or horizontal; vertical bars are more popular.

Illustration

The following table gives the birth rate per thousand of different countries over a certain period of time.

Country	Birth rate	Country	Birth rate
India	33	China	40
Germany	15	New Zealand	30
U.K.	20	Sweden	15

Represent the above data by a suitable diagram.

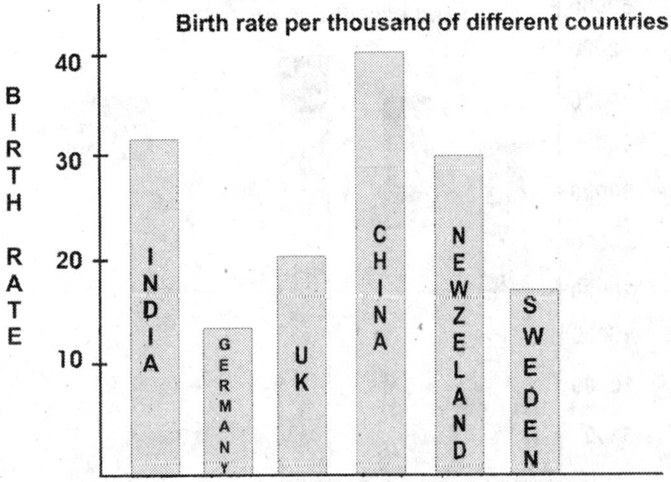

Comparing the size of bars, you can easily see that China's birth rate is the highest while Germany and Sweden equal in the lowest positions. Such diagrams are also known as component bar diagrams.

2. Sub-divided Bar Diagram

While constructing such a diagram, the various components in each bar should be kept in the same order. A common and helpful arrangement is that of presenting each bar in the order of magnitude with the largest component at the bottom and the smallest at the top. The components are shown with different shades or colors with a proper index.

Illustration

During 1968 - 71, the number of students in University ' X ' are as follows. Represent the data by a similar diagram.

Year	Arts	Science	Law	Total
1968-69	20,000	10,000	5,000	35,000
1969-70	26,000	9,000	7,000	42,000
1970-71	31,000	9,500	7,500	48,000

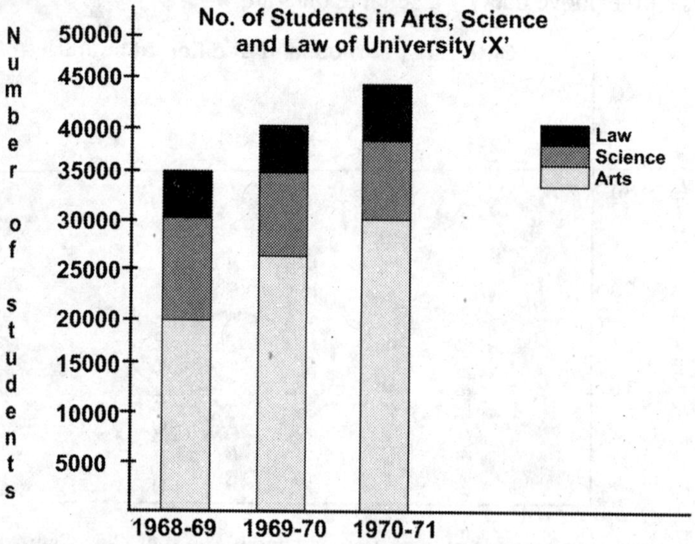

3. Multiple Bar Diagram

This method can be used for data which is made up of two or more components. In this method the components are shown as separate adjoining bars. The height of each bar represents the actual value of the component. The components are shown by different shades or colors. Where changes in actual values of component figures only are required, multiple bar charts are used.

Illustration

The table below gives data relating to the exports and imports of a certain country X (in thousands of dollars) during the four years ending in 1930–31.

Year	Export	Import
1927 - 28	319	250
1928 - 29	339	263
1929 - 30	345	258
1930 - 31	308	206

Represent the data by a suitable diagram

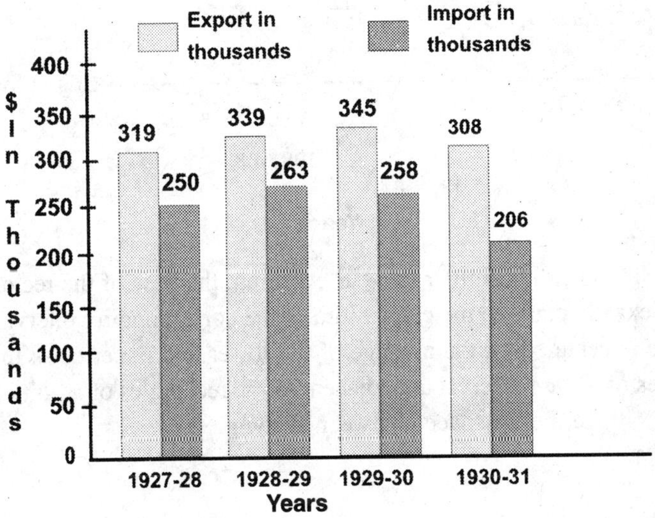

4. Deviation Bar Charts

Deviation bars are used to represent net quantities excess or deficit i.e. net profit, net loss, net exports or imports, swings in voting etc. Such bars have both positive and negative values. Positive values lie above the base line and negative values lie below it.

Illustration

Years	Sales	Net Profits
1985–86	10%	50%
1986–87	14%	–20%
1987-88	12%	– 10%

Present the above data by a suitable diagram showing the sales and net profits of private industrial companies.

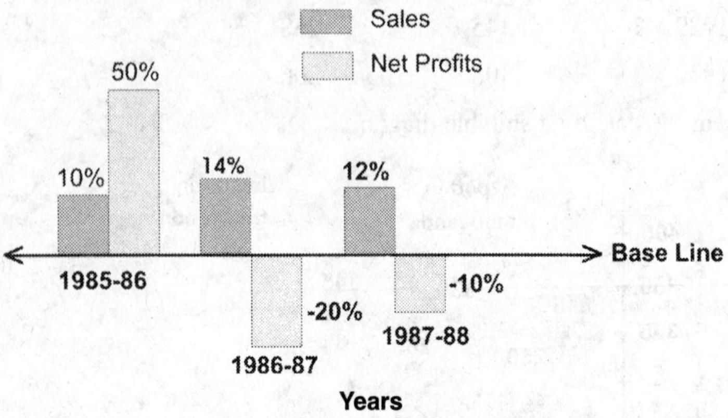

A **histogram** is similar to a bar chart, but the base of the rectangle has a length exactly equal to the class width of the corresponding interval. As the rectangle is centered on the average of the lower and upper class limits, the rectangles of a class-interval are adjacent to the rectangles of adjoining class-intervals—there are no spaces between rectangles.

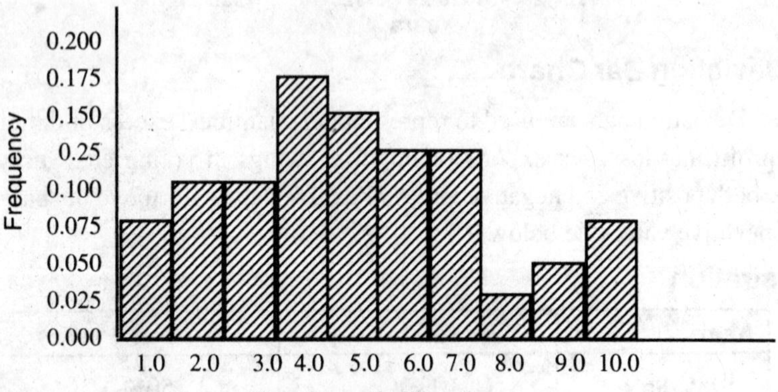

Class Intervals Histogram

Example

A stock broker, keeps a daily list of the number of transactions where his customers buy the stocks on margin. The following numbers of stocks were bought on margin by his customers during the first weeks of 2002.

30	28	16	23	22	10	8	15	16	23
29	30	22	15	24	9	5	4	15	24
21	24	16	14	21	13	6	2	23	22
24	21	27	13	20	8	4	3	24	20
22	18	23	23	17	7	6	1	16	17

Construct a frequency distribution for the preceding data and then draw a histogram.

Solution

Fix the number of class = 10 (say)

The largest number in 30 and smallest is 1

Class Size = Range/number of classes = (30 – 1)/10 = 29/10 = 2.9 or 3

Thus the group size is 3

No. of Stocks	Class Frequency
1 – 4	3
4 – 7	5
7 – 10	4
10 – 13	1
13 – 16	6
16 – 19	7
19 – 22	5
22 – 25	14
25 – 28	1
28 – 31	4

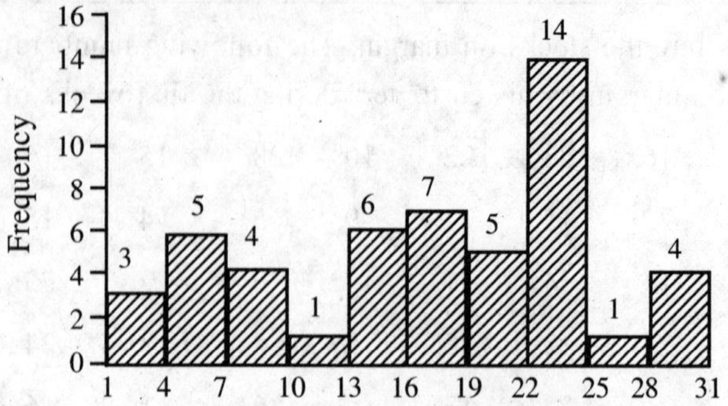

Histogram of number of Stocks

Construction of Histogram When Class-intervals are Unequal

In a Histogram, a rectangle is proportional to the frequency of the concern class-interval. Naturally, if the class-intervals are of unequal widths, we have to adjust the heights of the rectangle accordingly. We know that the area of a rectangle = l. h. Now suppose the width (l) of a class is double that of a normal class-interval, its height and thus the corresponding frequency must be halved. After this precaution has been taken, the construction of the Histogram of classes of unequal intervals is the same as before.

Note: The smallest class-interval should be assumed to be "NORMAL"

Illustration

Represent the following data by means of Histogram.

Classes :	11-14	16-19	21-24	26-29	31-39	41-59	61-79
Frequencies :	7	19	27	15	12	12	8

Solution

Note that class-intervals are unequal and also they are of inclusive type. We have to make them equal and of the exclusive type.

Correct factor = (16 – 14) / 2 = 1. Using it we have

Classes :	10-15	15-20	20-25	25-30	30-40	40-60	60-80
Frequencies :	7	19	27	15	12	12	8
Adjusted Heights: (Frequencies)	7	19	27	15	12/2 = 6	12/4 = 3	12/4 = 3

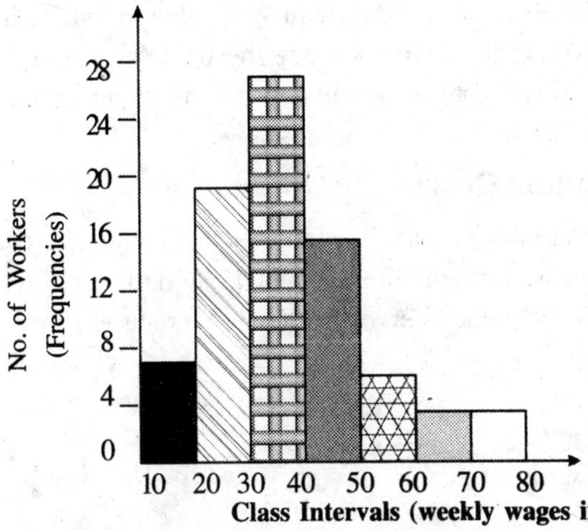

Frequency Polygon

If the midpoints (class marks) of the tops of the bars or histograms are joined together by straight lines, then the resulting figure without the bars, is a frequency polygon.

Example

Height in cm.	150–154	154–158	158–162	162–166	166–170
No. of children	10	15	20	12	8

The polygon is closed at the base by extending it on both its sides (ends) to the midpoints of two hypothetical classes, at the extremes of the distribution, with zero frequencies.

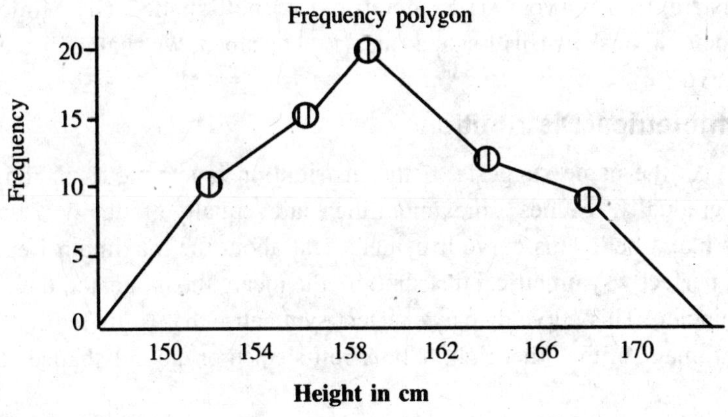

On comparing the Histogram and a frequency polygon, you will notice that, in frequency polygons the points replace the bars (rectangles). Also, when several distributions are to be compared on the same graph paper, frequency polygons are better than Histograms.

Frequency Distribution Curve

Frequency distribution curves are like frequency polygons. In frequency distribution, instead of using straight line segments, a smooth curve is used to connect the points. The frequency curve for the above data is shown as:

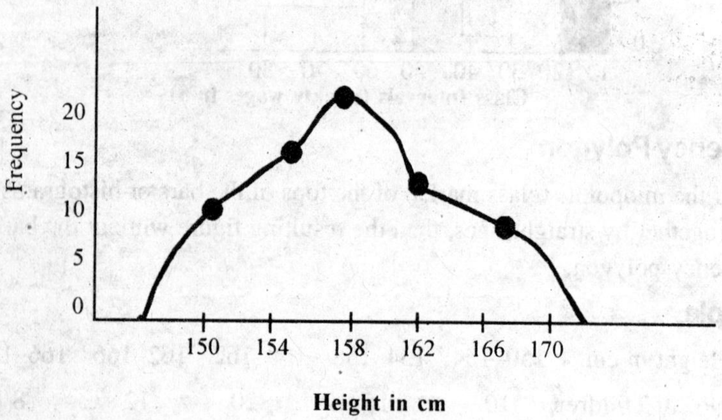

Shape of Distribution Curves

We have seen what a distribution curve looks like. There are four types of distribution curves: (i) Symmetrical or bell-shaped (ii) Moderately symmetrical or skew (iii) J-shaped and (iv) U-shaped. We shall only study the first two.

i. Symmetrical Distribution

As the name suggests, if the distribution is symmetrical, the curve rises gradually, reaches a maximum then falls equally gradually. The curve looks like a bell. This curve is symmetrical about the maximum frequency. For a perfectly symmetrical distribution, the mean, the mode and the median all coincide. This curve displays perfect symmetry, that is, its left half is the mirror image of the other right half. A bell-shaped or mound-shaped curve is also known as the normal curve, giving it special properties. This is an ideal situation and therefore, rarely found in practice.

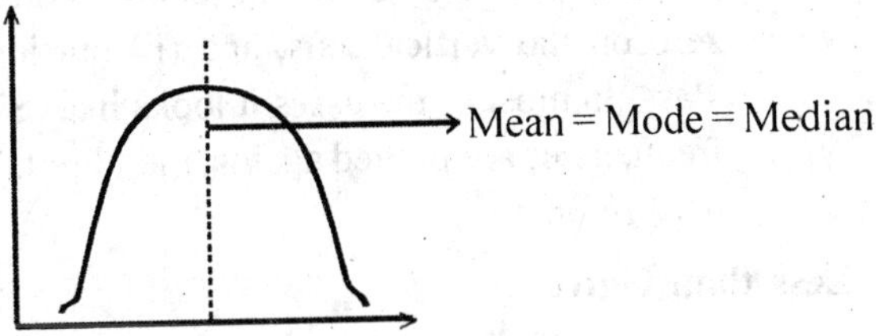

ii. Moderately Symmetrical or Skew

The curve is symmetrical but only moderately. If it rises rapidly, reaches a maximum and then falls slowly, it is a called a positively skewed curve. If it rises slowly, reaches a maximum and then falls rapidly, it is called a "negatively skewed curve". For these curves; the mean, the median and the mode do not coincide. In much of the economic and social phenomenon, we come across such curves.

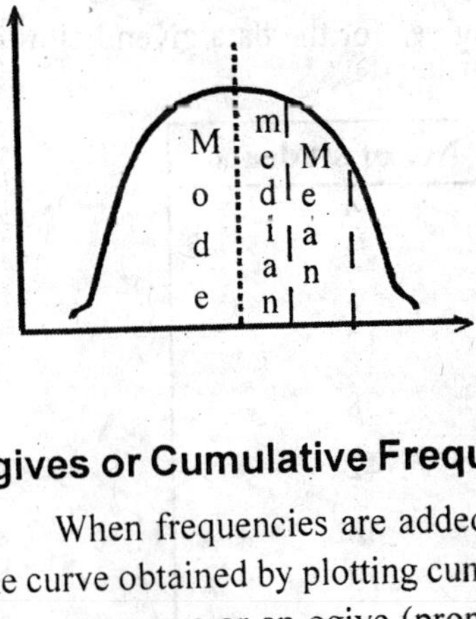

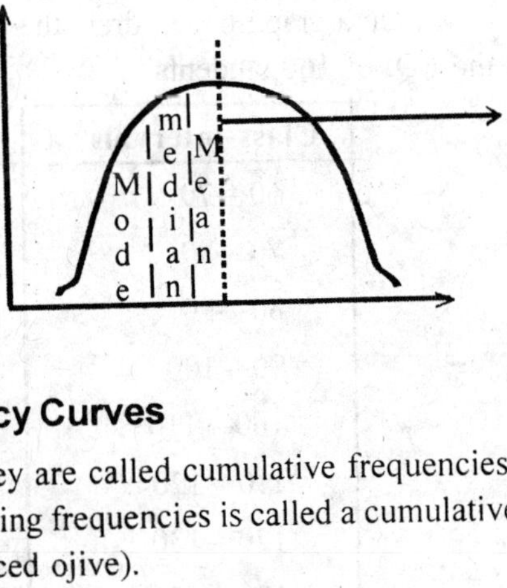

Ogives or Cumulative Frequency Curves

When frequencies are added, they are called cumulative frequencies. The curve obtained by plotting cumulating frequencies is called a cumulative frequency curve or an ogive (pronounced ojive).

To Construct an Ogive

1. Add up the progressive totals of frequencies, class by class, to get the cumulative frequencies.

2. Plot classes on the horizontal (x-axis) and cumulative frequencies on the vertical (y-axis).

3. Join the points by a smooth curve. Note that Ogives start at (i) zero on the vertical axis, and (ii) outside class limit of the last class. In most of the cases it looks like 'S'. Note that cumulative frequencies are plotted against the 'limits' of the classes to which they refer.

(A) Less than Ogive

To plot a less than ogive, the data is arranged in ascending order of magnitude and the frequencies are cumulated starting from the top. It starts from zero on the y-axis and the lower limit of the lowest class interval on the x-axis.

(B) Greater than Ogive

To plot this ogive, the data are arranged in the ascending order of magnitude and frequencies are cumulated from the bottom. This curve ends at zero on the y-axis and the upper limit of the highest classinterval on the x-axis.

Illustrations

On a graph paper, draw the two ogives for the data given below of the I.Q. of 160 students.

Class-intervals	No. of students
60—70	2
70—80	7
80—90	12
90—100	28
100—110	42
110—120	36
120—130	18
130—140	10
140—150	4
150—160	1

Solution

classes	f	c.f. less than	c. f. greater than
60—70	2	2	159 + 1 = 160
70—80	7	2 + 7 = 9	151 + 7 = 158
80—90	12	9 + 12 = 21	139 + 12 = 151
90—100	28	21 + 28 = 49	111 + 28 = 139
100—110	42	49 + 42 = 91	69 + 42 = 111
110—120	36	91 + 36 = 127	33 + 36 = 69
120—130	18	127 + 18 = 145	15 + 18 = 33
130—140	10	145 + 10 = 155	5 + 10 = 15
140—150	4	155 + 4 = 159	1 + 4 = 5
150—160	1	159 + 1 = 160	1
	$\sum f = 160$		

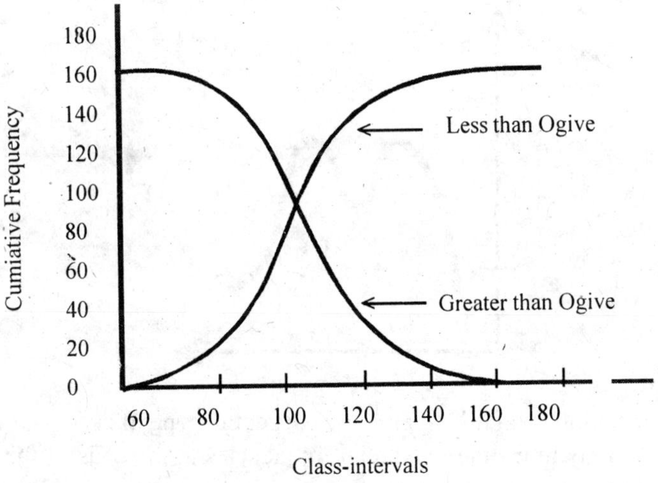

Uses

Certain values like median, quartiles, deciles, quartile deviation, coefficient of skewness etc. can be located using ogives. It can be used to find the percentage of items having values less than or greater than certain value. Ogives are helpful in the comparison of the two distributions.

J-Shaped Curve

These curves are so called, as they have the shape of a 'J' or a' U'. The distributions are extremely asymmetrical.

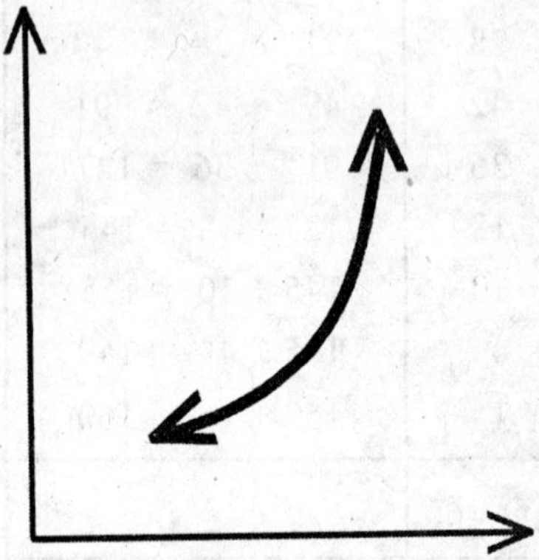

Biomodal Curve

Unlike a normal curve (symmetric distribution), a bimodal curve has two peaks or humps.

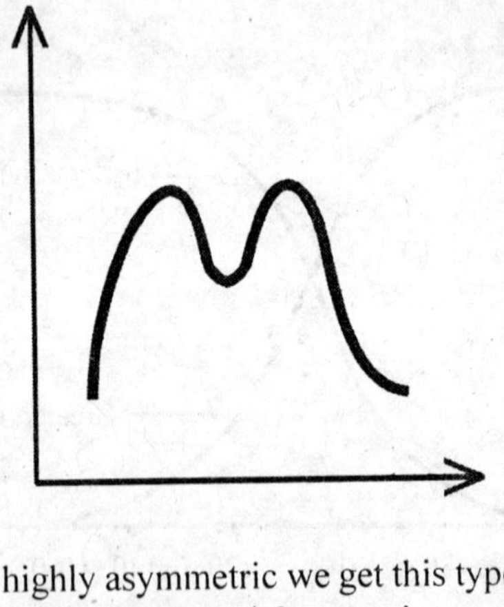

When a distribution is highly asymmetric we get this type of curve (U - type). U-Shaped curve exhibits the maximum frequencies at the ends of the range and the minimum towards the center.

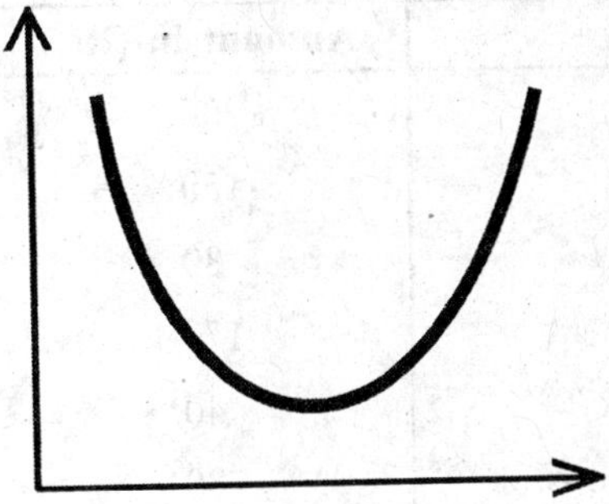

PIE CHARTS

A circle is broken up into various categories of interest in the same way as one may slice a pie. Each category is assigned a certain percentage of the 360 degree of the total circle, depending upon the data.

Steps required to construct a pie chart are as follows:

1. Determine all the categories that are of interest from the data.
2. For each category determined in step 1, calculate its relative frequency.
3. Draw a circle and assign a slice of the circle to each category. The size of each slice should be proportional to the fraction of observations in that category. Also, the central angle should be an angle whose measure is 360 degree times the relative frequency of that category. The sum of the measures of the central angles should be 360 degree.
4. Place an appropriate label in each category and indicate the percentage of the total number of observations in the category. This can be found by using the fact that for each category.

   Percentage = Relative Frequency * 100.
5. The sum of all percentages must always be 100% (except for possible rounding errors).

Example

The following table shows the monthly living expenses in 2002 for an employee of a company.

Item	Amount in (Rs.)
Food	200
Apartment	150
Transport	80
Entertainment	170
Maintenance	40
Miscellaneous	80
Total	720

Draw a pie chart of monthly expenses.

Solution

Since the total expenditure was Rs. 720 and there are 360 degree in a circle. We have to convert the percentage in degrees.

Conversion to % (Relative Frequency)

Item	Amount	R.F.
Food	200	200 / 720 = 0.2778 or 27.78
Apartment	150	0.2083
Transport	80	0.1111
Entertainment	170	0.2361
Maintenance	40	0.05561
Misc.	30	0.1111
Total	720	

Conversion to Degrees

Item	R.F.	Degree
Food	0.2778	0.2778 x 360 = 100
Apartment	0.2083	0.2083 x 360 = 75
Transport	0.1111	0.1111 x 360 = 40
Entertainment	0.2361	0.2361 x 360 = 85
Maintenance	0.0556	0.0556 x 360 = 20
Misc.	0.111	0.1111 x 360 = 40

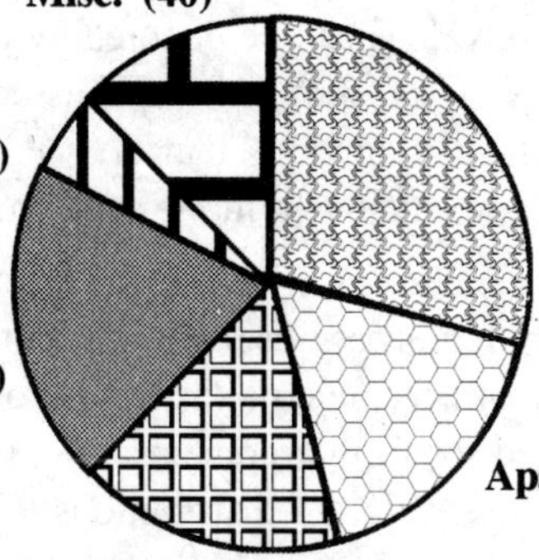

Percentiles

Percentiles are values in a given set of observations that divide the data into 100 equal parts. These values can be denoted by $P_1, P_2 ... P_{99}$, where 1% of the data falls below (is less than or equal to) P_1, 2% of the data falls below P_2, 99% of the data falls below P_{99}. Percentiles can be calculated using a sorted list of observations or the cumulative frequency distribution table corresponding to the observations. In the latter method, it is assumed that the values in a class interval are uniformly distributed within it; extrapolation is then used to calculate the percentiles. As this assumption is often untrue, percentile values can differ depending on whether raw data or frequency distributions were used in the computation. Therefore, percentiles are often treated as estimates for the value below which certain percentages of the observations fall. Some percentiles have special names:

Percentile	Special Name
25th	Lower Quartile (LQ)
50th	Median (M or MED)
75th	Upper Quartile (UQ)

Deciles are values in a given set of observations that divide the data into 10 equal parts. These values can be denoted by $D_1, D_2 ... D_9$, where 10% of the data falls below D_1, 20% of the data falls below D_2, 90% of the data falls below D_9.

It is easy to see that

$D_1 = P_{10}, D_4 = P_{40}, D_7 = P_{70}$

$D_2 = P_{20}, D_5 = P_{50}, D_8 = P_{80}$

$D_3 = P_{30}, D_6 = P_{60}, D_9 = P_{90}$

Quartiles are values in a given set of observations that divide the data in 4 equal parts. These values can be denoted by Q_1, Q_2 and Q_3, where 25% of the data falls below Q_1, 50% of the data falls below Q_2 75% of the data falls below Q_3. Again, it is obvious that $Q_1 = P_{25}$, $Q_2 = P_{50}$, and $Q_3 = P_{75}$. Deciles and quartiles are calculated in the same manner as percentiles.

In the previous section, we have studied how to collect raw data, its classification and tabulation in a useful form, which contributes in solving many problems of statistical concern. Yet, this is not sufficient, for in practical purposes, there is need for further condensation, particularly when we want to compare two or more different distributions. Statisticians utilize various kinds of measurements based on the collected data as an initial step towards developing inferences on the population from which observations were taken. Some measures reflect, in a sense, the center or middle point of a set of data; others provide a measure of the variability of the data. These measures can apply to either the population as a whole or to a sample taken from the population.

1.4 MEASURE OF THE CENTRAL TENDENCY

Measure of central tendency gives us an idea about the concentration of the values in the central part of distribution. In fact, measure of central tendency of a statistical data is the value which is representative of the entire data. A single value which can be considered as typical or representative of a set of observations and around which the observations can be considered as centered is called an 'Average' (or average value) or a center of location. Since such typical values tend to lie centrally within a set of observations when arranged according to magnitudes, averages are called measures of central tendency.

The fundamental measures of tendencies are:

(1) Arithmetic mean
(2) Median
(3) Mode
(4) Geometric mean
(5) Harmonic mean
(6) Weighted averages

However the most common measures of central tendencies or locations are **Arithmetic** mean, median and mode.

Arithmetic Mean

The statistical **mean** of a set of observations is the average of the measurements in a set of data. The population mean and sample mean are defined as: Given the set of data values $x_1, x_2, ... x_N$ from a finite population of size N, the population mean μ is calculated as

$$\mu = \frac{1}{N}\sum_{i=0}^{N} x_i$$

Given the set of data values $x_1, x_2... x_n$ from a sample of size n, the sample mean $\overline{x}$ is calculated as:

$$\overline{x} = \frac{1}{n}\sum_{i=0}^{n} x_i$$

The sample mean is often used as an estimator of the mean of the population from whence the sample was taken. In fact, the sample mean is statistically proven to be a most effective estimator for the population mean. An interesting property of the arithmetic mean is that the sum of deviations of the individual values from their mean is always equal to zero, that is:

$$\sum_{i=0}^{n}\left(x_i - \overline{x}\right) = 0$$

Example

A variable takes the values as given below. Calculate the arithmetic mean of 110, 117, 129, 195, 95, 100, 100, 175, 250 and 750.

Solution

$$\text{Arithmetic mean} = \frac{\Sigma X_i}{n}$$

$$\sum x_i = 110 + 117 + 129 + 195 + 95 + 100 + 100 + 175 + 250 + 750 = 2021$$

and n = 10, so mean = 202.1

Indirect Method (Assumed Mean Method)

$$\overline{\mu} = \frac{\Sigma \mu_i}{n} \quad \text{Where } \mu_i = x_i - A$$

A = Assumed Mean = $A + \bar{\mu}$

Calculations

Let A = 175 then

$\sum \mu_{ii}$ = – 65, –58, – 46, +20, – 80, – 75, – 75, +0, +75, + 575

= 670 – 399

= 271/10 = 27.1

$\therefore \bar{x} = A + \bar{\mu}$

= 175 + 27.1 = 202.1

Example

The weights (in gms) of 29 articles are given below :

14, 16, 16, 14, 22, 13, 15, 24, 23, 14, 20, 17, 21, 18, 18, 19, 20, 17, 16, 15, 11, 22, 21, 20, 17, 18, 19, 22, 23.

Form a grouped frequency table, by dividing the variate range into intervals of equal width, one class being 11-13 and then compute the arithmetic mean.

Solution

Weight	Mid-Values x_i	Frequency f_i	Direct Method f_ix_i	Short-cut method A =18 $u_i = x_i$ -A	f_iu_i
11–13	12	3	36	–6	–18
13–15	14	4	56	–4	–16
15–17	16	5	80	–2	–20
17–19	18	6	108	0	0
19–21	20	5	100	+2	+10
21–23	22	4	88	+4	+16
23–25	24	3	72	+6	+18
Total		$\sum f_i$=30	$\sum f_ix_i$=540		$\sum f_iu_i$=0

Direct methods

Arithmetic mean

$$\bar{(x)} = \frac{\sum f_i x_i}{\sum f_i}$$

$$\bar{x} = \frac{540}{30} = 18$$

Short-cut methods

Arithmetic mean

$$\bar{(x)} = A + \frac{\sum f_i u_i}{\sum f_i}$$

$$\bar{(x)} = 18 + \frac{0}{30} = 18$$

Mean weight = 18 gms

Example

From the following data of the calculation of arithmetic mean, find the missing item:

Wages in:	110	112	113	117	?	125	129	130
No. of workers:	25	17	13	15	14	8	7	2

Mean wage Rs. 115.86

Solution

Wages in Rs. (x_i)	Number of workers (f_i)	$f_i x_i$
110	25	2750
112	17	1904
113	13	1496
117	15	1755
x	14	14x
125	8	1000
128	6	768
130	2	260
Total	$\sum f_i = 100$	$\sum f_i x_i = 9906 + 14x$

Now the arithmetic mean $(\bar{x}) = \frac{\sum f_i x_i}{\sum f_i}$

Therefore $115.86 = \frac{9906 + 14x}{100}$

or $115.86 \times 100 = 9906 + 14x$

$11586 - 9906 = 14x$

$1680 = 14x$

or $x = 1680/14$

$x = 120$

Therefore the missing item is 120.

Properties of Arithmetic Mean

1. The sum of the deviations, of all the values of x, from their arithmetic mean, is zero.

   Justification: $\sum f_i(x_i - \bar{x}) = \sum f_i x_i - \bar{x}\sum f_i = 0$

   Since $\bar{x}$ is a constant, $\bar{x} = \frac{\sum f_i x_i}{\sum f_i} \therefore \sum f_i x_i = \bar{x}\sum f_i$

2. The product of the arithmetic mean and the number of items gives the total of all items.

   $$\bar{x} = \frac{\sum f_i x_i}{\sum f_i} \Rightarrow \sum f_i x_i = \bar{x}\sum f_i$$

   Justification:

   or $\bar{x} = \frac{\sum x_i}{N} \Rightarrow \bar{x}.N = \sum x_i$

3. If $\bar{x}_1$ and $\bar{x}_2$ are the arithmetic mean of two samples of sizes n_1 and n_2 respectively then, the arithmetic mean $\bar{x}$ of the distribution combining the two can be calculated as:

$$\bar{x} = \frac{n_1\overline{x_1} + n_2\overline{x_2}}{n_1 + n_2}$$

This formula can be extended for still more groups or samples.

$$\overline{x_1} = \frac{\sum x_{1i}}{n_1} \Rightarrow \sum x_{1i} = n_1\overline{x_1}$$

Justification: $\overline{x_1} = \frac{\sum x_{1i}}{n_1} \Rightarrow \sum x_{1i} = n_1\overline{x_1}$ = total of the observations of the first sample.

Similarly $\sum x_{2i} = n_2\overline{x_2}$ = total of the observations of the second sample.

The combined mean of the two samples:

$$= \frac{\text{Combined Total}}{n_1 + n_2}$$

$$\bar{x} = \frac{n_1\overline{x_1} + n_2\overline{x_2}}{n_1 + n_2}$$

Example

The average marks of three batches of students having 70, 50 and 30 students respectively are 50, 55 and 45. Find the average marks of all the 150 students taken together.

Solution

Let x be the average marks of all 150 students taken together.

	Batch - I	Batch - II	Batch - III
marks :	$\overline{x_1} = 50$	$\overline{x_2} = 55$	$\overline{x_3} = 45$

No. of students $n_1 = 70$ $n_2 = 50$ $n_3 = 30$

$$\bar{x} = \frac{n_1\bar{x}_1 + n_2\bar{x}_2 + n_3\bar{x}_3}{n_1 + n_2 + n_3} = \frac{70\times 50 + 50\times 55 + 30\times 45}{70+50+30} = \frac{7600}{150}$$

$$\bar{x} = 50.67$$

Example

The mean of a certain number of observations is 40. If two or more items with values 50 and 64 are added to this data, the mean rises to 42. Find the number of items in the original data.

Solution

Let 'n' be the number of observations whose mean $\bar{x} = 40$.

$$\bar{x} = \frac{\sum x_i}{n} \therefore \sum x_i = n\bar{x} = n(40) = 40n \text{ Total of n values.}$$

Two more items of values 50 and 64 are added therefore, total of (n + 2) values:

$$= \sum x_i + 50 + 64$$

$$= 40\,n + 50 + 64$$

$$= 40n + 114$$

Now new mean is 42.

$$\therefore \text{New } \bar{x} = \frac{\text{New total of (n + 2) values}}{n+2}$$

$$\therefore 42 = \frac{40n + 14}{n+2}$$

$$\therefore 42n + 84 = 40n + 114$$

$$\therefore 2n = 30$$

$$\therefore n = 15$$

Therefore, the number of items in the original data = 15.

Example

The mean weight of 98 students is found to be 50 lbs. It is later discovered that the frequency of the class interval (30- 40) was wrongly taken as 8 instead of 10. Calculate the correct mean.

Solution

$$\text{Incorrect mean } (\bar{x}) = 50 \text{ Kg and } \sum f_i = 98$$

$$\therefore \text{Incorrect } \bar{x} = \frac{Incorrect \sum f_i x_i}{\sum f_i}$$

$$50 = \frac{\text{Incorrect} \sum f_i x_i}{\sum f_i}$$

Therefore, incorrect $\sum f_i x_i = 98 \times 50 = 4900$

Now correct

$$\sum f_i x_i = \text{Incorrect} \sum f_i x_i - (8 \times 35) + (10 \times 35)$$

Note that the class-mark of classinterval (30 - 40) is 35 and for the calculation of the mean we consider class marks.

$$\text{The Correct} \sum f_i x_i = 4900 - 280 + 350 = 4970$$

Also the correct $\sum f_i = 98 + 2 = 100$

Therefore, the correct mean

$$\bar{x} = \frac{\text{correct} \sum f_i x_i}{\text{correct} \sum f_i} = \frac{4970}{100}$$

$$\bar{x} = 49.701b$$

Example

The average marks obtained by male students in CPMT examination are 80 and that of their counterpart was 70 the mean marks obtained by the students of CPMT were 78. Find the percentage of Male and Female students.

Solution

$\bar{x}_1 = 80,\ \bar{x}_2 = 70,\ \bar{x} = 78$

$\bar{x} = (n_1 x_1 + n_2 x_2)/(n_1 + n_2)$

$78 = (80\, n_1 + 70\, n_2)/(n_1 + n_2)$

$78\,(n_1 + n_2) = 80n_1 + 70n_2$

$8n_2 = 2n_1$

$n_1/n_2 = 8/2 = 4/1$

Percentage of male students in the class $= 4 / 4 + 1 \times 100 = 400 / 5$
$= 80\%$

Percentage of female student in class $= 1 / 4 + 1 \times 100 = 100 / 5$
$= 20\%$

Merits of Mean

1. It is rigidly defined. Its value is always definite.
2. It is easy to calculate and easy to understand. Hence it is very popular.
3. It is based on all the observations; so that it becomes a good representative.
4. It can be easily used for comparison.
5. It is capable of further algebraic treatment.
6. It is not affected much by sampling fluctuations.

Demerits

1. It is affected by outliers or extreme values. For example, the average (A) mean of 10, 15, 25 and 500 is:

$$\bar{x} = \frac{10 + 15 + 25 + 500}{4} = 137.5$$

Now observe first three values whose A mean is:

$$\frac{10 + 15 + 25}{3} = 16.67\text{(approx)}$$

Due to the outlier 500 the A mean of the four numbers is raised to 137.5. In such a case A mean is not a good representative of the given data.

2. It is a value which may not be present in the given data.
3. Many a times it gives absurd results like 4.4 children per family.
4. It is not possible to take out the averages of ratios and percentages.
5. We cannot calculate it when open-end class intervals are present in the data.

Median

It is the value of the size of the central item of the arranged data (data arranged in the ascending or the descending order). Thus, it is the value of the middle item and divides the series in to two equal parts.

Median in Individual Series (Ungrouped Data)

The **median** of a set of observations is that value that, when the observations are arranged in an ascending or descending order, satisfies the following condition:

If the total number of observations be 'n' then:

A. If 'n' is odd

$$\text{The median} = \text{size of } \left(\frac{n+1}{2}\right)^{th} \text{ observation}$$

B. If 'n' is even, the median

$$= \frac{1}{2}\left[\text{size of } \left(\frac{n}{2}\right)^{th} \text{ observation} + \text{size of } \left(\frac{n+2}{2}\right)^{th} \text{ observation}\right]$$

The median is the same as the 50th percentile of a set of data. It is denoted by $\bar{x}$.

Example

The following figures represent the number of books issued at the counter of a medical library on 11 different days. 96, 180, 98, 75, 270, 80, 102, 100, 94, 75 and 200. Calculate the median.

Solution

Arrange the data in the ascending order as 75, 75, 80, 94, 96, 98, 100, 102,180, 200, 270.

Now the total number of items 'n'= 11 (odd)

Therefore, the median = size of $(\frac{n+1}{2})^{th}$ item

$= \text{size of } (\frac{11+1}{2})^{th} \text{ item}$

$= \text{size of } 5^{th} \text{ item}$

= 98 books per day

Median in Discrete Series

Steps:

1. Arrange the data in ascending or descending order of magnitude.
2. Find the cumulative frequencies.
3. Apply the formula:

A. If $n = \sum f_i$ (odd) then,

$$\text{Median} = \text{size of } (\frac{n+1}{2})^{th} \text{ item}$$

B. If $n = \sum f_i$ (even) then,

$$\text{Median} = \frac{1}{2}\left[\text{size of } (\frac{n}{2})^{th} \text{ observation} + \text{size of } (\frac{n+2}{2})^{th} \text{ observation}\right]$$

Example

Locate the median in the following distribution.

Size :	8	10	12	14	16	18	20
Frequency :	7	7	12	28	10	9	6

Solution

Size (x_i)	Frequency (f_i)	Cumulative frequency (c.f.)
8	3	3
10	7	3 + 7 = 10
12	12	12+ 10 = 22
14	28	28+ 22 = 50
16	10	50 + 10 = 60
18	9	60 + 9 = 69
20	6	69 + 6 = 75
	$n = \sum f_i = 75$ (odd)	

Therefore, the median = size of $\left(\frac{n+1}{2}\right)$ item

= size of $\left(\frac{75+1}{2}\right)$ item

= size of 38th item

In the order of the cumulative frequency, the 38th term is present in the 50th cumulative frequency, whose size is 14.

Therefore, the median = 14

Median in Continuous Series (Grouped Data)

Consider the situation when the data is given in the form of a frequency distribution. Steps for calculating the median:

Step 1: Find $\frac{N}{2}$, Where $N = \sum_{i=1}^{n} f_i$

Step 2: Locate the cumulative frequency just greater than N / 2.

Step 3: The corresponding class gives idea about the median class, i.e., the class where the median will lie.

Step 4: After ascertaining the class in which median lies, the following formula is used for determining the exact value of the median.

$$\text{Median} = l_1 + \left[\frac{N/2 - c.f.}{f}\right](l_1 - l_2)$$

where, l_1 = lower limit of the median class, the class in which the middle item of the distribution lies.

l_2 = upper limit of the median class

c.f. = cumulative frequency of the class preceding the median class

f = sample frequency of the median class

It should be noted that while interpolating the median value of frequency distribution it is assumed that the variable is continuous and that there is an orderly and even distribution of items within each class.

Example

Calculate the median for the following data.

Age (years) :	20-25	25-30	30-35	35-40	40-45
No. of person :	70	80	180	150	20

Solution

Age (year) C.I:	No. of persons f_i	Cumulaative frequency (c.f.)
20-25	70	70
25-30	80	70+ 80 = 150
30-35	180	150+180 = 330
35-40	150	330 + 150 = 480
40-45	20	480 + 20 = 500
	$n = \sum f_i = 500$	

Now Median = size of $\left(\frac{n}{2}\right)$ item

$$= \text{size of} \left(\frac{500}{2}\right)^{th}$$

= size of 250th item which lies in (30 – 35) class interval

$$\text{Median} = l_1 + \left[\frac{n/2 - C.f.}{f}\right](l_2 - l_1)$$

Here $l_1 = 30$, $l_2 = 35$, $n/2 = 250$, c.f. = 150 and f = 180

Therefore, Median

$$= 30 + [\frac{250 - 150}{180}](35 - 30)$$

$$= 30 + \frac{100}{180} \times 5$$

= 32.78 years

Merits of Median

1. It is also rigidly defined.
2. It is easy to calculate.
3. It can be used for qualitative studies.
4. It is not affected by the extreme values but is affected by the middle one or two values.
5. In case of grouped data, it can be calculated even if the end intervals are open or not clearly specified.
6. It can be obtained graphically.

Demerits of Median

1. If the series is comparatively long then re-arranging the data in order of magnitude (ascending or descending) is time consuming.
2. In case of even number of observations median can not be determined exactly, since it involves only the mean of two middle terms.

3. It is comparatively more effective by the fluctuation of sampling as far as mean is concerned.

Mode

The **mode** of a set of observations is the specific value that occurs with the greatest frequency. There may be more than one mode in a set of observations, if there are several values that all occur with the greatest frequency. A mode may also not exist; this is true if all the observations occur with the same frequency. For distributions which are symmetrical (that is, where the corresponding frequency polygons or histograms are symmetrical), mean, mode and median coincide. For slightly asymmetric distributions, it has been empirically found that:

3 (Mean–Median) = (Mean – Mode) or Mode = 3 Median – 2 Mean

Ungrouped Data

Individual Series

The mode of this series can be obtained by mere inspection. The number which occurs most often is the mode.

Example

Locate mode in the data 7, 12, 8, 5, 9, 6, 10, 9, 4, 9, 9

Solution

On inspection, it is observed that the number 9 has maximum frequency. Therefore 9 is the mode.

Note that if in any series, two or more numbers have the maximum frequency, then the mode will be difficult to calculate. Such series are called as Bi-modal, Tri-modal or Multi-modal series.

Grouped Data

Steps:

1. Determine the modal class which has the maximum frequency.
2. By interpolation the value of the mode can be calculated as -

$$\text{Mode} = l_1 + \left[\frac{f_1 - f_0}{2f_1 - f_0 - f_2}\right](l_2 - l_1)$$

where

l_1 = lower limit of the modal class

l_2 = upper limit of the modal class

f_1 = frequency of the modal class

f_0 = frequency of the class preceding to the modal class

f_2 = frequency of the class succeeding the modal class

Example

Calculate the modal wages.

Daily wages in Rs. :	20 -25	25-30	30-35	35-40	40-45	45-50
No. of workers :	1	3	8	12	7	5

Verify it graphically.

Solution

Here the maximum frequency is 12, corresponding to the class interval (35 - 40) which is the modal class.

Therefore $l_1 = 35$, $l_2 = 40$, $f_0 = 8$, $f_1 = 12$, $f_2 = 7$

By interpolation

$$\text{Mode} = l_1 + [\frac{f_1 - f_0}{2f_1 - f_0 - f_2}](l_2 - l_1)$$

$$= 40 + [\frac{12-8}{24-8-7}](40-35)$$

$$= 40 + [\frac{4}{9}] \times 5$$

$$= 40 + 2.22$$

$$= 37.22$$

Modal wages is Rs. 37.22

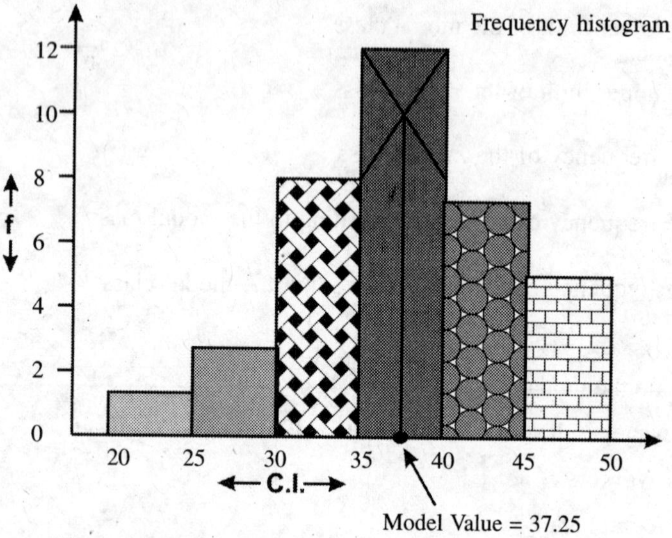

Uses of the Mode

The mode, like the median, can be used as a central location for quantitative as well as qualitative data. If a printing press turns out 5 impressions, which we rate "Very sharp", "Sharp", "Sharp", "Sharp" and "blurred", then the modal value is "Sharp". Like the median the mode is not unduly affected by extreme values. Even if the high values are very high and the low values very low, we choose the most frequent value of the data set to be the modal value. Also, mode can be used even when one or more of the classes are open-ended. However, the mode is not used as often to measure central tendency as are the mean and median. Too often, there is no modal value because the data set contains no values that are repeated more than once.

For example in the case of this example, the mode of size of shoes used in this set of data

Size of shoes:	5	6	7	8	9
No. of customer:	14	25	45	20	21

Maximum frequency is 45; size of shoes corresponding to this is 7. Hence mode is shoe of size 7.

In case of **grouped data**, the mode can be calculated by the following process.

Step 1: Locate the maximum frequency, the corresponding class is the modal class, then use the formula to obtain

$$\text{Mode} = L + h\,(f_0 - f_{-1}) / (2f_0 - f_{-1} - f_{+1})$$

Where

L = Lower limit of the modal class.
h = Magnitude of the modal class
f_0 = Frequency of the modal class.
f_{-1} = Frequency of the class preceding the modal class.
f_{+1} = Frequency of the class succeeding the modal class.

Example

The income of 80 families are given below

Income (Rs.):	400-600	600-800	800-1000	1000-1200
No. of families:	10	15	35	20

Find the mode.

Solution

The maximum frequency is 35. So 800-1000 is the modal class

$L - 800 \quad f_0 - 35$

$h = 200 \quad f_{-1} = 15$

$f_{+1} = 20$

Mode = $(800 + 200\,(35 - 15)) / (2\,'\,35 - 15 - 20)$

$= (800 + 200 \times 20) / (70 - 35) = 900$

MERITS OF MODE

1. It is simple to calculate.
2. In individual or discrete distribution it can be located by mere inspection.
3. It is easy to understand. Everyone is used to the idea of average
4. It is not isolated like the median as it is the most common item.
5. Like the average mean, it is not a value which cannot be found in the series.

6. It is not necessary to know all the items. What we need the point of maximum density frequency.
7. It is not affected by sampling fluctuations.

DEMERITS

1. It is ill defined.
2. It is not based on all observations.
3. It is not capable of further algebraic treatment.
4. It is not a good representative of the data.
5. Sometimes there are more than one values of mode.

Another measure of central location that is occasionally used is the **midrange**. It is computed as the average of the smallest and largest values in a set of data.

Empirical Relation Between Mean, Median and Mode

A distribution in which the values of mean, median and mode coincide (i.e. mean = median = mode) is known as a symmetrical distribution. Conversely, when values of mean, median and mode are not equal the distribution is known as asymmetrical or skewed distribution. In moderately skewed or asymmetrical distribution a very important relationship exists among these three measures of central tendency. In such distributions the distance between the mean and median is about one-third of the distance between the mean and mode, as will be clear from the Figures 1 and 2. Karl Pearson expressed this relationship as:

$$\text{Mode} = \text{mean} - 3\ [\text{mean} - \text{median}]$$

$$\text{Mode} = 3\ \text{median} - 2\ \text{mean}$$

$$\text{and Median} = \text{mode} + \frac{2}{3}\ (\text{mean} - \text{mode})$$

Knowing any two values, the third can be computed.

Example

Given median = 20.6, mode = 26 Find mean.

Solution

$$\text{Mode} = 3\ \text{median} - 2\ \text{mean}$$

$$\therefore \text{mean} = \frac{1}{2}[3 \text{ median - mode}]$$

$$\therefore \text{mean} = \frac{1}{2}[3(20.6) - (26)]$$

$$\therefore \text{mean} = \frac{1}{2}[35.8]$$

$$\therefore \text{mean} = 17.9$$

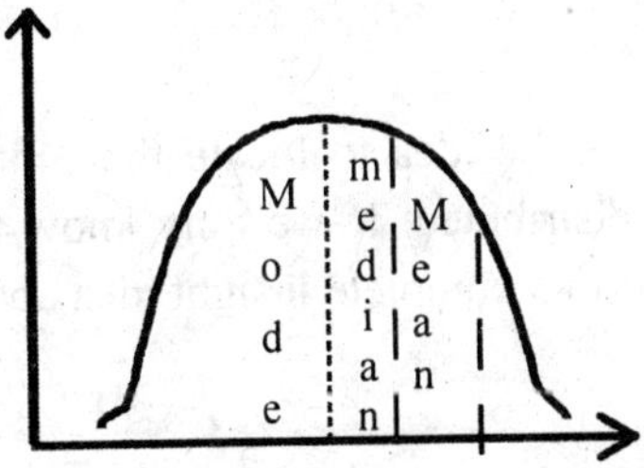

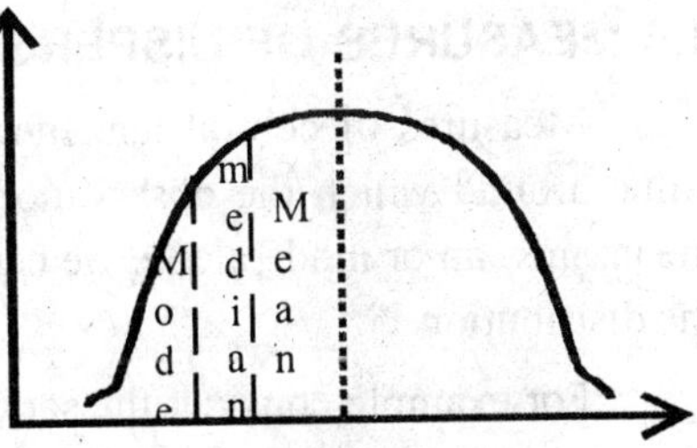

Geometric Mean

$$\text{GM} = \sqrt[n]{x_1 x_2 \ldots\ldots x_n}$$

Used for:

A: to average percents, indexes

B: to determine the average % increase in case of sales, production or other business or economic series from one time period to another.

Example

Profit earned by a company on four projects were 3%, 2%, 4% and 6%

$$\text{Average profit} = \text{GM} = \sqrt[4]{3 \times 2 \times 4 \times 6} = 3.46\%$$

$$\text{Average \% increase} = \text{n} - 1\sqrt{\frac{\text{Value at the end of period}}{\text{Value at the begnning of period}}}$$

AM ≥ GM

Harmonic Mean

Harmonic mean is the reciprocal of the AM of the reciprocals of the values of its various items.

$$HM = \frac{1}{\frac{1}{n}\left(\frac{1}{x_1} + \frac{1}{x_2} + \ldots\ldots\ldots + \frac{1}{x_n}\right)}$$

AM ≥ GM ≥ HM

1.5 MEASURES OF DISPERSION

Measures of central tendency give us the idea to locate the central value around which the observations are distributed. If we only know the mean, median or mode alone, we cannot form a complete insight idea about the distribution.

For example consider the series:

1. 4, 6, 12, 10, 18
2. 4, 10, 7, 16, 13
3. 10, 11,12, 13, 4

All the above three series we see that the number of observations are same and the mean is 10.

If it is given that the mean of the observations is 10, we may fail to form an idea as to whether it is the average of the first series, second series or third series. Hence, measure of central tendency is inadequate to give a complete idea.

A further description about the degree of **scatter ness** is must to get a better description of data. One such measure is **Measures of dispersion**. In the above quoted example series three is more homogenous (i.e. less scattered) as respect to other two series.

The following are the most common measures of dispersions:

1. Range
2. Quartile deviation

3. Mean deviation
4. Variance
5. Standard deviation
6. Coefficient of variation
7. Coefficient of dispersion.

Out of these six measures of dispersion first five measures the absolute variation, whereas the last two measures the relative dispersion of a given set of data. Statistical **measures of dispersion / variation** are numerical values that indicate the variability inherent in a set of data measurements. The most common measures of variation are the range, variance and standard distribution.

1. Range

It is the simplest but a crude measure of dispersion. The range of a set of observation is the difference between the largest and the smallest value of the set of observation. If A and B are the largest and the smallest, value in the set of observations, then its range

$$\mathbf{R = A - B}$$

Range, as it is seen here that it is based only on the two extreme values, so it is not at all a reliable measure of dispersion, nevertheless the range gives us a quick measure. It is widely used in statistical quality control to see the variation in the production unit. The range is also used frequently by stock brokers to describe the prices of certain stock.

In any statistical series, the difference between the largest and the smallest values is called as the range.

$$\text{Thus Range (R)} = L - S = \begin{Bmatrix} L = \text{Largest value of the series} \\ S = \text{Smallest value of the series} \end{Bmatrix}$$

Coefficient of Range

The relative measure of the range. It is used in the comparative study of the dispersion co-efficient of Range = $= \dfrac{L - S}{L + S}$

Example

(Individual series) Find the range and the co-efficient of the range of the following items:

110, 117, 129, 197, 190, 100, 100, 178, 255, 790.

Solution

R = L - S = 790 - 100 = 690

$$\text{Co-efficient of Range} = \frac{L-S}{L+S} = \frac{790-100}{790+100} = \frac{690}{890} = 0.78$$

Example

(Continuous series) Find the range and its co-efficient from the following data.

Size	10-20	20-30	30-40	40-50	50-10
Frequency	2	3	5	4	2

Solution

R = L - S = 100 - 10 = 90

$$\text{Co-efficient of range} = = \frac{L-S}{L+S} = \frac{100-10}{100+10} = \frac{90}{110} = 0.82$$

2. Quartile Deviation

$Q = (Q_3 - Q_1)/2$, where Q_1 and Q_3 are the first and third quartiles

3. Mean Deviation

If x_i (I = 1, 2…*n*) are the observations of a variable with frequencies f_i then mean deviation from the mean is:

$$\text{M.D.} = \frac{1}{n}\sum_{1}^{n} f_i \,|x_i - \bar{x}| \qquad \text{where,} \quad N = \sum_i f_i$$

Mean deviation is least when taken from median.

4. Variance

Given the set of data values $x_1, x_2 \ldots x_N$ from a finite population of size N, the variance is calculated as

$$\sigma^2 = \frac{1}{n}\sum_{1}^{n} f_i(x_i - \bar{x})^2$$

5. Standard Deviation (S.D.)

The **standard deviation σ** of a set of data is the positive square root of the variance. **S.D. is least when taken from mean.** For any discrete distribution S.D. ≥ M.D. from mean.

Mathematically, it is the square root of the arithmetic mean of the square deviations of various values from their arithmetic mean. It is denoted by S.D. or σ.

Thus, S.D. $(\sigma x) = \sqrt{\frac{\Sigma(x_i - \bar{x})^2}{n}}$ for the un grouped data

$\sqrt{\frac{\Sigma f_i(x_i - \bar{x})^2}{n}}$ for the grouped data

where n = Σ fi

Merits

1. It is rigidly defined and based on all observations.
2. It is amenable to further algebraic treatment.
3. It is not affected by sampling fluctuations.
4. It is less erratic.

Demerits

1. It is difficult to understand and calculate.
2. It gives greater weight to extreme values.

Note that variance $V(x) = \frac{\Sigma(x_i - \bar{x})^2}{n}$

and S.D. $(\sigma x) = \frac{\Sigma(x_i - \bar{x})^2}{n}$ and $(\sigma x) = \frac{\Sigma f_i(x_i - \bar{x})^2}{n}$

Then $V(x) = \sigma_x^2$

6. Co-efficient of Variation (C. V.)

To compare the variations (dispersion) of two different series, relative measures of standard deviation must be calculated. This is known as co-efficient of variation or the co-efficient of S.D. Its formula is:

$$C.V. = \frac{\sigma x}{\bar{x}} \times 100$$

Thus it is defined as the ratio of S.D. to its mean.

Remark: It is given as a percentage and is used to compare the consistency or variability of two more series. The higher the C.V., the higher the variability and lower the C.V., the higher is the consistency of the data.

Example

Calculate the standard deviation and its co-efficient from the following data:

A	10
B	12
C	16
D	8
E	25
F	30
G	14
H	11
I	13
J	11

Solution

No	x_i	$(x_i - \bar{x})$	$(x_i - \bar{x})^2$
A	10	-5	25
B	12	-3	9

C	16	+1	1
D	8	-7	49
E	25	+10	100
F	30	+15	225
G	14	-1	1
H	11	-5	16
I	13	-2	4
J	11	-4	16
n= 10	$\Sigma xi = 150$		$\Sigma(x_i - x)^2$
			=446

Calculations

i. $\bar{x} = \frac{\Sigma x_i}{n} = \frac{150}{10} = 15$

ii. $\text{S.D. } (\sigma x) = \sqrt{\frac{\Sigma(x_i - \bar{x})^2}{n}} = \sqrt{\frac{446}{10}} = 6.7$

iii. Co-efficient of S.D. = $\frac{\sigma x}{\bar{x}} = \frac{6.7}{15} = 0.45$

Example

Find the mean and S.D. of the expenditure on the drugs while taking TB treatment from the data given below:

Class interval	Mid Expenditure	No. of patients	$d_i = x_i - A$	$f_i d_i$	d_i^2	$f_i d_i^2$
790-810	800	7	-100	-700	10000	70000
810-830	820	4	-80	-320	6400	25600
830-850	840	10	-60	-600	3600	36000
850-870	860	10	-40	-400	1600	16000
870-890	880	9	-20	-180	400	3600

890-910	900	25	0	0	0	0
910-930	920	10	20	200	400	4000
930-950	940	10	40	400	1600	16000
950-970	960	20	60	1200	3600	72000
970-990	980	10	80	800	6400	64000
990-1010	1000	5	100	500	10000	50000
Total		N=Σfi=100		900		357200

Here A (assumed mean) is 900, therefore, Mean $\bar{x}$ = A+ ($\sum$ fi di)/N

i.e. Mean = 900+900/100 = 909 and

Standard Deviation S.D. = $\sqrt{\sum fi\ di^2/n}$ = 597.6/100 =5.9

Hence mean expenditure is Rs. 909± 5.9

Use of Standard Deviation

1. It helps us to compare the degree of variation of two or more sets by comparing their standard deviation. The set of data having smaller SD will have less dispersion.
2. It helps us to decide whether the mean will be representative or not. If SD is comparatively low their mean becomes the representative of the distribution.
3. The standard deviation along with the mean gives a fairly good amount of information about the distribution. These help in the summarization of data.

Coefficient of Variation and Coefficient of Dispersion

It has been told earlier that Range, Standard deviation, Variance and Mean deviation are the measure of absolute dispersion. To compare the variations (dispersion) of two different series, relative measures of standard deviation must be calculated. This is known as:

1. Coefficient of dispersions, and
2. Coefficient of variation

Coefficient of Dispersion

Based on Range

$$C.D. = \frac{A - B}{A + B}$$

Based on Q.D.

$$C.D. = \frac{Q_3 - Q_1}{Q_3 + Q_1}$$

Based on M.D.

$$C.D. = \frac{M.D.}{\overline{X}}$$

Based on S.D.

$$C.D. = \frac{\sigma}{\overline{X}}\%$$

Coefficient of Variation

The coefficient of variation is a measure of relative dispersion and is given by

$$\text{Coefficent of Variation} = \frac{\text{Standard Deviation}}{\text{Mean}}$$

It is generally expressed as a percentage. The use of coefficient of variation lies partly in the fact that the mean and standard deviation tend to change together in many experiments.

Example

After analyzing the wage pattern of the workers of two medical firmsA and B following results were obtained.

	Firm A	**Firm B**
No. of workers:	400	500
Average monthly income:	350	225
Standard deviation :	8	9

Find which of these have the larger variation.

Solution

C.V. for firm A= 8 / 350 × 100 = 2.28%.

C. V. for firm B = 9 / 225 × 100 = 4.0%.

Hence we see that the firm B has slightly greater variation.

Combined Standard Deviation

If two sets containing n_1 and n_2 items having means x_1 and x_2 and standard deviations s_1 and s_2 respectively are taken together then:

(1) Mean of the combined data is $\bar{x} = \dfrac{n_1 \bar{x}_1 + n_2 \bar{x}_2}{n_1 + n_2}$

(2) S.D. of the combined set is

$$\sigma = \sqrt{\frac{n_1(\sigma^2_1 + d^2_1) + n_2(\sigma^2_2 + d^2_2)}{n_1 + n_2}}$$

Where $d_1 = \bar{x}_1 - \bar{x}$ and $d_2 = \bar{x}_2 - \bar{x}$

Moments

Moment is a familiar mechanical term for the measure of a force with reference to its tendency to produce rotation. In statistics moments are used to describe the various characteristics of a frequency distribution like central tendency, variation, skewness and kurtosis. The moments about mean are called the "central moment" and are denoted by $\mu_1, \mu_2, \mu_3, \mu_4$....

The rth moment of a variable x about any point x=A is

$$\mu_r = \frac{1}{N}\sum_1^n f_i (x_i - A)^r$$

rth moment about mean is (also called Central Moments)

$$\mu_r = \frac{1}{N}\sum_1^n f_i (x_i - \bar{x})^r$$

Pearson's Co-efficient

$\beta_1 = \mu_3^2 / \mu_2^3, \quad \gamma_1 = \beta_1$

$\beta_2 = \mu_4 / \mu_2^2, \quad \gamma_2 = \beta_2 - 3$

For discrete distribution $\beta_2 > 1$, and $\beta_2 > \beta_1 + 1$

1.6 MEASURE OF SKEWNESS AND KURTOSIS

So far we have seen that measures of location and dispersion are two important characteristics of the distribution of mass of data. Besides these two there are two other characteristics of a distribution. They are skewness, also known as Asymmetry and Kurtosis, also known as peakedness.

The voluminous raw data cannot be easily understood. Hence, we calculate the measures of central tendencies and obtain a representative figure. From the measures of variability, we can know that whether most of the items of the data are close to our away from these central tendencies. But these statistical means and measures of variation are not enough to draw sufficient inferences about the data. Another aspect of the data is to know its symmetry. In the chapter "Graphic display" we have seen that a frequency may be symmetrical about mode or may not be. This symmetry is well studied by the knowledge of the "skewness". Still one more aspect of the curve that we need to know is its flatness or otherwise its top. This is understood by what is known as "Kurtosis".

Skewness

It may happen that two distributions have the same mean and standard deviations. For example, see the following diagram.

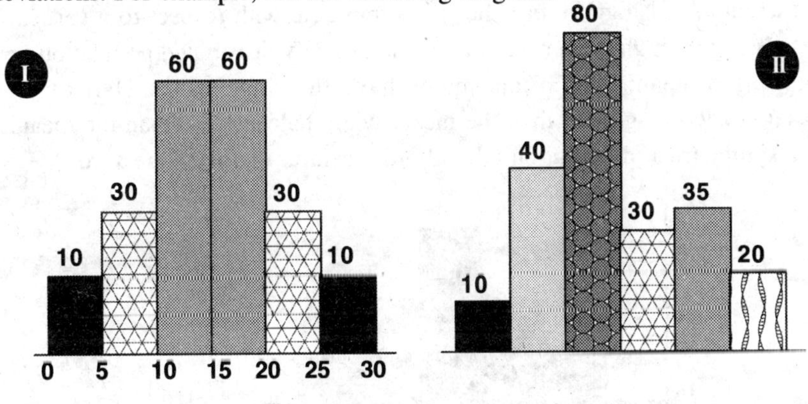

Although the two distributions have the same means and standard deviations they are not identical. Where do they differ?

They differ in symmetry. The left-hand side distribution is symmetrical one where as the distribution on the right-hand is asymmetrical or skewed. For a symmetrical distribution, the values, of equal distances on either side of the mode, have equal frequencies. Thus, the mode, median and mean–all coincide. Its curve rises slowly, reaches a maximum (peak) and falls equally slowly (Figure). But for a skewed distribution, the mean, mode and median do not coincide. Skewness is positive or negative as per the positions of the mean and median on the right or the left of the mode.

A positively skewed distribution curve rises rapidly, reaches the maximum and falls slowly. In other words, the tail as well as median on the right-hand side. A negatively skewed distribution curve rises slowly reaches its maximum and falls rapidly. In other words, the tail as well as the median are on the left-hand side.

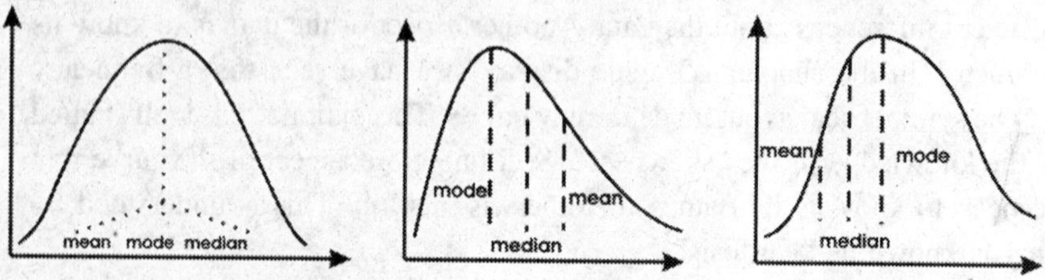

Symmetry and Skewness

A set of observations is **symmetrically distributed** if its graphical representation (histogram, bar chart) is symmetric with respect to a vertical axis passing through the mean. For a symmetrically distributed population or sample, the mean, median and mode have the same value. Half of all measurements are greater than the mean, while half are less than the mean. For a symmetrical distribution all odd order central moments are zero.

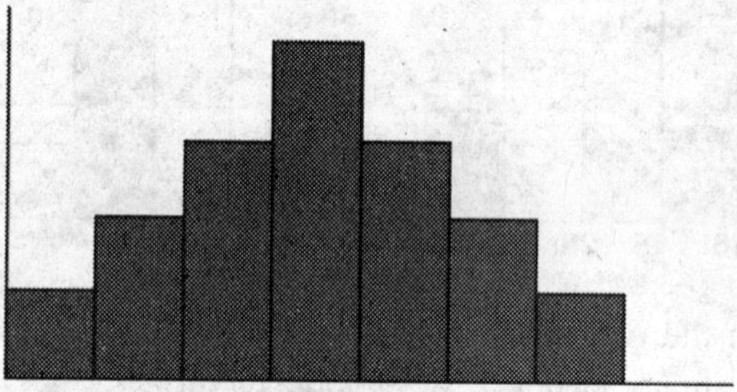

Symmetric distribution histogram

A set of observations that is not symmetrically distributed is said to be **skewed**. It is **positively skewed** if a greater proportion of the observations are less than or equal to (as opposed to greater than or equal to) the mean; this indicates that the mean is larger than the median. The histogram of a positively skewed distribution will generally have a long right tail; thus, this distribution is also known as being **skewed to the right.** On the other hand, a **negatively skewed** distribution has more observations that are greater than or equal to the mean. Such a distribution has a mean that is less than the median. The histogram of a negatively skewed distribution will generally have a long left tail; thus, the phrase **skewed to the left** is applied here.

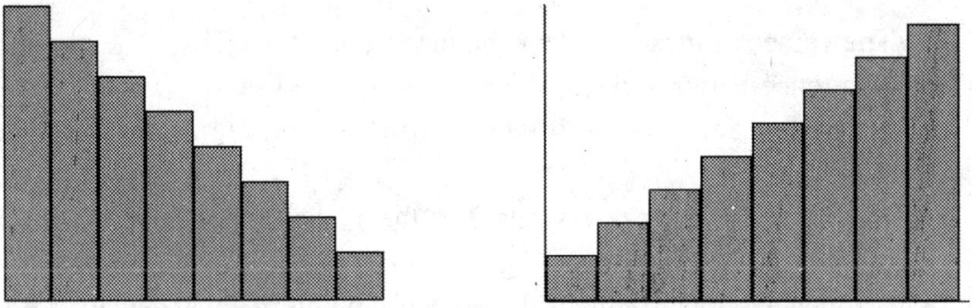

Positively Skewed Histogram **Negatively Skewed Histogram**

The figure on the left illustrates the effect in both negative and positive skewed distributions on the measures of central tendency.

Measure of Skewness

1. First measure of skewness is given by Karl Pearson. The Pearson coefficient of skewness provides a numerical measure of the skewness of a distribution. Denoted by SK, it is calculated as follows:

   SK = (Mean– Mode) / σ = 3 (Mean - Median) / σ.

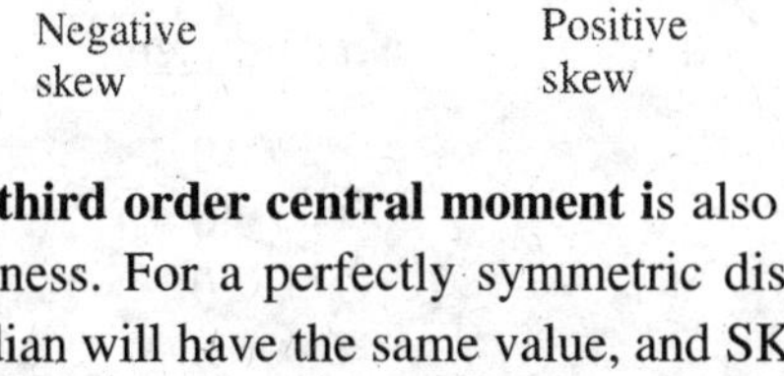

Negative skew Positive skew

μ_3, **the third order central moment is** also taken as coefficient of skewness. For a perfectly symmetric distribution, the mean and median will have the same value, and SK will have the value of 0. A distribution that is skewed to the right will have a mean that is larger than the median, and thus SK will have a positive value; thus, the distribution is also known as being positively skewed. A distribution that is skewed to the left will have a mean that is less than the median, and so SK will have a negative value;

thus, the phrase "negatively skewed". In general, the values of SK will vary between – 3 and 3.

Tests of Skewness

1. The values of mean, median and mode do not coincide. The more the difference between them, the more is the skewness.
2. Quartiles are not equidistant from the median, i.e. $(Q_3 - Me)$ $(Me - Q_1)$.
3. The sum of positive deviations from the median is not equal to the sum of the negative deviations.
4. Frequencies are not equally distributed at points of equal deviation from the mode.
5. When the data is plotted on a graph they do not give the normal bell-shaped form.

Note

i. Although the co-efficient of skewness is always within ± 1, but Karl Pearson's co-efficient lies within ± 3.
ii. If J = 0, then there is no skewness.
iii. If J is positive, the skewness is also positive.
iv. If J is negative, the skewness is also negative.

Unless and until no indication is given, you must use only Karl Pearson's formula.

Example

Find Karl Pearson's coefficient of skewness from the following data:

Marks above:	No.of students:
0	10
10	40
20	20
30	0
40	10
50	40
60	16
70	14
80	150

Marks (x_i)	Mid-Value (x_i)	No. Students (f_i)	Deviation $u_i = x_i\text{-}A/10$	f_iu_i	$f_iu_i^2$
0–10	5	10	-4	-40	160
10–20	15	40	-3	-120	360
20–30	25	20	-2	-40	80
30–40	35	0	-1	0	0
40–50	45⇒A	10	0	0	0
50–60	55	40	+1	+40	40
60–70	65	16	+2	+32	64
70–80	75	14	+3	+42	126
		$n=\sum f_i=150$		$n=\sum f_i=150$	$\sum f_i u_i=830$

Karl Pearson co-effiencient of skewness is j= (M –M0)/M , where M is the mean and is 18.7

j = (18.7- 40) /18.7 = -1.139, the skewness is negative.

Note

You will always find the different values of J when calculated by Karl Pearson's and Bowley's formula. But the value of J by Bowley's formula always lies with ± 1.

Kurtosis

It has its origin in the Greek word "Bulginess". In statistics it is the degree of flatness or "peakedness" in the region of mode of a frequency curve. It is measured relative to the 'peakedness' of the normal curve. It tells us the extent to which a distribution is more peaked or flat-topped than the normal curve. If the curve is more peaked than a normal curve it is called 'Lepto Kurtic'. In this case items are more clustered about the mode. If the curve is more flat-topped than the more normal curve, it is Platy-Kurtic. The normal curve itself is known as "Meso Kurtic".

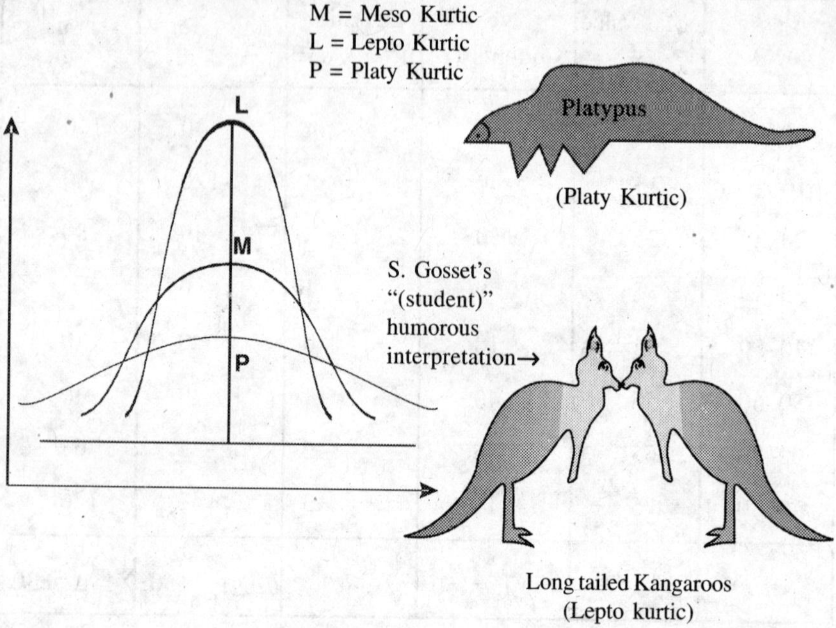

Kurtosis is measured by a similar to skewness dimensionless number which is called a **coefficient of kurtosis,** β_2 ($\beta_2 = \mu_4 / \mu_2^2$ or $\gamma_2 = \beta_2 - 3$). A flat topped distribution tends to have a low value of β_2 and is called to be **platykurtic** (flat bulging).

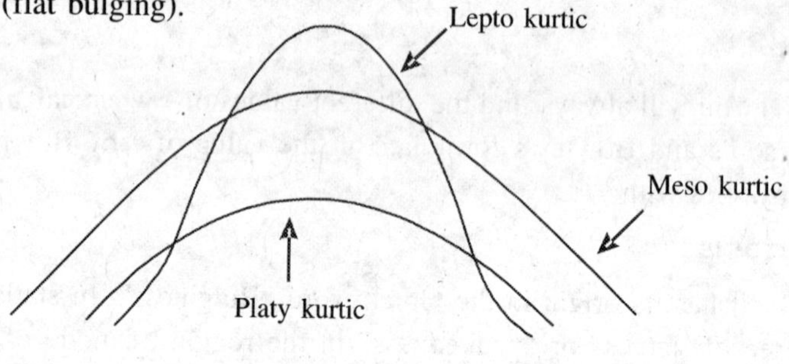

A sharp-peaked distribution will tend to have a high value of β_2 and is called **leptokurtic** (thin bulging).

If $\beta_2 = 3$ then the distribution curve is called Mesokurtic.

If $\beta_2 > 3$ then the distribution curve is called Leptokurtic.

If $\beta_2 < 3$ then the distribution curve is called Platykurtic.

1.7 NORMAL DISTRIBUTION

The normal distribution with parameters μ and σ^2, denoted as N (μ, σ^2), is the continuous probability distribution with the following probability density function:

$$f_x(x;\mu,\sigma)=\frac{1}{\sigma\sqrt{2\pi}}e^{-0.5[(x-\mu)/\sigma]^2} \quad -\infty < x < \infty \quad \text{where } \pi = 3.14159.....$$

and e = 2.71828.....

A random variable that has a normal distribution is called a **normal random variable** and is said to be normally distributed. Also known as the Gaussian distribution, the normal distribution is the cornerstone of the field of statistical inference, and definitely the most important continuous probability distribution in the study of statistics.

PROPERTIES OF THE NORMAL DISTRIBUTION

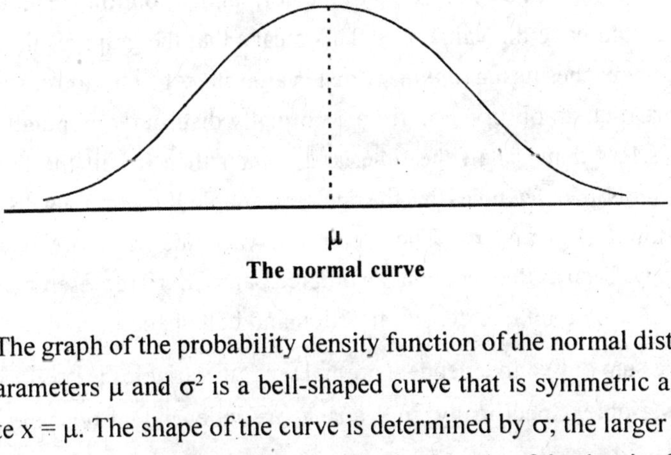

The normal curve

The graph of the probability density function of the normal distribution with parameters μ and σ^2 is a bell-shaped curve that is symmetric about the ordinate x = μ. The shape of the curve is determined by σ; the larger σ is, the greater is the variation among the values in the domain of the density function, and the flatter the curve is. The bell-shaped curve approaches the horizontal axis asymptotically in both directions. Because the normal distribution is a continuous probability distribution, the area bounded by its graph and the x-axis is equal to 1; also, the probability that a normally distributed variable assumes a value in the interval (a, b) is equal to the area bounded by the curve of its density function, the x-axis, and the two ordinates x = a and x = b.

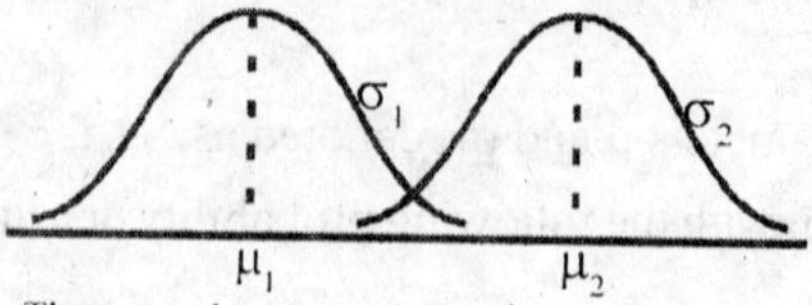

The normal curves with $\mu_1 = \mu_2$ and $\sigma_1 = \sigma_2$

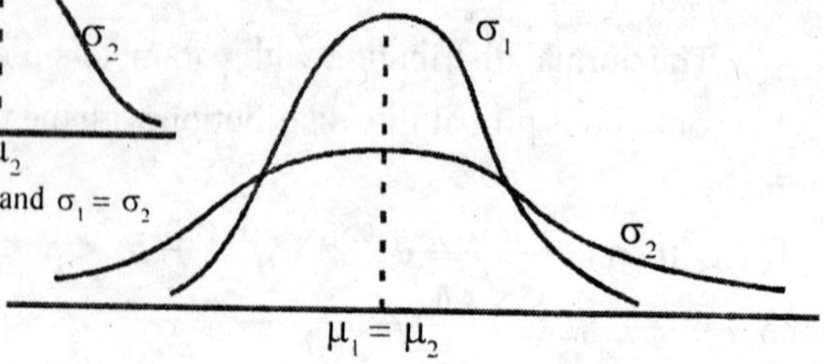

The normal curves with $\mu_1 = \mu_2$ and $\sigma_1 < \sigma_2$

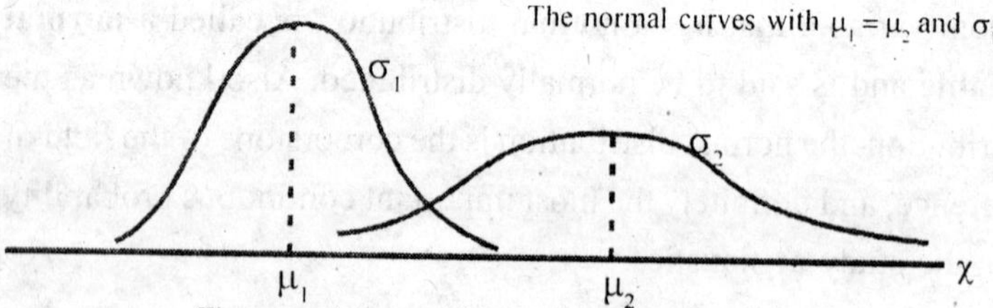

The normal curves with $\mu_1 \neq \mu_2$ and $\sigma_1 < \sigma_2$

The mean, mode and median of the normal distribution are all equal to each other and have the value of μ. This means that the graph of the normal distribution reaches its maximum ordinate value at $x = \mu$. The above statement also asserts that an observation from a normally distributed population with mean μ is less than μ half the time, and greater than μ half the time. The notation $X \sim N(\mu, \sigma^2)$ denotes that the random variable X is normally distributed with parameters μ and σ^2. The mean and variance of X are μ and σ^2, respectively. Each of the uncountable ordered pairs (μ, σ^2) represents a normal distribution with a unique density function and bell-shaped curve.

The sum of two independent normal random variables is itself a normal random variable. Specifically, if X and Y are independent normal random variables,

$$X \sim N(\mu_1, \sigma_1^2), Y \sim N(\mu_2, \sigma_2^2) \subset X+Y \sim N(\mu_1+\mu_2, \sigma_1^2+\sigma_2^2)$$

The following are the properties of normal p.d.f.:

(a) f is symmetric about $x = \mu$.

(b) f is increasing for $x < \mu$ and decreasing for $x > \mu$.

(c) The mode occurs at $x = \mu$.

(*d*) f is concave upward for $x < \mu - \sigma$ and for $x > \mu + \sigma$ and is concave downward for $\mu - \sigma < x < \mu + \sigma$.

(*e*) The inflection points of f occur at $x = \mu \pm \sigma$.

(*f*) $f(x) \to 0$ as $x \to 0$ and as $x \to -\infty$.

STANDARD NORMAL DISTRIBUTION

The **standard normal distribution** is the normal distribution having the parameters $\mu = 0$ and $\sigma = 1$. Thus, the standard normal distribution has the following density function:

$$f_x(X) = \frac{1}{\sqrt{2\pi}} e^{-0.5x^2} \qquad -\infty < x < \infty$$

A random variable X that has a standard normal distribution is called a **standard normal random variable.** This can be denoted as X ~ N(0, 1).

The graph of the standard normal distribution is symmetric about the y-axis need not be limited to people. The mean, mode and median of this distribution is 0. Thus, half of the area between its graph and the x-axis is to the left of the y-axis, while the other half is to the right of the y-axis.

The probability that the value of a standard normal random variable is less than a real number z is equal to the area of the region to the left of the ordinate x = z that is bounded by the graph of its density function and the x-axis. These probability values have been tabulated for selected values of z in the interval [– 3.09, 0.0] in any Standard Distribution Table. For X ~ N(0, 1).

P(X < – z) = P(X > z) because of the symmetry of the N(0, 1) distribution.,

P(X < z) = 1 – P(X > z) = 1 – P(X < – z) and the above probability values can be computed for z $\in$[0.0, 3.09] using the values in a Standard Distribution Table.

CHAPTER 2

SAMPLING THEORY

2.1 SAMPLING: POPULATION AND SAMPLE

In statistics, **survey sampling** is random selection of a sample from a finite population. It is an important part of planning statistical research and design of experiments. Sophisticated sampling techniques that are both economical and scientifically reliable have been developed. An entire industry of public opinion polling as well as the technical activities of the any country's. Bureau of the Census depends on these techniques.

The most elementary methodology is called simple random sampling. Most of the theory of statistics assumes this kind of sampling unless otherwise noted. In theory it ensures that all subsets of the population are given a balanced probability of selection.

The possibility of very expensive or very atypical samples has led to a variety of modifications such as stratified sampling, cluster sampling, and multistage sampling.

In public opinion polling by private companies or organizations unable to require response, the resulting sample is self-selected rather than random. Volunteering for the sample may be determined by characteristics such as submissiveness or availability. The samples in such surveys are therefore non-probability samples of the population, and the validity of estimates of parameters based on them is unknown. Generally, the survey is designed to minimise such bias, such that it can reasonably be assumed that the sample is close enough to random, to be treated as such.

Population

Any well defined set (group) of objects about which a statistical enquiry is being made is called a population or universe. The total number of objects (individuals or members) in a population is known as the size of the population which may be finite or infinite.

The population can refer to things as well as people. For example,

- All members of the cultural society of any city.
- All students of medical college.
- All Indians who saw 'TITANIC' last year.
- Heights of all students of a school.
- Weights of all the citizens of New Delhi above 20 years of age.
- Mileages of automobiles tiers of Dunlop, etc.

A population is finite if it contains finite numbers of individuals. For example, the ages of 20 boys of your class. A population is infinite if it contains infinite number of individuals. For example, the pressures at various points in the atmosphere.

Often, statisticians want to know things about population, but they fail to do so almost because in every case such data for every individual of the population is not available. Suppose I am a researcher in the field of 'Tuberculosis' (TB). I want to learn how many Indians suffer from it. It would not be practical (or perhaps even impossible) to contact every Indian. Thus whenever we want to study the characteristic of a certain population, it is difficult to study the whole population. It is often expensive and time consuming and many times we lack resources for the study of the whole population. In any science we cannot study more than a part of population. A part or small section selected from the population is called a sample.

Sample

A finite set of objects drawn from the population with an aim is called a sample.

Even in every day life we make many of our decisions based on samples taken, though we are not aware of it. I met **Shrishti** yesterday first time for an hour or two, I concluded that "Shrishti is intelligent" which may or may not be true. We just take a little from a gunny bag of rice, we judge its quality and then we purchase the whole bag. If we want to taste milk, we just take a glassful of milk from the can and taste it. Note that taking a sample is easy in many cases where the population is uniform or homogeneous. When the population is heterogeneous (not uniform), the selection of a sample is not very easy.

The fundamental assumption underlying most of the theory of sampling is **random sampling**. This consists of the selection of individuals from the population in such a way that each individual of the population has an equal chance of being selected i.e. a sample so selected must be a **true representative** of the population. The process of such selection is called random sampling.

The aim of the theory of sampling is to get as much information as possible, ideally all the information about the population from which the sample has been drawn. From the parent population, in particular, we would like to estimate the parameters of the population or specify the limits or ranges within which the population parameters are expected to lie with a specified degree of confidence.

The logic of the sampling theory is the logic of induction, that is, we go from particular (i.e. sample) to general (i.e. population). Naturally all results will have to be expressed in terms of probability. In the theory of sampling, we often come across two words, '**parameters**' and '**statistics**'.

Parameters and Statistics

The word '**Parameters**' is associated with the population and it is understood as the measure of the characteristics of the population, such as mean and standard deviation etc.

The word '**Statistics**' is used for a random sample and it is understood as the measure of the characteristics of the random sample, such as mean and standard deviation etc.

Note: Different symbols are used to denote parameters and statistics.

Characteristic	**Mean**	**Standard deviation**
Sample Statistics	x	δ or S.D.
Parameters of the population	μ (Read : Mu)	σ (read : sigma) or S.D.

Inferential or inductive statistics helps us in making an educated guess about the population parameters based on the statistics of its random sample.

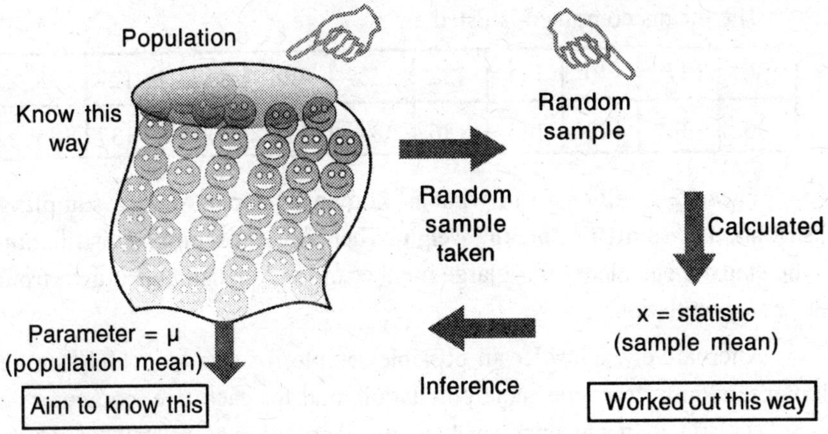

For instance, say

Aim to Know

The average (mean) income of families living in the area "Park avenue" in the year 1997-1998. i.e. the population parameter μ (in Rupees).

Work Out This Way

Draw a random sample of 200 families and compute their mean income, i.e. the statistic of sample x say Rs. 120000.

Conclusion (or Inference)

The population mean (parameter) is close to sample mean (statistic) i.e. mean income of the families living in the area 'Park Avenue' is Rs. 120000.

Sampling Distribution

Consider a finite population of 4000 students of a medical college. Of this 200 students are selected randomly and their mean weight is calculated. It was computed as x = 135 lbs. If we draw 20 different samples of 200 students, instead of just one as we did previously. We can't expect the same mean weight of these 20 samples chosen randomly. It is due to sampling variability i.e. each sample drawn randomly from the same population differs from each other in their computed '**statistic**'.

The means computed is listed as:

130	137	140	131	132	133	128	125	129	138
133	134	142	145	136	134	128	143	137	136

These 20 values form what is known as a part of the sampling distribution of a **statistic "mean" weight**. Therefore, the sampling distribution is the statistic calculated for a large number of random samples drawn from the same population.

Alternatively, consider all possible samples of size 'n' which can be drawn randomly from the same population, and for each one, compute the aimed statistic. In this manner we obtain the distribution of the statistic, which is the sampling distribution.

Now we compute mean of this sampling distribution which is 134.55 lb note that is obtained using the formula

$$\bar{x} = \frac{\Sigma x_i}{n} = \frac{2691}{20} = 134.55$$

Now we are told that the population mean (μ) i.e. mean weight of 4000 students is 134.21 lb (In case of infinite population, this is not known). Therefore, 135 lb is not a bad estimate of the population mean. But 134.55 lb is a still better estimation. We thus conclude that the more the sample means (statistics) included in the sampling distribution, the more correct the chances of the mean of the sampling distribution becoming an estimate of the population mean (parameter). The following graphical representation, supports this argument.

Now recall the list of means computed for 20 random samples. We observe that the 20 sample means differed from the true population mean m = 134.21 lbs. The means 137, 140, 138, 133, 142, 142, 136, 143, 147, 136 are clearly above the true mean while 130, 131, 133, 132, 128, 125, 129, 133, 134, 134, 128 are below the true mean. These deviations or differences from true value is due to the variability of samples. This is known as 'Random error' in statistical estimation. Note that the mean of 20 random sample means is slightly greater than the true population mean. If we take 20 more samples of 200 students, the mean of this new sampling distribution might be lower than the true population mean.

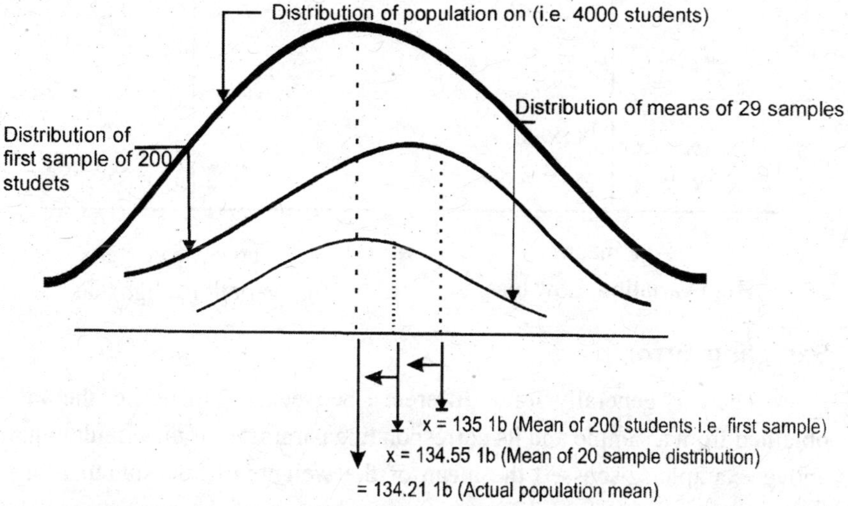

Graphical Reprenstation

Other than random error, error arises due to the tendency of consistent under estimating or over estimating a true value. This is known as systematic error or bias. Suppose, in the example discussed above, an investigator is investigating only those students who are healthy and fit. He would most likely overestimate the population mean. Generally healthy bodies have reasonable weights. Clearly the investigator's choice is one of bias.

This is an example from one of the bias that occurs in estimation.

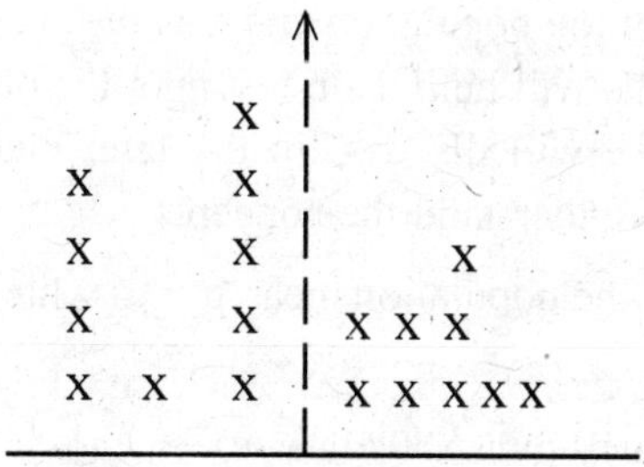

True mean

Less variation, Low bias

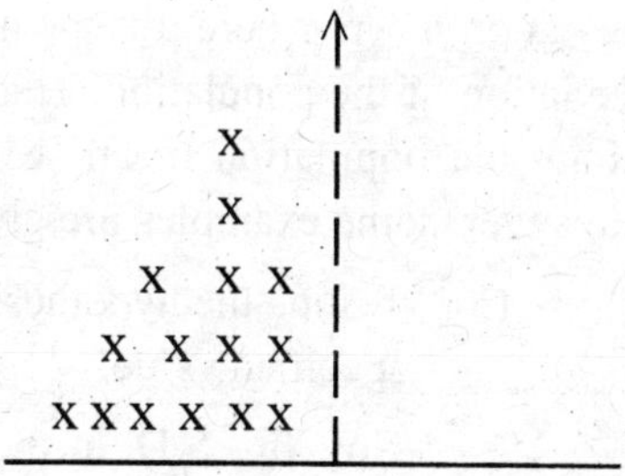

True mean

Less variation, High bias

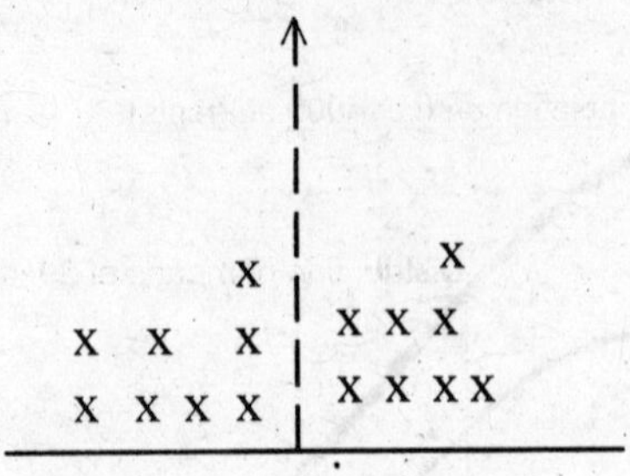

True mean
High variation, Low bias

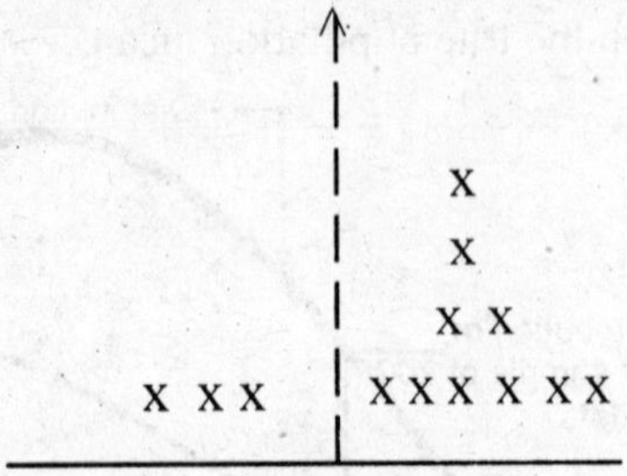

True mean
High variation, High bias

Sampling Error

There is generally some difference between a statistic i.e. the value obtained from a sample and its corresponding parameter of the population. In above example, discussed the mean of the weights of 200 students taken (first sample) is slightly different from the mean of the weights of 4000 students i.e. the population. This difference is called **sampling error** (whose types and situations are discussed). This error can be minimized by increasing the size of the sample and by taking sample of extremely random in nature. If the size of sample is large the sampling error is small. The accuracy of the sample increases as the square root of the size 'n' of the sample i.e. according to $\sqrt{n}$. Hence we take samples of sufficiently large in size.

Sampling of Variables

The sample mean $\overline{x}$ is normally distributed with mean μ and standard deviation $\sigma/\sqrt{n}$ where μ is the mean of the population and σ is the standard deviation of the population. This results will help us in testing a hypothesis about the population mean (which we will discuss in the later chapter. However, some examples are given to understand the concept).

1. Testing the hypothesis that the population mean $\mu = \mu_0$ which is a specified value.

   Now σ = S.D. of the population is known.

   In notations:

   The null hypothesis: $\mu = \mu_0$ i.e. $\mu - \mu_0 = 0$. First calculate:

$$|z| = \left|\frac{\overline{x}-\mu}{\sigma/\sqrt{n}}\right|$$

i. If $|z| < 1.96$, the difference is not significant at 5% level and H_0 is accepted, otherwise rejected.

ii. If $|z| < 2.58$, the difference is not significant at 1% level and H_0 is accepted, otherwise rejected.

Note : We have assumed that σ is known. If however σ is not known, we take σ to be equal to the S.D. of the sample.

Example: A random sample of 400 male students have average weight of 55 kg. Can we say that the sample comes from a population with mean 58 kg. with a variance of 9 kg.?

Solution : The null hypothesis H_0 is that the sample comes from the given population.

In notations : $H_0 : \mu = 58$ kg. and $H\alpha : \mu \neq 58$ kg.

$$|z| = \left|\frac{\overline{x}-\mu}{\sigma/\sqrt{n}}\right| \text{ Insert } \overline{X} = \text{sample mean} = 55 \text{ kg.}$$

Now

μ – population mean = 58 kg. n = 400 and σ = population S.D. = 3

$$\text{Therefore } |z| = \left|\frac{55-58}{3/\sqrt{400}}\right| = 20 > 2.58$$

This value is highly significant. We will reject H_0 on the basis of this sample. The sample therefore, is not likely to be from the given population.

Example : A random sample of 400 tins of vegetable oil and labeled "5 kg. net weight" has a mean net weight of 4.98 kg. with standard deviation of 0.22 kg. Do we reject the hypothesis of net weight of 5 kg. per tin on the basis of this sample at 1% level of significance?

Solution : The null hypothesis H_0 is that the net weight of each tin is 5 kg.

In notations H_0: $\mu = 5$ kg.

Inserting, = 4.98 kg., μ = 5 kg. σ = 0.22 kg. and n = 400

$$|Z| = \left|\frac{\bar{x} - \mu}{\sigma/\sqrt{n}}\right| \quad \text{We get}$$

In $$|z| = \left|\frac{4.98-5}{0.22/\sqrt{400}}\right| = 1.8 < 2.58$$

Hence H_o is accepted at 1% level of significance.

Example : A stenographer claims that she can take dictation at the rate of 120 words per minute. Can we reject her claim on the basis of 100 trials in which she demonstrated a mean of 116 words with standard deviation of 15 words?

Solution : The hypothesis to be tested is that her claims to be accepted.

In notations H_o: $\mu = 120$ and $H\alpha$: $\mu \neq 120$

Substituting, $\bar{x}$ = 116, σ = 15, n = 100 in

$$|Z| = \left|\frac{\bar{x} - \mu}{\sigma/\sqrt{n}}\right| \quad \text{we get}$$

$$|z| = \left|\frac{116-120}{15/\sqrt{100}}\right| = 2.67 > 1.96$$

The difference is not significant at both 5% and 1% level of significance i.e. the value of z - score 2.67 is highly significant. Hence H_o is rejected i.e. her claim is to be rejected.

If somebody is interested in the number of trials on the basis of which, with the same figure, her claim would not have been rejected, he can proceed as

$$|z| = \left|\frac{116-120}{15/\sqrt{n}}\right| = \left|\frac{-4}{15/\sqrt{n}}\right| \leq 1.96$$

$$\text{i.e.} \quad = \frac{4\sqrt{n}}{15} \leq 1.96$$

$$\sqrt{n} \leq 0.49 \times 15$$

$$\leq 7.35$$

$$\text{i.e.} \quad n \leq (7.35)^2$$

$$\text{i.e.} \quad n = 54 \text{ trials.}$$

Example: An automatic machine was designed to pack exactly 2 kg. of salt. A sample of 100 packs was examined to test the machine. The average weight was found to be 1.94 kg. with standard deviation of 0.10 kg. is the machine working properly?

Solution: The null hypothesis to be tested is that the machine is working properly.

In notations $H_o : \mu = 2$ kg. and $H_a : \mu \neq 2$ kg.

Substituting, $\bar{x} = 1.94$, $s = 0.10$, $n = 100$ in

$$|Z| = \left| \frac{\bar{x} - \mu}{\sigma / \sqrt{n}} \right|$$

$$= \left| \frac{1.94 - 2}{0.10/\sqrt{100}} \right| = 6.1 > 2.58$$

The z-score is highly significant, hence, we reject H_0 on the basis of this sample i.e. the machine is not working properly.

Sampling of Attributes

Characteristics like religion, language, locality etc. cannot be measured in numbers as they are attributes. We can only say whether a particular attribute is present or absent in an individual. The sampling of attributes means drawing a sample from the population, of which every member possesses a particular attribute or does not have it. In many cases, we are interested in knowing how many in the population possess the attribute. For instance, **Shashwat** wants to know how many from his area are smokers i.e. he is interested in the number or proportion of smokers in his area. Now we shall see how to test a hypothesis about the number or proportion of the individuals of the population possessing an attribute.

Testing the hypothesis that population proportion $p = P_o$

In notations: H_o: population proportion $= P_o$

Now P' = sample proportion is normally distributed with mean P_o and standard deviation $\sqrt{\frac{p_0 q_0}{n}}$

$$\text{Hence } z = \left| \frac{P' - P_0}{\sqrt{\frac{p_0 q_0}{n}}} \right|$$

i. If $|z| > 1.96$ a rare event has taken place.

If $P(|z| > 1.96) = 0.05$ we reject the hypothesis $= P_o$ at 5% level of significance.

ii. If $|z| > 1.96$ a usual event has happened and accept the hypothesis that $P = P_o$ at 5% level of significance.

iii. If $|z| > 2.58$ a rare (unusual) event has taken place. Now $P(|z| > 2.58) = 0.01$. We then reject the hypothesis $P = P_o$ at 1% level of significance.

iv. If $|z| > 2.58$, an unusual event occurred and we accept the hypothesis at 1% level of significance.

Example : A sample of 600 persons selected at random from a large city shows that there are 53% smokers. Is there any reason to doubt the hypothesis that smokers and non-smokers are equal in number in the city?

Solution : The null hypothesis is that the smokers and nonsmokers are equal in numbers.

$H_o : P = P_o$ and

$Ha : P \neq P_o$

where $P_o = 0.5 \Rightarrow q_o = 1 - P_o = 0.5$

Also the sample proportion is $P' = 53\% = 0.53$ and $n = 600$.

$$\therefore \quad |z| = \left| \frac{P' - P_0}{\sqrt{\frac{P_0 q_0}{n}}} \right| = \left| \frac{0.53 - 0.5}{\sqrt{\frac{0.5 \times 0.5}{600}}} \right|$$

$$= 1.5 < 1.96$$

Hence the hypothesis H_o is accepted at 5% level of significance. i.e. we can undoubtedly say that both smokers and non-smokers are equal in numbers in that city.

Example: A patented medicine claimed that it is effective in curing 90% of the patients suffering from malaria. From a sample of 200 patients using this medicine, it was found that only 170 were cured. Determine whether the claim is right or wrong. (Take 1% level of significance).

Solution: The null hypothesis is that the claim is quite right.

i.e. $H_o : P = P_o$ where $P_o = 90\% = 0.9$ and $H_\alpha : P \neq 0.9$.

Also $q_o = 0.1$ and $n = 200$.

The sample proportion $P' = 170/200 = 0.85$

$$|z| = \left| \frac{P^1 - P_0}{\sqrt{\frac{P_0 q_0}{n}}} \right| = \left| \frac{0.85 - 0.9}{\sqrt{\frac{0.9 \times 0.1}{200}}} \right| = 2.36 < 2.58$$

The null hypothesis H_o is quite right at 1% level of significance and that the claim is justified.

2.2 SURVEYS AND SAMPLING

In this section we'll learn how sample surveys can be organised, and how samples can be chosen in such a way that they will give statistically reliable results. We will also see how, with a certain amount of knowledge of what is being surveyed, to decide on an appropriate sample size.

Cost-Effective Survey Sampling: Tailor Your Sample Design to Your Survey Objectives

Right now, somewhere, a survey research study is failing. Sponsors are spending too much, and analysts are drawing wrong conclusions–all because the sampling plan did not fit the research needs.

- Which sampling method should I use?
- How large a sample size do I need?
- What is the margin of error?
- What is the power of the design?
- How can I get the best results at the lowest cost?

On completion of this section we should be able to:

- Describe the relationship between censuses and samples.
- List the sequences of stages involved in developing a sample survey.
- Explain the formulation and operation of a sample frame .
- Define the major types of sampling methods, using both probability and non-probability techniques.
- Describe the major forms of spatial sampling for selecting samples from phenomena that vary across the landscape.
- Explain the major factors that govern the calculation of minimum sample size, and the basic formulae for deriving sample sizes.

Censuses and Samples

In simple terms, we could call any data collection process that is not a controlled experiment a *survey*. Given the ethical problems associated with studying people (and the different issues in studying animals) much research in these fields is based on surveying rather than experimentation. In these terms a census is a survey whose domain is the characteristics of an entire *population*; a census is any study of the entire population of a particular set of 'objects'.

If we are only able (or we choose) to collect, analyse or study only some members of a population then we are carrying out a survey. If the total population is finite and known, or continuous (infinite) then what we are doing is defining some proportion of the total population to study; we are therefore creating a *sample*.

Sample Surveys

Why do we use sample surveys? We have no choice when the population is continuous (that is, effectively infinite), but we can define a sample from either a finite or an infinite population. Surveys are done for several reasons. A sample survey costs less than a census of the equivalent population, assuming that relatively little time is required to establish the sample size. Whatever the sample size, there are 'establishment costs' associated with any survey. Once the survey has begun, the marginal costs associated with gathering more information, from more people, are proportional to the size of the sample. But remember that surveys aren't conducted simply because they are less expensive than a census: they are carried out to answer specific questions, and sample surveys answer questions about the whole population. Researchers are not interested in the sample itself, but in what they can learn from it than can be applied to the whole population.

A sample survey will usually offer greater *scope* than a census. This may mean, for example, that it's possible to study the population of a larger (geographical) area, or to find out more about the same population by asking a greater variety of questions, or to study the same area in greater depth.

Development of a Sample Survey

Of course, whatever the potential advantages of sample surveys, they will not be realised unless the sample survey is correctly defined and organised. If we ask the wrong 'people' the wrong 'questions' we will not get a useful estimate of the characteristics of the population. Sample surveys have advantages provided they are properly designed and conducted. The first component is to plan the survey (and select the sample if this is a sample survey) using the correct methods. The following are the main stages in survey and sample design:

- *State the objectives of the survey*

  If you cannot state the objectives of the survey you are unlikely to generate usable results. You have to be able to formulate something quite detailed, perhaps organised around a clear statement of a testable hypothesis. Clarifying the aims of the survey is critical to its ultimate success.

- *Define the target population*

  Defining the *target population* can be relatively simple, especially for finite populations (for example, 'all male students enrolled in the unit SCC 171 at Delhi University in 1994'). For some finite populations, however, it may be more difficult to define what constitutes 'natural' membership of the population; in that case, arbitrary decisions have to be made. Thus we might define the population for a survey of voter attitudes in a particular town as 'all men or women currently on the electoral roll' or 'all people old enough to vote, whether they are enrolled or not' or 'all current voters (on the electoral roll) and those who will be old enough to vote at the next election'. Each of these definitions might be acceptable but, depending on the aims of the survey, one might be preferable.

  As suggested earlier, the process of defining the population is quite different when dealing with *continuous* (rather than *discrete*) phenomena. As you will see, it is still possible to define a sample size even if you don't know the proportion of the population that the sample represents.

- *Define the data to be collected*

  If we are studying, for example, the effect of forest clearance on the breeding process of a particular animal species, we obviously want to collect information about the actual changes in population size, but we will also want to know other things about the survey sample: how is the male/female ratio affected, is the breeding period changed, how are litter sizes affected, and so on. In searching for relationships (particularly those that may be causal) we may find interesting patterns in data that do not, at first glance, seem immediately relevant. This is why many studies are 'fishing expeditions' for data.

- *Define the required precision and accuracy*

  The most subjective stage is defining the precision with which the data should be collected. Strictly speaking, the precision can only be correctly estimated if we conduct a census. The precision provided by a sample survey is an estimate the 'tightness' of the range of estimates of the population characteristics provided by various samples.

  When we estimate a population value from a sample we can only work out how accurate the sample estimate is if we actually know the correct value –which we rarely do–but we can estimate the 'likely' accuracy. We need to design and select the sample in such a way that we obtain results that have acceptable precision and accuracy.

- *Define the measurement 'instrument'*

  The measurement instrument is the method–interview, observation, questionnaire – by which the survey data is generated . You will look in detail at the development of these (and other) methods in later chapters.

- *Define the sample frame, sample size and sampling method, then select the sample*

  The *sample frame* is the list of people ('objects' for inanimate populations) that make up the target population; it is a list of the individuals who meet the 'requirements' to be a member of that population. The sample is selected from the sample frame by specifying the *sample size* (either as a finite number, or as a proportion of the population) and the *sampling method* (the process by which we choose the members of the sample).

  The process of generating a sample requires several critical decisions to be made. Mistakes at this stage will compromise–and possibly invalidate– the entire survey. These decisions are concerned with the *sample frame*, the *sample size*, and the *sampling method.*

The Sample Frame

The creation of a sample frame is critical to the sampling process; if the frame is wrongly defined the sample will not be representative of the target population. The frame might be 'wrong' in three ways:

- It contains too many individuals, so that the sample frame contains the target population plus others who should *not* be included; we say that the membership has been *under-defined*

- It contains too few individuals, so that the sample frame contains the target population minus some others who *ought* to be included; we say that the membership has been *over-defined*
- It contains the wrong set of individuals, so that the sample frame does not necessarily contain the target population; we say that the membership has been *ill-defined*

Creating a Sample Frame is Done in Two-Stages

1. Divide the target population into sampling units. Examples of valid sampling units might include people (individuals), households, trees, light bulbs, soil or water samples and cities.
2. Create a finite list of sampling units that make up the target population. For a discrete population this will literally be a list (for example, of names, addresses or identity numbers). For a continuous population this 'list' may not specifiable except in terms of how each sample is to be collected. For example, when collecting water samples for a study of contaminant levels, we are only able to say that the sample frame is made up of a specific number of 50 millilitre sample bottles, each containing a water sample.

Definitions

Before examining sampling methods in detail, we need to be aware of some more formal definitions of some terms used so far, and some that will be used in subsequent sections.

Population	A finite (or infinite) set of 'objects' whose properties are to be studied in a survey.
Target population	The population whose properties are estimated via a sample; usually the same as the 'total' population.
Sample	A subset of the target population chosen so as to be representative of that population.
Sampling Unit	• A member of the sample frame. • A member of the sample.

Cont..

Probability sample	Any method of selecting a sample such that each sampling unit has a specific probability of being chosen. These probabilities are usually (but not always) equal. Most probability sampling employs some form of random sample to generate equal probabilities for each unit of being selected.
Non-probability	A method in which sample units are collected with no sample specific probability structure.

2.3 SAMPLING TECHNIQUES FOR CONDUCTING SURVEYS

The general aim of all sampling methods is to obtain a sample that is *representative* of the target population. By this we mean that, as much as possible, the information derived from the sample survey is the same (allowing for inevitable variations in the estimates due to imprecision) as we would find if we carried out a census of the target population.

When selecting a sampling method we need some minimal prior knowledge of the target population; with this and some reasonable assumptions we can estimate a sample size required to achieve a reasonable estimate (with acceptable precision and accuracy) of population characteristics.

How we actually decide which sampling units will be chosen makes up the sampling method. Sampling methods can be categorised according to the approach they take to the probability of a particular unit being included. Most sampling methods attempt to select units such that each has a definable probability of being chose. Moreover, most of these methods also attempt to ensure that each unit has the same chance of being included as every other unit in the sample frame. All methods that adopt this general approach are called *probability sampling methods*.

Alternatively, we can ignore the probability of selection issue and choose the sample on some other criterion, such as accessibility or voluntary participation; we call all methods of this type *non-probability sampling methods*.

Non-Probability Sampling

Non-probability methods are all sampling procedures in which the units that make up the sample are collected with no specific probability structure in mind. This might include, for example, the following:

- The units are *self-selected*; that is, the sample is made up of 'volunteers'.
- The units are the most easily accessible (in geographical terms).
- The units are selected on economic grounds.
- The units are considered by the researcher as in some way 'typical' of the target population.
- The units are chosen without no obvious design ("the first fifty who come in this morning").

It is clear that such methods depend on unreliable and unquantifiable factors, such as the researcher's experience, or even on luck. They are correctly regarded as 'inferior' to probability methods because they provide no statistical basis upon which the 'success' of the sampling method (that is, whether the sample was representative of the population and so could provide accurate estimates) can be evaluated.

On the other hand, in situations where the sample cannot be generated by probability methods, such sampling techniques may be unavoidable, but they should really be regarded as a 'last resort' when designing a sample scheme.

Probability Sampling

The basis of probability sampling is the selection of sampling units to make up the sample based on defining the chance that each unit in the sample frame will be included. If we have 100 units in the frame, and we decide that we should have a sample size of 10, we can define the probability of each unit being selected as one in ten, or 0.1 (assuming each unit has the same chance). As we shall see next, there are various sampling methods that we can use to select the units.

It is important feature of probability sampling that each time we apply the same method to the same sample frame we will generate a *different* sample.

For a finite population we can use simple combinatorial arithmetic to calculate how many samples we can draw from a particular sample frame such that no two samples are identical. It turns out that, from any population of N objects we can draw ${}_NC_n$ different samples, each of which contains n sampling units.

In fact, in probability sampling we are concerned with the probability of each *sample* being chosen, rather than with the probability of choosing individual units. If each sample is as likely to be selected as every other sample (assuming equal probabilities), then each sampling unit automatically has the same chance of being included as every other sampling unit.

Simple Random Sampling

The simplest way of selected sampling units using probability is the simple random sample. This method leads us to select n units (from a population of size N) such that every one of the ${}_NC_n$ possible samples has an equal chance of being chosen.

To actually implement a random sample, however, we 'reverse' the process so that we generate a sample by selecting from the sample frame by any method that guarantees that each sampling unit has a specified (usually equal) probability of being included. How we actually do the sampling (using dice, random number tables, or whatever) is of no significance, provided the technique ensures that each unit retains its specified probability of being selected.

Stratified Sampling

On occasion we may suspect that the target population actually consists of a series of separate 'sub-populations', each of which may have, on average, different values for the properties we are studying. If we ignore this possibility the population estimates we derive will be a sort of 'average of the averages' for the sub-populations, and may therefore be meaningless.

In these circumstances we should apply sampling methods that take such sub-populations into account. It may turn out, when we analyse the results, that the sub-populations do not exist, or they exist but the differences between them are not significant; in which case we will have wasted a certain (minimal) amount of time during the sampling process.

If, on the other hand, we do not take this possibility into account, we will have reduced confidence in the accuracy of our population estimates.

The process of splitting the sample to take account of possible sub-populations is called *stratification*, and such techniques are called *stratified sampling methods*. In all stratified methods the total population (N) is first divided into a set of L mutually exclusive sub-populations $N_1, N_2 \ldots N_L$, such that

$x_s = \Sigma W_t . \bar{x}_t$, over t=1, 2, ..L (strata), and $\bar{x}_t$ is $\Sigma X_{it}/n_t$.

Its variance is:

$\Sigma W^2_t /(N_t - n_t)S^2_t/[n_t(N_t - 1)]$

Population total T is estimated by $N. \bar{x}_s$, its variance is

$\Sigma N^2_t (N_t - n_t) S^2_t/[n_t(N_t - 1)]$.

Since the survey usually measures several attributes for each population member, it is impossible to find an allocation that is simultaneously optimal for each of those variables. Therefore, in such a case we use the popular method of allocation which use the same sampling fraction in each stratum. This yield optimal allocation given the variation of the strata are all the same.

Determination of sample sizes (n) with regard to binary data: Smallest integer greater than or equal to:

$[t^2 N p(1-p)] / [t^2 p(1-p) + \alpha^2 (N-1)]$

With N being the size of the total number of cases, n being the sample size, α the expected error, t being the value taken from the t distribution corresponding to a certain confidence interval, and p being the probability of an event.

Usually the strata are of equal sizes ($N_1 = N_2 = \ldots = N_L$) but we may also decide to use strata whose relative sizes reflect the estimated proportions of the sub-populations within the whole population.

Within each stratum we select a sample ($n_1, n_2, \ldots n_L$), usually ensuring that the probability of selection is the same for each unit in each sub-population. This generates a *stratified random* sample.

Systematic

Sometimes too much emphasis is placed on the significance of the equal probability of sampling unit selection, and consequently on random sampling. In most cases the estimates provided by such techniques are no better than those provided by *systematic* sampling techniques, which are often simpler to design and administer. In a systematic sample (as in other probability methods) we decide the sample size n from a population of size N. In this case, however, the population has to be organised in some way, such as points along a river, or in simple numerical order (the order of sample units is irrelevant in simple random or stratified random samples). We choose a starting point along the sequence by selecting the rth unit from one 'end' of the sequence, where r is less than n, and is usually chosen randomly. We then take the rest of the sample by adding *k* to r, where *k* is an integer number equal to $^N/_n$, or to the next lowest integer below $^N/_n$ if this division produces a real number. We do this repeatedly until we reach the end of the sequence.

One way of envisioning a systematic sample is think of the sample frame as a 'row' of units, and the sample as a sequence of equal-spaced 'stops' along the row, as shown in figure given below:

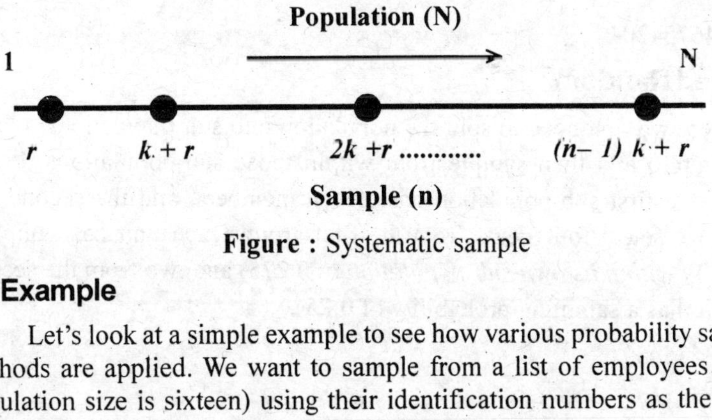

Figure : Systematic sample

An Example

Let's look at a simple example to see how various probability sampling methods are applied. We want to sample from a list of employees (whose population size is sixteen) using their identification numbers as the sample frame, and we want to select a sample size of six units.

Simple Random

We select the units by random sampling from the frame. We might use random number tables, or use a short computer program to generate six random numbers between one and sixteen.

94407382

94409687 <========

93535459 <========

93781078

94552345

94768091 <========

93732085

94556321

94562119

93763450 <========

94127845

94675420

94562119 <========

93763450 <========

94127845

94675420

Stratified Random

Here we first need to split the population into sub-populations (two in this example) and then sample from within those sub-populations. In the example the first sub-population has eleven members, and the second has five; so we select four items from the first group (each unit has sampling probability *within its own sub-population* of 0.275) and two from the second (each unit has a sampling probability of 0.25).

93535459

93781078

93732085 <========

93763450

93763450 <========

94407382

93427890

94409687 <========

94552345

94768091 <========

94556321

94562119 <========

94127845

94675420

94562119 <========

94127846

Systematic

Here we first need to order the sample units (in this case in increasing numerical order). We then select the first point (the value of r) between one and three (${}^N/_n = {}^{16}/_6$); in the example this turns out to be two. We then take every third sample after this (2, 5, 8, 11, 14). Depending on the size of the sample frame this may (as it does here) produce a sample that is too small or too large by a single unit.

93535459

93781078 <========

93732085

93763450

93763450 <========

94407382

94409687

94552345 <========

94768091

94556321

94562119 <========

94127845

94675420

94562119 <========

94127846

94675420

Quota Sampling

Interviews, mail surveys and telephone surveys (which you'll examine quite often) are often used in conjunction with *quota sampling*. Quota sampling is based on defining the distribution of characteristics required in the sample, and selecting respondents until a 'quota' has been filled. For example, if a survey requires a sample of fifty men and fifty women, a quota sample will 'tick off' respondents until the right number of each type has been surveyed. This process can been extended to cover several characteristics ('males under fifty years of age', 'females with children'). Quota sampling can be regarded as a form of stratification, although formal stratified sampling has major statistical advantages.

Questionnaire Design and Surveys Management

This part of the section is aimed at students who need to perform basic statistical analyses on data from sample surveys, especially those in the medical science. Students are expected to have a basic knowledge of statistics such as descriptive statistics and the concept of hypothesis testing.

When the sampling units are human beings, the main methods of collecting information are:

- Face-to-face interviewing.
- Postal surveys.
- Telephone surveys.
- Direct observation.
- Internet.

The main questions are:

* What is the purpose of the survey?
* What kinds of questions the survey would be developed to answer?
* What sorts of actions is the company considering based on the results of the survey?

Step 1: Planning Questionnaire Research

Consider the advantages and disadvantages of using questionnaires.

Prepare written objectives for the research.

Have your objectives reviewed by others.

Review the literature related to the objectives.

Determine the feasibility of administering your questionnaire to the population of interest.

Prepare a time-line.

Step 2: Conducting Item Try-Outs and An Item Analysis

Have your items reviewed by others.

Conduct "think-aloud" with several people.

Carefully select individuals for think-aloud.

Consider asking about 10 individuals to write detailed responses on a draft of your questionnaire.

Ask some respondents to respond to the questionnaire for an item analysis. In the first stage of an item analysis, tally the number of respondents who selected each choice.

In the second stage of an item analysis, compare the responses of high and low groups on individual items.

Step 3: Preparing a Questionnaire for Administration

Write a descriptive title for the questionnaire.

Write an introduction to the questionnaire.

Group the items by content, and provide a subtitle for each group.

Within each group of items, place items with the same format together.

At the end of the questionnaire, indicate what respondents should do next.

Prepare an informed consent form, if needed.

If the questionnaire will be mailed to respondents, avoid having your correspondence look like junk mail.

If the questionnaire will be mailed, consider including a token reward.

If the questionnaire will be mailed, write a follow-up letter.

If the questionnaire will be administered in person, consider preparing written instructions for the administrator.

Step 4: Selecting a Sample of Respondents

Identify the accessible population.

Avoid using samples of convenience.

Simple random sampling is a desirable method of sampling.

Systematic sampling is an acceptable method of sampling.

Stratification may reduce sampling errors.

Consider using random cluster sampling when every member of a population belongs to a group.

Consider using multistage sampling to select respondents from large populations.

Consider the importance of getting precise results when determining sample size.

Remember that using a large sample does not compensate for a bias in sampling.

Consider sampling non-respondents to get information on the nature of a bias.

The bias in the mean is the difference of the population means for respondents and non-respondents multiplied by the population non-response rate.

Step 5: Preparing Statistical Tables and Figures

Prepare a table of frequencies.

Consider calculating percentages and arranging them in a table with the frequencies.

For nominal data, consider constructing a bar graph.

Consider preparing a histogram to display a distribution of scores.

Consider preparing polygons if distributions of scores are to be compared.

Step 6: Describing Averages and Variability

Use the median as the average for ordinal data.

Consider using the mean as the average for equal interval data.

Use the median as the average for highly skewed, equal interval data.

Use the range very sparingly as the measure of variability.

If the median has been selected as the average, use the interquartile range as the measure of variability.

If the mean has been selected as the average, use the standard deviation as the measure of variability.

Keep in mind that the standard deviation has a special relationship to the normal curve that helps in its interpretation.

For moderately asymmetrical distributions the mode, median and mean satisfy the formula: mode=3*median-2*mean.

Step 7: Describing Relationships

For the relationship between two nominal variables, prepare a contingency table.

When groups have unequal numbers of respondents, include percentages in contingency tables.

For the relationship between two equal interval variables, compute a correlation coefficient.

Interpret a Pearson r using the coefficient of determination.

For the relationship between a nominal variable and an equal interval variable, examine differences among averages.

Step 8: Estimating Margins of Error

It is extremely difficult, and often impossible, to evaluate the effects of a bias in sampling.

When evaluating a percentage, consider the standard error of a percentage.

When evaluating a mean, consider the standard error of the mean.

When evaluating a median, consider the standard error of the median.

Consider building confidence intervals, especially when comparing two or more groups.

Step 9: Writing Reports of Questionnaire Research

In an informal report, variations in the organization of the report are permitted.

Academic reports should begin with a formal introduction that cites literature.

The second section of academic reports should describe the research methods.

The third section of academic reports should describe the results.

The last section of academic reports should be a discussion. Acknowledge any weakness in your research methodology.

Missing Values on a Sensitive Topic

A natural way to get answers is to, as much as possible, assure people that the surveys are anonymous, and to find a way to make the respondent at least minimally comfortable. So, according to US General Accounting Office book, "Developing and Using Questionnaires" (Oct 1983) chapter 9, you should do the following:

1. Explain to respondent the reasons for asking the questions.
2. Make response categories as broad as possible.
3. Word the question in a non-judgemental style that avoids the appearance of censure, or, if possible, make the behavior in question appear to be socially acceptable.
4. Present the request as factual matter as possible.
5. Guarantee confidentiality or anonymity.
6. Make sure the respondent knows the info will not be used in any threatening way.
7. Explain how the info will be handled.
8. Avoid cross classification that will allow for pinpointing responses.

2.4 Source of Sampling Errors

1. The use of an inadequate frame.
2. A poorly designed questionnaire.
3. Recording and measurement errors.
4. Non-response problems.

For example consider the following question: "Over the last twelve months would you say your health has on the whole been : Good? / Fairly good? / Not good?". The respondent is required to tick one of 3 thus-labeled boxes.

What is Wrong With the Following?

It is the ONLY question on the form, which asks about a matter of opinion rather than fact, but this distinction is not in any way represented in its layout or wording.

Whereas for a question about opinion there should be a response option of 'Don't Know' this is not provided. In some cases, such as the Census Form and the Census advisory staff are adamant that the question must be answered. Thus a person with no opinion on the matter is in a quandary and threatened with possible legal action.

This particular question is highly ambiguous as regards the qualitative nature of what is being asked about (your health). Is one to respond in terms of how one feels, how one can perform, comparisons with peer groups, comparisons with other periods of one's life, or what?

Relatively recent innovations surrounding the Internet have spawned new ways for conducting surveys: most notably electronic mail (e-mail) surveys and WWW surveys. While still in its infancy, it is clear that the Internet is here to stay and this new medium is going to be used for survey data collection. The main question is how the Internet can be used for survey data collection by some effective and efficient design considerations.

Survey Non-Sampling Errors

The widely used measure of the total error in a survey estimated is the mean squared error (MSE). The MSE consists of two components: variance and the square of the bias. Survey researchers are able to obtain a good quantitative estimated of the variance component of mean squared error. Unfortunately, the theory and methods of estimating the bias (non-sampling error) component are underdeveloped. Because the non-sampling error is usually much greater than the sampling error in estimates from large sample surveys, it is imperative that we learn more about it. In recent years U.S. Bureau of Labor Statistics measures various aspects of non-sampling error by means of behavioral science among others.

A sample is generally selected for study because the population is too large to study in its entirety. The sample should be representative of the general population. This is often best achieved by random sampling. Also, before collecting the sample, it is important that the researcher carefully and completely defines the population, including a description of the members to be included.

Random Sampling

Random sampling of size n from a population size N. Unbiased estimate for variance of is Var (x) = $S^2(1\text{-}n/N)/n$, where n/N is the sampling fraction.

For sampling fraction less than 10% the finite population correction factor (N-n)/(N-1) is almost 1.

The total T is estimated by N. $\overline{X}$, its variance is N^2 Var (x). For 0, 1 (binary) type variables, variation in estimated proportion p is:

$$S^2 = p.(1-p).(1-n/N)/(n-1).$$

For ratio $r = \Sigma x_i / \Sigma y_i = x / y$, the variation for r is

$$[(N-n)(r^2 S^2_x + S^2_y - 2\, r\, Cov(x, y)]/[n(N-1).x^2].$$

Stratified Sampling

Stratified sampling can be used whenever the population can be partitioned into smaller sub-populations, each of which is homogeneous according to the particular characteristic of interest.

Cross-Sectional Sampling

Cross-Sectional Study is the study where the observation of a defined population at a single point in time or time interval. Exposure and outcome are determined simultaneously.

Quota Sampling

Quota sampling is availability sampling, but with the constraint that proportionality by strata be preserved. Thus the interviewer will be told to interview so many white male smokers, so many black female non-smokers, and so on, to improve the representatives of the sample. Maximum variation sampling is a variant of quota sampling, in which the researcher purposively and non-randomly tries to select a set of cases, which exhibit maximal differences on variables of interest. Further variations include extreme or deviant case sampling or typical case sampling.

What is a Statistical Instrument?

A statistical instrument is any process that aim at describing a phenomena by using any instrument or device, however the results may be used as a control tool. Examples of statistical instruments are questionnaire and surveys sampling.

What is Grab Sampling Technique?

The grab sampling technique is to take a relatively small sample over a very short period of time, the result obtained are usually instantaneous.

However, the **Passive Sampling** is a technique where a sampling device is used for an extended time under similar conditions. Depending on the desirable statistical investigation, the Passive Sampling may be a useful alternative or even more appropriate than grab sampling. However, a passive sampling technique needs to be developed and tested in the field.

What is the Margin of Error?

Estimation is the process by which sample data are used to indicate the value of an unknown quantity in a population. Results of estimation can be expressed as a single value; known as a point estimate, or a range of values, referred to as a confidence interval. Whenever we use point estimation, we calculate the margin of error associated with that point estimation. For example; for the estimation of the population proportion, by the means of sample proportion (P), the margin of errors calculated *often* as follows:

$$\pm 1.96\ [P(1-P)/n]^{1/2}$$

In newspapers and television reports on public opinion pools, the margin of error is often appears in ***small font*** at thc bottom of a table or screen, respectively. However, reporting the amount of error only, is not informative enough by itself, what is missing is the **degree of the confidence** in the findings. The more important missing piece of information is the sample size n. that is, how many people participated in the survey, 100 or 100000? By now, you know it well that the larger the sample size the more accurate is the finding, right?

The reported margin of error is the margin of "sampling error". There are many nonsampling errors that can and do affect the accuracy of polls. Here we talk about sampling error. The fact that subgroups have larger sampling error than one must include the following statement: "Other sources of error include but are not limited to, individuals refusing to participate in the interview and inability to connect with the selected number. Every feasible effort is made to obtain a response and reduce the error, but the reader (or the viewer) should be aware that some error is inherent in all research."

If you have a yes/no question in a survey, you probably want to calculate a proportion P of Yes's (or No's). Under simple random sampling survey, the variance of P is P(1-P)/n, ignoring the finite population correction, for large n, say over 30. Now a 95% confidence interval is

$$P - 1.96\ [P(1-P)/n]^{1/2},\ P + 1.96\ [P(1-P)/n]^{1/2}.$$

A conservative interval can be calculated, since P(1-P) takes its maximum value when P = 1/2. Replace 1.96 by 2, put P = 1/2 and you have a 95% consevative confidence interval of $1/n^{1/2}$. This approximation works well as long as P is not too close to 0 or 1. This useful approximation allows you to calculate approximate 95% confidence intervals.

2.5 RESEARCH PROTOCOLS

Statistical investigations are those in which observations are made on group of individuals by the presence of random variation, for example: if the blood pressure were an exact function of age, varying neither from person to person nor between occasion on the same person. The blood pressure at age 55 could be determined by one observation only. For this type of situation statistical analysis would not be required. But for this particular example, blood pressure vary both between individuals and between occasions. Comparisons of the effects of different medical treatments must therefore be made on group of patients; studies of physiological norms require population surveys.

In the planning of a statistical study a number of administrative and technical problems are likely to arise. These will be characteristics of the particular field of research and cannot be discussed in present context. Two aspects of the planning will almost invariably be present and are of particular concern to the statistician. (A) the inference from the study to be sufficiently precise; (B) the results to be relevant to the question of the study. Discussions of the statistical design of the investigation are concerned especially with the general consideration which bear on these two objectives. Some of the questions arises are (1) how to select the individuals on which observations are to be made, (2) how to decide on the numbers of observations falling into different groups, and (3) how to allocate observations between different possible categories of individuals, such as groups of individuals receiving different treatments or groups of people living in different areas.

It is useful to make a conceptual distinction between two different types of statistical investigations, the experiment and the survey.

What is an experiment? Experimentation involves a planned interference with the natural cause of events so that its effect can be observed.

What is survey? In a survey, on the other hand, the investigator is a more passive observer, interfering as little as possible with the phenomena he wishes to record. It is easy to think of extreme example to illustrate this antithesis but in practice the distinction is sometimes hard to draw. Examples are :

1. A public opinion poll.
2. A survey to find out tuberculosis among general population.
3. A study of the respiratory function (as measured by various tests) of men working in glass industries.
4. Observations of the survival times of mice of three different strains after inoculation with the same dose of a toxic substance.
5. A clinical trial to compare the merits of surgery and conservative treatment for patients with a certain condition, the subjects being allocated randomly to the two treatments.

Study 1, 2 and 3 are clearly surveys, although they involve an increasing amount of interference with nature. Study 5 is clearly equalized as experiment. Study 4 occupies an equivocal position. In its statistical aspects it is conceptually a survey as the object is to observe and compare certain characteristics of these strains of mice. But on the other side, the characteristics of interest requires the most extreme form of interference – the death of the animal and the non-statistical techniques involved are more akin to those of a laboratory experiment than to those required in most survey work.

In population based health research, despite the fact that many of studies are observation rather than experimental, it remains essentials to elaborate and follow a research protocol for the same reason as in the laboratory. Doing so will increase the likelihood that the conclusions drawn from the research are scientifically sound.

The first step before embarking and developing a detailed protocol is to select a research topic. The topic should be able to stand alone as an explanation of the study. In doing so we need to understand prevailing operational realities and how to work within their limits. The protocols should explain the study in terms of answers to the following questions:

WHY? Sets out the study questions and the relevant background information: that why we should embark on this particular research problem.

HOW? Describes the study design and the rational for choosing it. Also describes instruments/techniques to be used.

WHO? Defines the targets and the study population and sample size.

WHAT? Identifies the variables to be measured and outcomes to be analysed.

SO WHAT? Comments on the expected significance of results and contribution to knowledge.

FORMAT OF A RESEARCH PROTOCOL

PROTOCOL SUMMARY

INTRODUCTION

- **Study question**
- **Rationales and previous knowledge on the subject**

OBJECTIVES

DESIGN AND METHODS

- **Study design**
- **Study population**
- **Sample size and sampling**
- **Study subject : selection, definitions**
- **Study questionnaires, formats**
- **Data collection methods**
- **Data management and statistical analysis**

PROJECT MANAGEMENT

- **Personnel**
- **Action-plan**

STRENGTHS AND LIMITATIONS

ETHICAL CONSIDERATIONS

EXPECTED OUTCOME

BUDGET SUMMARY

REFERENCES

ANNEXURE

- **Study formats**
- **Budget details**
- **Curriculum–vitae of chief investigator and co-investigator**

2.6 RECORD LINKAGE

Record linkage (RL) refers to the task of finding entries that refer to the same entity in two or more files. Record linkage is an appropriate technique when you have to join data sets that do not have a unique database key in common. A data set that have been through record linkage is said to be **linked.**

Record linkage is a useful tool when performing data mining tasks, where the data originated from different sources or different organizations. Most commonly, performing RL on datasets involves joining records of persons based on name, since no national identification number or similar is recorded in the data.

Naming conventions: Record linkage is the term used by statisticians, epidemiologists and historians among others. Commercial mail and database applications refer to it as **merge/purge processing** or **list washing**. Computer scientists often refer to it as **data matching** or as the **object identity problem**. Other names used to describe the same concept include **entity resolution**, **entity disambiguation**, **duplicate detection**, **record matching**, **instance identification**, **deduplication**, **coreference resolution**, **reference reconciliation** and **database hardening**. This confusion of terminology has led to few cross-references between these research communities.

Methods: There are several approaches to record linkage. The most straightforward is a *rules-based* approach, in which reasonable rules are developed and then refined as common exceptions are found. The advantage to this approach is that it is possible to get a good deal of accuracy without needing a lot of labeled data to train or test the rules on. The disadvantage is that to obtain very high accuracy, more and more exceptions and special cases would need to be handled, and eventually the list of rules gets too complex to be built by hand.

A very popular approach has been *Probabilistic Record Linkage* (*PRL*). In this approach, a large set of pairs of records are human-labeled as being matching or differing pairs. Then statistics are calculated from the agreement of fields on matching and differing records to determine weights on each field. During execution, the agreement or disagreement weight for each field is added to get a combined score that represents the probability that the records refer to the same entity. Often there is one threshold above which a pair is considered a match, and another threshold below which it is considered not to be a match. Between the two thresholds a pair is considered to be "possibly a match", and dealt with accordingly (e.g., human reviewed, linked, or not linked, depending on the application).

In recent years, a variety of machine learning techniques have been used in record linkage. It has been recognized that Probabilistic Record Linkage is equivalent to the "Naive Bayes" algorithm in the field of machine learning, and suffers from the same assumption of the independence of its features, which is typically not true. Higher accuracy can often be achieved by using various other machine learning techniques, including a single-layer Perceptron.

Regardless of whether rule-based, PRL or machine learning techniques are used, *normalization* of the data is very important. Names are often spelled differently in different sources (e.g., "Wm. Smith", "William Smith", "William J. Smith", "Bill Smith", etc.), dates can be recorded various ways ("1/2/73", "1973.1.2", "Jan 2, 1973"), and places can be recorded differently as well ("Berkeley, CA", "Berkeley, Alameda, California, USA", etc.). By normalizing these into a common format and using comparison techniques that handle additional variation, much more consistency can be achieved, resulting in higher accuracy in any record linkage technique.

Applications in Historical Research

Record linkage is important to social history research since most data sets, such as census records and parish registers were recorded long before the invention of national identification numbers. When old sources are digitized, linking of data sets is a prerequisite for longitudinal study. This process is often further complicated by lack of standard spelling of names, family names that changes according to place of dwelling, changing of administrative boundaries and problems of checking the data against other sources. Record

Linkage was among the most prominent themes in the history and computing field in the 1980s, but has since been subject to less attention in research.

Applications in Medical Practice and Research

Record linkage is an important tool in creating data required foı examining the health of the public and of the health care system itself. It can be used to improve data holdings, data collection, quality assessment, and the dissemination of information. Data sources can be examined to eliminate duplicate records, to identify underreporting and missing cases (e.g., census population counts), to create person-oriented health statistics, and to generate disease registries and health surveillance systems. Some cancer registries link various data sources (e.g., hospital admissions, pathology and clinical reports, and death registrations) to generate their registries. Record linkage is also used to create health indicators. For example, fetal and infant mortality is a general indicator of a country's socioeconomic development, public health, and maternal and child services. If infant death records are matched to birth records, it is possible to use birth variables, such as birth weight and gestational age, along with mortality data, such as cause of death, in analyzing the data. Linkages can help in follow-up studies of cohorts or other groups to determine factors such as vital status, residential status, or health outcomes. Tracing is often needed for follow-up of industrial cohorts, clinical trials, and longitudinal surveys to obtain the cause of death and/or cancer.

CHAPTER 3

ESTIMATION

3.1 INTRODUCTION

The problems of statistical inferences are divided into problems of estimation and test of hypotheses, though actually they are all decision problems and, hence, could be handled by the unified approach which is presented in this chapter. The main difference between the two kinds of problems is that in estimation we must determine the value of the parameter (or the value of the several parameters) from a possible continuum of alternatives, while in testing of hypotheses we must decide whether or not to accept or reject a specific value of a parameter (or those of several parameters).

When we use the value of statistics to estimate a population parameter, we call this point estimation and we refer to the value of the statistics as a point estimate of the parameter. For example we use a value of xi to estimate the mean of a population, an observed sample proportion to estimate the parameter of a binomial population we are using a point estimate of the parameter in question.

In statistics, interval estimation is the use of sample data to calculate an interval of possible (or probable) values of an unknown population parameter. The most prevalent forms of interval estimation are confidence intervals (a frequentist method) and credible intervals (a Bayesian method). In statistics, a confidence interval (CI) is an interval estimate of a population parameter. Instead of estimating the parameter by a single value, an interval of likely estimates is given. How likely the estimates are is determined by the confidence coefficient. The more likely it is for the interval to contain the parameter, the wider the interval will be.

Confidence intervals are used to indicate the reliability of an estimate. For example, a CI can be used to describe how reliable survey results are. All other things being equal, a survey result with a small CI is more reliable than a result with a large CI.

In a narrower sense, a CI for a population parameter is an interval with an associated proportion p that is generated from a random sample of an underlying population such that if the sampling was repeated numerous times and the confidence interval recalculated from each sample according to the same method, a proportion p of the confidence intervals would contain the population parameter in question. Confidence intervals are the most prevalent form of interval estimation.

If U and V are statistics (i.e., observable random variables) whose probability distribution depends on some unobservable parameter θ, and

$Pr(U < \theta < V / \theta) = x$ (where x is a number between 0 and 1) then the random interval (U, V) is a "100x% confidence interval for θ".

The number x (sometimes reported as a percentage (100%·x)) is called the confidence level or confidence coefficient. In modern applied practice, most confidence intervals are stated at the 95% level (Zar 1984).

Various statistical properties of estimators can, thus, be used to decide which estimator is most appropriate in a given situation, which will expose us to the smallest risk, and give the most information at the lowest cost, and so forth.

Properties of a Good Estimator

Unbiased

Thus, an estimator should do so at least on the average – namely, that its expected value should equal to the parameter which it is supposed to estimate. If this is the case, the estimator is said to be unbiased; otherwise, biased. Mathematically

A statistic $\hat{\theta}$ is an unbiased estimator of the parameter $\hat{\theta}$ if and only if $E(\theta) = \theta$.

Efficient: If we have to choose one of the several unbiased estimators of a given parameter, we usually take the one whose sampling distribution has smallest variance. We say that the estimator with the smaller variance is "more reliable". To check that whether a given estimator has at the smallest possible variance, namely, whether it is a minimum variance unbiased estimator (also called a best unbiased estimator) is unbiased, we make use of the fact that if θ must satisfy the inequality

$$\text{Var}(\hat{\theta}) \geq \frac{1}{n.E\left[\left(\frac{\partial \ln f(x)}{\partial \theta}\right)^2\right]}$$

where f(x) is the value of the population density at x and n is the size of the random sample.

Consistence

Consistence is nothing but is the concept of closeness and is expressed by the following:

A statistic $\hat{\theta}$ is a consistent estimator of the parameter θ if and only if for each c > 0

$$\lim_{n \to \infty} P(|\hat{\theta} - \theta| < c) = 1$$

Sufficient

An estimator $\hat{\theta}$ is said to be sufficient if it utilizes all the information in a sample relevant to the estimation of θ, that is, if all the knowledge about θ that can be gained from the individual sample values and their order can just as well be gained from the value

$\hat{\theta}$ alone.

The statistics $\hat{\theta}$ is a sufficient estimator of the parameter θ if and only if for each

value of $\hat{\theta}$ the conditional probability distribution or density of random sample

$x_1, X_2 \ldots X_n$ given $\hat{\theta} = \theta$ is independent of θ.

3.2 ESTIMATION OF MEANS

Interval estimation involves using sample data to determine a range (interval) that, at an established level of confidence, that is expected to contain the mean of the population.

Steps

1. Determine confidence level (df = n—1; alpha .05, 2-tailed)
2. Use either z distribution (if n>120) or t distribution (for all sizes of n).
3. Use the appropriate table to find the critical value for a 2-tailed test.
4. Multiple hypotheses can be compared with the estimated interval for the population to determine their significance. In other words, differing values of population means can be compared with the interval estimation to determine if the hypothesized population means fall within the region of rejection.

Estimation Formula

$$CI = \overline{X} \pm CV(S_{\bar{x}})$$

where

$\overline{X}$ = Sample mean

CV = Critical value (consult distribution table for df = n-1 and chosen alpha–commonly .05)

$S_{\bar{x}}$ = Standard error of the mean = $S/\sqrt{n}$

Note: Assumes sample standard deviation was calculated using:

$$S = \sqrt{\frac{\Sigma(X_i - \bar{X})2}{n-1}}$$

Interval Estimation for Means

Example A random sample of 30 incoming college freshmen revealed the following statistics: mean age 19.5 years; sample standard deviation 1.2. Based on a 5% chance of error, estimate the range of possible mean ages for all incoming college freshmen.

Estimation

Critical value (CV)

Df=n-1 or 29

Consult t-distribution for alpha .05, 2-tailed

CV=2.045

Standard error

$$S_{\bar{x}} = \frac{S}{\sqrt{n}}$$

$$S_{\bar{x}} = \frac{1.2}{\sqrt{30}}$$

$$S_{\bar{x}} = .218$$

Estimate

$$CI_{95} = \overline{X} \pm CV\,(S_{\bar{x}})$$

$$CI_{95} = 19.5 \pm 2.045\,(.218)$$

$$CI_{95} = 19.5 \pm .446$$

Interpretation

We are 95% confident that the actual mean age of the all incoming freshmen will be somewhere between 19 years (the lower limit) and 20 years (the upper limit) of age.

3.3 ESTIMATION OF DIFFERENCE BETWEEN MEANS

This chapter describes how to construct a confidence interval for the difference between two means.

Estimation Requirements

The approach described in this section is valid whenever the following conditions are met:

- Both samples are simple random samples.
- The samples are independent.
- Each population is at least 10 times larger than its respective sample.
- The sampling distribution of the difference between means is approximately normally distributed.

Generally, the sampling distribution will be approximately normally distributed if each sample is described by at least one of the following statements.

- The population distribution is normal.
- The sampling distribution is symmetric, unimodal, without outliers, and the sample size is 15 or less.
- The sampling distribution is moderately skewed, unimodal, without outliers, and the sample size is between 16 and 40.
- The sample size is greater than 40, without outliers.

The Variability of the Difference Between Sample Means

To construct a confidence interval, we need to know the variability of the difference between sample means. This means we need to know how to compute the standard deviation and/or the standard error of the sampling distribution of the difference.

- If the population standard deviations are known, the standard deviation of the sampling distribution is:

  $$\sigma_{x_1-\dot{x}_2} = \text{sqrt}(\sigma_1^2 / n_1 + \sigma_2^2 / n_2)$$

  where σ_1 is the standard deviation of the population 1, σ_2 is the standard deviation of the population 2, and n_1 is the size of sample 1, and n_2 is the size of sample 2.
- When the standard deviation of either population is unknown, the standard deviation of the sampling distribution cannot be calculated. Under these circumstances, use the standard error. The standard error (SE) provides an unbiased estimate of the standard deviation. It can be calculated from the equation below.

  $$SE_{X_1 - X_2} = \text{sqrt}\,[\,S^2{}_1/n_1 + S^2{}_2/\,n_2]$$

  where s_1 is the standard deviation of the sample 1, s_2 is the standard deviation of the sample 2, and n_1 is the size of sample 1, and n_2 is the size of sample 2.

  Note: In real-world analyses, the standard deviation of the population is seldom known. Therefore, the standard error is used more often than the standard deviation.

Some texts present additional options for calculating standard deviations and standard errors. These formulas, which should only be used under special circumstances, are described below.

- Standard deviation. Use this formula when the population standard deviations are known and are equal.

$$\sigma_{x_1 - x_2} = \sigma_d = \sigma^* \text{ sqrt } [(1/n_2) + (1/n_2)] \text{ Where } \sigma = \sigma_1 = \sigma_2$$

- Pooled standard error. Use this formula when the population standard deviations are unknown, but assumed to be equal; and the samples sizes (n_1) and (n_2) are small (under 30).

$$SE_{Pooted} = \text{sqrt } \{[(n_1 - 1)^* S_1^2 + (n_2 - 1)^* S_2^2]/(n_1 + n_2 - 1)\}$$

Where $\sigma_1 = \sigma_2$

Remember, these two formulas should be used only when the various required underlying assumptions are justified.

How to Find the Confidence Interval for a Mean?

Previously, we described how to construct confidence intervals. For convenience, we repeat the key steps below:

- Identify a sample statistic. Use the difference between sample means to estimate the difference between population means.
- Select a confidence level. The confidence level describes the uncertainty of a sampling method. Often, researchers choose 90%, 95%, or 99% confidence levels; but any percentage can be used.
- Find the margin of error. Previously, we showed how to compute the margin of error, based on the critical value and standard deviation.

  When the sample size is large, you can use a t score or a z score for the critical value. Since it does not require computing degrees of freedom, the z score is a little easier. When the sample sizes are small (less than 40), use a t score for the critical value.

  If we use a t score, we will need to compute degrees of freedom (DF). Here's how.

- The following formula is appropriate whenever a t score is used to analyze the difference between means.

  $DF = (s_1^2/n_1 + s_2^2/n_2)2 /\{ [(s_1^2 / n_1)^2 / (n_1 - 1)]+[(s_2^2 / n_2)^2/ (n_2- 1)] \}$

- If you are working with a pooled standard error (see above), $DF = n_1 + n_2 - 2$.

  In this section examples that illustrate the use to z scores and t scores as critical values are given.

- Specify the confidence interval. The range of the confidence interval is defined by the sample statistic $\pm$ margin of error. And the uncertainty is denoted by the confidence level.

Example Small Samples

Suppose that simple random samples of college freshman are selected from two universities–15 students from school A and 20 students from school B. On a standardized test, the sample from school A has an average score of 1000 with a standard deviation of 100. The sample from school B has an average score of 950 with a standard deviation of 90.

What is the 90% confidence interval for the difference in test scores at the two schools, assuming that test scores came from normal distributions in both schools? (Hint: Since the sample sizes are small, use a t score as the critical value.)

(A) 50 $\pm$ 1.70

(B) 50 $\pm$ 28.49

(C) 50 $\pm$ 32.74

(D) 50 $\pm$ 55.66

(E) None of the above

Solution

The correct answer is (D). The approach that we used to solve this Example is valid when the following conditions are met:

- The sampling method must be simple random sampling. This condition is satisfied; the problem statement says that we used simple random sampling.

- The samples must be independent. Since responses from one sample did not affect responses from the other sample, the samples are independent.
- The sampling distribution should be approximately normally distributed. The problem states that test scores in each population are normally distributed, so the difference between test scores will also be normally distributed.

Since the above requirements are satisfied, we can use the following four-step approach to construct a confidence interval.

- Identify a sample statistic. Since we are trying to estimate the difference between population means, we choose the difference between sample means as the sample statistic. Thus, $x_1 - x_2 = 1000 - 950 = 50$.
- Select a confidence level. In this analysis, the confidence level is defined for us in the problem. We are working with a 90% confidence level.
- Find the margin of error. Elsewhere on this site, we show how to compute the margin of error when the sampling distribution is approximately normal. The key steps are shown below.
- Find standard deviation or standard error. Since we do not know the standard deviation of the populations, we cannot compute the standard deviation of the difference between sample means; instead, we compute the standard error (SE).

$$SE = \text{sqrt}\,[s^2_1/n_1 + s^2_2 / n_2]$$

$$SE = \text{sqrt}\,[(100)^2/15 + (90)^2 / 20] = \text{sqrt}\,(10{,}000/15 + 8100/20)$$

$$= \text{sqrt}\,(666.67 + 405) = 32.74$$

- Find critical value. The critical value is a factor used to compute the margin of error. Because the sample sizes are small, we express the critical value as a **t score** rather than a **z score**. To find the critical value, we take these steps:
  - Compute alpha (α): $\alpha = 1 - (\text{confidence level} / 100) = 1 - 90/100 = 0.10$
  - Find the critical probability (p^*): $p^* = 1 - \alpha/2 = 1 - 0.10/2 = 0.95$

- Find the degrees of freedom (DF):

DF = $(s_1^2/n_1 + s_2^2/n_2)^2$ / { [$(s_1^2 / n_1)^2$ / $(n_1 - 1)$]+[$(s_2^2 / n_2)^2$/ $(n_2 - 1)$] }

DF = $(100^2/15 + 90^2/20)^2$ / { [$(100^2 /15)^2$ / 14] + [(90^2 /20)2 / 19] }

DF = $(666.67 + 405)^2$ / (31746.03 + 8632.89)

= 1150614.5 / 40378.92 = 28.495

Rounding off to the nearest whole number, we conclude that there are 28 degrees of freedom.

- The critical value is the t score having 28 degrees of freedom and a cumulative probability equal to 0.95. From the t Distribution Calculator, we find that the critical value is 1.7.
- Compute margin of error (ME): ME = critical value * standard error = 1.7 * 32.74 = 55.66.
- Specify the confidence interval. The range of the confidence interval is defined by thc sample statistic + margin of error. And the uncertainty is denoted by the confidence level.

Therefore, the 90% confidence interval is -5.66 to 100.66. That is, we are 99% confident that the true difference in population means is in the range defined by 50 $\pm$ 55.66.

Example Large Samples

The local baseball team conducts a study to find the amount spent on refreshments at the ball park. Over the course of the season they gather simple random samples of 50 men and 100 women. For men, the average expenditure was \$20, with a standard deviation of \$3. For women, it was \$15, with a standard deviation of \$2.

What is the 99% confidence interval for the spending difference between men and women? Assume that the two populations are independent and normally distributed.

(A) \$5 $\pm$ \$0.47

(B) \$5 $\pm$ \$1.21

(C) \$5 $\pm$ \$2.58

(D) \$5 $\pm$ \$5.00

(E) None of the above

Solution

The correct answer is (B). The approach that we used to solve this Example is valid when the following conditions are met:

- The sampling method must be simple random sampling. This condition is satisfied; the problem statement says that we used simple random sampling.
- The samples must be independent. Again, the problem statement satisfies this condition.
- The sampling distribution should be approximately normally distributed. The problem states that test scores in each population are normally distributed, so the difference between test scores will also be normally distributed.

  Since the above requirements are satisfied, we can use the following four-step approach to construct a confidence interval.
- Identify a sample statistic. Since we are trying to estimate the difference between population means, we choose the difference between sample means as the sample statistic. Thus, $\bar{x}_1 - \bar{x}_2$ = \$20 - \$15 = \$5.
- Select a confidence level. In this analysis, the confidence level is defined for us in the problem. We are working with a 99% confidence level.
- Find the margin of error. Elsewhere on this site, we show how to compute the margin of error when the sampling distribution is approximately normal. The key steps are shown below:
- Find standard deviation or standard error. Since we do not know the standard deviation of the populations, we cannot compute the standard deviation of the difference between sample means; instead, we compute the standard error (SE).

  SE $= \text{sqrt} [\, s^2_1 / n_1 + s^2_2 / n_2 \,]$

  SE $= \text{sqrt} [(3)^2 / 50 + (2)^2 / 100] = \text{sqrt} (9/50 + 4/100)$

  $= \text{sqrt} (0.18 + 0.04) = 0.47$
- Find critical value. The critical value is a factor used to compute the margin of error. Because the sample sizes are large enough, we express

the critical value as a z score. To find the critical value, we take these steps:

- Compute alpha (α): $\alpha = 1 - (\text{confidence level}/100)$

  $= 1 - 99/100 = 0.01$

- Find the critical probability (p*): $p^* = 1 - \alpha/2 = 1 - 0.01/2 = 0.995$
- The critical value is the z score having a cumulative probability equal to 0.995. From the Normal Distribution Calculator, we find that the critical value is 2.58.
- Compute margin of error (ME): ME = critical value * standard error = 2.58 * 0.47 = 1.21
- Specify the confidence interval. The range of the confidence interval is defined by the sample statistic + margin of error. And the uncertainty is denoted by the confidence level.

  Therefore, the 99% confidence interval is \$3.79 to \$6.21. That is, we are 99% confident that men outspend women at the ballpark by about \$5 + \$1.21.

3.4 ESTIMATION OF PROPORTIONS

This chapter describes how to construct a confidence interval for a sample proportion, p.

Estimation Requirements

The approach described in this lesson is valid whenever the following conditions are met:

- The sampling method is simple random sampling.
- The sample includes at least 10 successes and 10 failures. (Some texts say that 5 successes and 5 failures are enough.)

The Variability of the Sample Proportion

To construct a confidence interval for a sample proportion, we need to know the variability of the sample proportion. This means we need to know how to compute the standard deviation and/or the standard error of the sampling distribution.

- Suppose k possible samples of size n can be selected from the population. The standard deviation of the sampling distribution is the "average" deviation between the k sample proportions and the true population proportion, P. The standard deviation of the sample proportion σ_p is:

$$\sigma_p = \text{sqrt} [P^* (1 - P) / n]^* \text{sqrt} [(N - n) / (N - 1)]$$

where P is the population proportion, n is the sample size, and N is the population size. When the population size is much larger (at least 10 times larger) than the sample size, the standard deviation can be approximated by:

$$\sigma_p = \text{sqrt} [P * (1 - P) / n]$$

- When the true population proportion P is not known, the standard deviation of the sampling distribution cannot be calculated. Under these circumstances, use the standard error. The standard error (SE) provides an unbiased estimate of the standard deviation. It can be calculated from the equation below:

$$SEp = \text{sqrt}[p^* (1 - p) / n]^* \text{sqrt}[(N - n) / (N - 1)]$$

where p is the sample proportion, n is the sample size, and N is the population size. When the population size at least 10 times larger than the sample size, the standard error can be approximated by:

$$SEp = \text{sqrt}[p^* (1 - p) / n]$$

How to Find the Confidence Interval for a Proportion?

Previously, we described how to construct confidence intervals. For convenience, we repeat the key steps below:

- Identify a sample statistic. Use the sample proportion to estimate the population proportion.
- Select a confidence level. The confidence level describes the uncertainty of a sampling method. Often, researchers choose 90%, 95%, or 99% confidence levels; but any percentage can be used.
- Find the margin of error. Previously, we showed how to compute the margin of error.

- Specify the confidence interval. The range of the confidence interval is defined by the sample statistic + margin of error. And the uncertainty is denoted by the confidence level.

In the next section, we work through a problem that shows how to use this approach to construct a confidence interval for a proportion.

Example

A major metropolitan newspaper selected a simple random sample of 1,600 readers from their list of 100,000 subscribers. They asked whether the paper should increase its coverage of local news. Forty percent of the sample wanted more local news. What is the 99% confidence interval for the proportion of readers who would like more coverage of local news?

(A) 0.30 to 0.50

(B) 0.32 to 0.48

(C) 0.35 to 0.45

(D) 0.37 to 0.43

(E) 0.39 to 0.41

Solution

The answer is (D). The approach that we used to solve this problem is valid when the following conditions are met.

- The sampling method must be simple random sampling. This condition is satisfied; the problem statement says that we used simple random sampling.
- The sample should include at least 10 successes and 10 failures. Suppose we classify a "more local news" response as a success, and any other response as a failure. Then, we have 0.40 * 1600 = 640 successes, and 0.60 * 1600 = 960 failures–plenty of successes and failures.
- If the population size is much larger than the sample size, we can use an "approximate" formula for the standard deviation or the standard error. This condition is satisfied, so we will use one of the simpler "approximate" formulas.

Since the above requirements are satisfied, we can use the following four-step approach to construct a confidence interval.

- Identify a sample statistic. Since we are trying to estimate a population proportion, we choose the sample proportion (0.40) as the sample statistic.
- Select a confidence level. In this analysis, the confidence level is defined for us in the problem. We are working with a 99% confidence level.
- Find the margin of error. Now, we show how to compute the margin of error when the sampling distribution is approximately normal. The key steps are shown below:
  - Find standard deviation or standard error. Since we do not know the population proportion, we cannot compute the standard deviation; instead, we compute the standard error. And since the population is more than 10 times larger than the sample, we can use the following formula to compute the standard error (SE) of the proportion:

    SE = sqrt [p(1 - p) / n] = sqrt [(0.4)*(0.6) / 1600]

    = sqrt [0.24/1600] = 0.012
  - Find critical value. The critical value is a factor used to compute the margin of error. Because the sampling distribution is approximately normal and the sample size is large, we can express the critical value as a **z score** by following these steps:
    - Compute alpha (α):α = 1 – (confidence level / 100)

      = 1 – (99/100) = 0.01
    - Find the critical probability (p*): p* = 1 – α/2 = 1– 0.01/2

      = 0.995
    - The critical value is the z score having a cumulative probability equal to 0.995. From the Normal Distribution Calculator, we find that the critical value is 2.58.
  - Compute margin of error (ME): ME = critical value * standard error = 2.58 * 0.012 = 0.03

- Specify the confidence interval. The range of the confidence interval is defined by the sample statistic + margin of error. And the uncertainty is denoted by the confidence level.

Therefore, the 99% confidence interval is 0.37 to 0.43. That is, we are 99% confident that the true population proportion is in the range defined by 0.04 ± 0.03.

3.5 ESTIMATION OF DIFFERENCE BETWEEN PROPORTIONS

This chapter describes how to construct a confidence interval for the difference between two sample proportions, $p_1 - p_2$.

Estimation Requirements

The approach described in this lesson is valid whenever the following conditions are met:

- Both samples are simple random samples.
- The samples are independent.
- Each sample includes at least 10 successes and 10 failures. (Some texts say that 5 successes and 5 failures are enough.)

The Variability of the Difference Between Proportions

To construct a confidence interval for the difference between two sample proportions, we need to know about the sampling distribution of the difference. Specifically, we need to know how to compute the standard deviation or standard error of the sampling distribution.

- The standard deviation of the sampling distribution is the "average" deviation between all possible sample differences ($p_1 - p_2$) and the true population difference ($P_1 - P_2$). The standard deviation of the difference between sample proportions $\sigma_{p_1 - p_2}$ is:

$$\sigma_{p_1 - p_2} = \text{sqrt}\{ [P_1 * (1 - P_1) / n_1] * [(N_1 - n_1) / (N_1 - 1)] + [P_2 * (1 - P_2) / n_2] * [(N_2 - n_2) / (N_2 - 1)] \}$$

where P_1 is the population proportion for sample 1, where P_2 is the population proportion for sample 2, n_1 is the sample size from population 1, n_2 is the sample size from population 2, N_1 is the number of observations in population 1, and N_2 is the number of observations in population 2. When each sample is small (less than 10% of its population), the standard deviation can be approximated by:

$$\sigma_{p_1 - p_2} = \text{sqrt}\{ [P_1 * (1 - P_1) / n_1] + [P_2 * (1 - P_2) / n_2] \}$$

When the population parameters (P_1 and P_2) are not known, the standard deviation of the sampling distribution cannot be calculated. Under these circumstances, use the standard error. The standard error (SE) provides an unbiased estimate of the standard deviation. It can be calculated from the equation below:

$$SE_{p_1 - p_2} = \text{sqrt}\{ [p_1 * (1 - p_1) / n_1] * [(N_1 - n_1) / (N_1 - 1)] + [p_2 * (1 - p_2) / n_2] * [(N_2 - n_2) / (N_2 - 1)] \}$$

where p_1 is the sample proportion for sample 1, and where p_2 is the sample proportion for sample 2. When each sample is small (less than 10% of its population), the standard deviation can be approximated by:

$$SE_{p_1 - p_2} = \text{sqrt}\{ [p_1 * (1 - p_1) / n_1] + [p_2 * (1 - p_2) / n_2] \}$$

Some texts present a different, less general version of the approximate formulas. These formulas, which appear below, are valid when the proportions are equal.

$$\sigma_{p_1 - p_2} = \text{sqrt}[P * (1 - P)] * \text{sqrt}[(1 / n_2) + (1 / n_2)]$$

where $P = P_1 = P_2$

$$SE_{p_1 - p_2} = \text{sqrt}[p * (1 - p)] * \text{sqrt}[(1 / n_2) + (1 / n_2)]$$

where $p = p_1 = p_2$

Remember, these two formulas should be used only when the proportions from each group are equal, and when each sample size is small (less than of the population size).

How to Find the Confidence Interval for a Proportion?

Previously, we described how to construct confidence intervals. For convenience, we repeat the key steps below:

- Identify a sample statistic. Use the sample proportions ($p_1 - p_2$) to estimate the difference between population proportions ($P_1 - P_2$).

- Select a confidence level. The confidence level describes the uncertainty of a sampling method. Often, researchers choose 90%, 95%, or 99% confidence levels; but any percentage can be used.
- Find the margin of error. Previously, we showed how to compute the margin of error.
- Specify the confidence interval. The range of the confidence interval is defined by the sample statistic + margin of error. And the uncertainty is denoted by the confidence level.

In the next section, we work through a problem that shows how to use this approach to construct a confidence interval for the difference between proportions.

Example

Suppose the Cartoon Network conducts a nation-wide survey to assess viewer attitudes toward Superman. Using a simple random sample, they select 400 boys and 300 girls to participate in the study. Forty percent of the boys say that Superman is their favourite character, compared to thirty percent of the girls. What is the 90% confidence interval for the true difference in attitudes toward Superman?

(A) 0 to 20 percent more boys prefer Superman

(B) 2 to 18 percent more boys prefer Superman

(C) 4 to 16 percent more boys prefer Superman

(D) 6 to 14 percent more boys prefer Superman

(E) None of the above

Solution

The correct answer is (C). The approach that we used to solve this problem is valid when the following conditions are met:

- The sampling method must be simple random sampling. This condition is satisfied; the problem statement says that we used simple random sampling.
- Both samples should be independent. This condition is satisfied since neither sample was affected by responses of the other sample.
- The sample should include at least 10 successes and 10 failures.

Suppose we classify choosing Superman as a success, and any other response as a failure. Then, we have plenty of successes and failures in both samples.

- The sampling distribution should be approximately normally distributed. Because each sample size is large, we know from the central limit theorem that the sampling distribution of the difference between sample proportions will be normal or nearly normal; so this condition is satisfied.

Since the above requirements are satisfied, we can use the following four-step approach to construct a confidence interval.

- Identify a sample statistic. Since we are trying to estimate the difference between population proportions, we choose the difference between sample proportions as the sample statistic. Thus, the sample statistic is $p_{boy} - p_{girl} = 0.40 - 0.30 = 0.10$.
- Select a confidence level. In this analysis, the confidence level is defined for us in the problem. We are working with a 90% confidence level.
- Find the margin of error. Now, we show how to compute the margin of error when the sampling distribution is approximately normal. The key steps are shown below.
- Find standard deviation or standard error. Since we do not know the population proportions, we cannot compute the standard deviation; instead, we compute the standard error. And since each population is more than 10 times larger than its sample, we can use the following formula to compute the standard error (SE) of the difference between proportions:

  $SE = sqrt\{ [p_1 * (1 - p_1) / n_1] + [p_2 * (1 - p_2) / n_2] \}$

  $SE = sqrt\{ [0.40 * 0.60 / 400] + [0.30 * 0.70 / 300] \}$

  $SE\ sqrt[(0.24 / 400) + (0.21 / 300)] = sqrt (0.0006 + 0.0007)$

  $= sqrt (0.0013) = 0.036$

- Find critical value. The critical value is a factor used to compute the margin of error. Because the sampling distribution is approximately normal and the sample sizes are large, we can express the critical value as a z score by following these steps:

- Compute alpha (α): $\alpha = 1 - (\text{confidence level} / 100)$
  $= 1 - (90/100) = 0.10$
- Find the critical probability (p*): $p^* = 1 - \alpha/2 = 1 - 0.10/2 = 0.95$
- The critical value is the z score having a cumulative probability equal to 0.95. From the Normal Distribution Calculator, we find that the critical value is 1.645.

Compute margin of error (ME): ME = critical value * standard error = 1.645 * 0.036 = 0.06

- Specify the confidence interval. The range of the confidence interval is defined by the sample statistic + margin of error. And the uncertainty is denoted by the confidence level.

Therefore, the 90% confidence interval is 0.04 to 0.16. That is, we are 90% confident that the true difference between population proportion is in the range defined by 0.10 + 0.06. Since both ends of the confidence interval are positive, we can conclude that more boys than girls choose Superman as their favourite cartoon character.

Notation

The following notation is helpful, when we talk about the standard deviation and the standard error.

Population parameter	Sample statistic
N: Number of observations in the population	n: Number of observations in the sample
Ni: Number of observations in population i	ni: Number of observations in sample i
P: Proportion of successes in population	p: Proportion of successes in sample
Pi: Proportion of successes in population i	pi: Proportion of successes in sample i
μ : Population mean	x: Sample estimate of population mean

Cont..

μ_i : Mean of population i	x_i: Sample estimate of μ_i
σ : Population standard deviation	s: Sample estimate of σ
σ_p : Standard deviation of p	SE_p: Standard error of p
σ_x : Standard deviation of x	SE_x: Standard error of x

3.6 ESTIMATION OF STANDARD DEVIATION OF SAMPLE ESTIMATES

Statisticians use sample statistics to estimate population parameters. Naturally, the value of a statistic may vary from one sample to the next.

The variability of a statistic is measured by its standard deviation. The table below shows formulas for computing the standard deviation of statistics from simple random samples. These formulas are valid when the population size is much larger (at least 10 times larger) than the sample size.

Statistic	Standard Deviation
Sample mean, x	$\sigma_x = \sigma$ / sqrt(n)
Sample proportion, p	σ_p = sqrt [P(1 - P) / n]
Difference between means, $x_1 - x_2$	$\sigma_{x_1-x_2}$ =sqrt [$\sigma^2_1 / n_1 + \sigma^2_2 / n_2$]
Difference between proportions, p_1-p_2	$\sigma_{p_1 - p_2}$= sqrt [$P_1(1-P_1) / n_1$ + $P_2(1 - P_2) / n_2$]

Note: In order to compute the standard deviation of a sample statistic, you must know the value of one or more population parameters.

Standard Error of Sample Estimates

Sadly, the values of population parameters are often unknown, making it impossible to compute the standard deviation of a statistic. When this occurs, use the standard error.

The standard error is computed from known sample statistics, and it provides an unbiased estimate of the standard deviation. The table below shows how to compute the standard error for simple random samples, assuming the population size is at least 10 times larger than the sample size.

Statistic	Standard Deviation
Sample mean, x	$SE_x = s / sqrt(n)$
Sample proportion, p	$SE_p = sqrt [p(1 - p) / n]$
Difference between means, $x_1 - x_2$	$SEx_1 - x_2 = sqrt [s^2_1 / n_1 + s^2_2 / n_2]$
Difference between proportions, $p_1 - p_2$	$SEp_1 - p_2 = sqrt [p_1 (1-p_1) / n_1 + p_2(1-p_2) / n_2]$

The equations for the standard error are identical to the equations for the standard deviation, except for one thing–the standard error equations use statistics where the standard deviation equations use parameters. Specifically, the standard error equations use p in place of P, and s in place of σ.

CHAPTER 4

STATISTICAL METHODS IN PLANNING OF INVESTIGATIONS

4.1 INTRODUCTION

Decision on the management of a patient requires a clinical diagnosis, based on the history, examination and special investigations. In the same way the medical policy for a community requires a community diagnosis which rests on epidemiological information— routine health statistics and the results of special surveys. A community diagnosis is expressed in terms of rates which relates data on ill-health to data on the whole population. No single set of statistics describes the illness in a community, and our picture of the frequency and cause of illness is built up from studying the various ways in which disease alerts people's life expectancy and behaviour. Morbidity data are widely used because of their ready availability, certificate of death being a legal requirement in many countries: but unless a disease is usually be fatal, data on morbidity (the frequency of illness) are preferable, albeit often difficult to obtain.

In this chapter a brief description is given about the kinds of population. Morbidity and mortality statistics which are freely available in many countries. As discussed in the previous chapter that there are various sampling procedures for conducting surveys. In this chapter we will discuss the case-control and cohort studies for epidemiological surveys.

4.2 CASE-CONTROL STUDIES AND COHORT STUDIES

Case-control studies are one type of epidemiological study design. They are used to identify factors that may contribute to a medical condition by comparing a group of patients who have that condition with a group of patients who do not.

Case-control studies are a relatively inexpensive and frequently-used type of epidemiological study that can be carried out by small teams or individual researchers in single facilities in a way that more structured trials often cannot be. They have pointed the way to a number of important discoveries and advances, but their very success has led some to place excessive faith in them to the point where their credibility has been significantly undermined. This is largely the result of misconceptions regarding the nature of such studies. These misconceptions are particularly widespread in the medical community.

The great triumph of the **case-control study** was the demonstration of the link between tobacco smoking and lung cancer, by Sir Richard Doll and others after him. Doll was able to show a statistically significant association between the two in a large case control study. Opponents, usually backed by the tobacco industry, argued (correctly) for many years that this type of study cannot prove causation, but the eventual results of double-blind prospective studies confirmed the causal link which the **case-control studies** suggested, and it is now accepted that tobacco smoking is the cause of about 87% of all lung cancer mortality in the US.

While the 'gold standard' of study design is the double blind randomized controlled trial, randomized controlled trials cannot be used to evaluate the effects of toxic substances. **Studying infrequent events** such as death from cancer using randomized clinical trials or other controlled prospective studies requires that large populations be tracked for lengthy periods to observe disease development. In the case of lung cancer this could involve 20 to 40 years, longer than the careers of most epidemiologists. In addition, these studies, which generally rely on government funding, are unlikely to be supported because of the low likelihood that the population will develop the disease. **Case-control studies use patients who already have a disease or other condition and look back to see if there are characteristics of these patients that differ from those who don't have the disease.**

The case-control study provides a cheaper and quicker study of risk factors; if the evidence found is convincing enough, then resources can be allocated to more "credible" and comprehensive studies.

Cross-Sectional Studies

Cross-sectional studies (usually from "snapshot" surveys), sometimes called prevalence studies, can frequently be carried out on pre-existing data, such as that collected by the Census Bureau or the Centers for Disease Control.

Such studies can cover study groups as large as the entire population of the United States. However, others could be small and geographically limited.

Cross-sectional study can contain individual-level data (one record per individual, for example, in national health surveys). Others, however, might only convey group-level information; that is, no individual records are available to the researcher. Instead data are aggregated at the group level. For example, by zip code, urban zone, or even by states/provinces or country. For example, census will never give you individual-level data, as private information must be protected at all cost and individual data is never released. For example, although cross-sectional studies confirm that people who consume large amounts of alcohol also show high rates of many other diseases, they cannot determine with certainty which variable is the cause and which one is the effect. It only shows that these variables were "associated" at some point in time. The temporality or succession of events is not objectively certain. Another problem may occur if the survey or cross-sectional study gathers information at the group level (or the administrator of the survey provides you only with group-level data and no individual-level data). In this case, you may not be able to access information needed to assess the contributions of other variables. For instance, high alcohol consumption is also associated with improper nutrition and hygiene, high rates of smoking and abuse of illegal drugs, and many other risk factors for disease. Ecological design containing only group-level information cross-sectional studies cannot differentiate between these possible causes, but **case-control** studies can determine that gastrointestinal bleeding, say, is directly associated with high alcohol consumption, whereas memory deterioration is more associated with improper nutrition among alcoholics.

The advantage of **case-control** studies over cross-sectional studies that contain only group-level information, then, is the ability to determine the association between potential cause and effect on an *individual* basis. In the cross-sectional study individual variables are aggregated over the population as a whole, then an association is sought between the aggregated variables. These limitations, however, do not apply to case-control studies containing individual-level data. In this case, the "ecological fallacy" is not present. Cross-sectional design with individual-level data allows for computation of absolute risks (from prevalence) and relative risks or odds ratios.

In the **case-control** study, the association is determined for each individual **case-control** pair, then aggregated. This provides a more specific analysis of the possible associations, and potentially determines more accurately which possible causes are directly related to the effect being studies and which are merely related by a common cause.

One benefit of cross-sectional studies is that they are considered to be "hypothesis generating", such that clues to exposure/disease relationships can often be seen in these studies, and then other studies, such as case-control, cohort studies or even sometimes randomized trials can be implemented to study this relationship.

Problems with Case-Control Studies

One major disadvantage of **case-control studies** is that they do not give any indication of the absolute risk of the factor in question. For instance, a **case-control study** may tell you that a certain behaviour may be associated with a tenfold increased risk of death as compared with the control group. Although this sounds alarming, it would not tell you that the actual risk of death would change from one in ten million to one in one million, which is quite a bit less alarming. For that information, data from outside the **case-control study** must be consulted.

Another problem is that of confounding. The nature of case-control studies is such that it is difficult, often impossible, to separate the chooser from the choice. For example, studies of road accident victims found that those wearing seat belts were 80% less likely to suffer serious injury or death in a collision, but data comparing rates for those collisions involving two front-seat occupants of a vehicle, one belted and one unbelted, show a measured efficacy only around half that. Many case-control studies have shown a link between bicycle helmet use and reductions in head injury, but long-term trends - including from countries which have substantially increased helmet use through compulsion– show no such benefit. Analysis of the studies shows substantial differences between the 'case' and 'control' populations, with much of the measured benefit being due to fundamental differences between those who choose to wear helmets voluntarily and those who do not.

More controversially, a significant number of case-control studies identified a link between combined hormone replacement therapy (HRT) and reductions in incidence of coronary heart disease (CHD) in women. Credible mechanisms were advanced as to why this might be, and a consensus arose that HRT was protective against CHD (e.g. *Estrogen replacement therapy and coronary heart disease; a quantitive assessment of the epidemiological evidence* Stampfer M, Colditz G. Int Jour Epid 2004;33:445-53). The evidence was sufficiently compelling that a full clinical trial was initiated– and this indicated that the effect was both far smaller and *in the opposite direction* – combined HRT showed a small but significant *increase* in risk of CHD in the study population. Subsequent analysis has shown that the group of women opting for HRT were predominantly from higher socio-economic groups and therefore had, on average, better diet and exercise habits. The studies had falsely attributed the benefits of these confounding factors to the intervention itself (see *The hormone replacement - coronary heart disease conundrum: is this the death of observational epidemiology?* Lawlor DA, Smith GD & Ebrahim S, International Journal of Epidemiology, 2004;33:464-467). There have been similar controversies regarding links between vitamins and cancer; MMR and autism; antibiotics and asthma; cannabis and psychosis. All these have been identified through small-scale case-control studies but fail to show any effect in whole population time series or other investigations.

A comparison with the tobacco/cancer link is instructive. Here the case-control studies pointed the way, but further confirmation was available in the form of time series showing rates of lung cancer tracking levels of smoking in whole populations, and in the form of laboratory experiments on animals.

Recent research has shown that a substantial majority of highly cited case-control studies are subsequently contradicted or found to be substantially over ambitious when more rigorous investigations are conducted.

As a result the following guidelines have been proposed when assessing case control evidence:

- Do not turn a blind eye to contradiction. Do not ignore contradictory evidence but try to understand the reasons behind the contradictions.
- Do not be seduced by mechanism. Even where a plausible mechanism exists, do not assume that we know everything about that mechanism and how it might interact with other factors.

- Suspend belief of the researchers defending observational studies, Pettiti says this: "Belief caused them to be unstrenuous in considering confounding as an explanation for the studies". Do not be seduced by your desire to prove your case.
- Maintain scepticism. Question whether the factor under investigation can *really* be that important; consider what other differences might characterise the case and control groups. Do not extrapolate results beyond the limits of reasonable certainty (e.g. with grandiose forecasts of "lives saved").

Case-control studies are a valuable investigative tool, providing rapid results at low cost, but caution should be exercised unless results are confirmed by other, more robust evidence.

Cross-sectional studies (also known as **cross-sectional analysis**) form a class of research methods that involve observation of some subset of a population of items all at the same time, in which, groups can be compared at different ages with respect of independent variables, such as IQ and memory. The fundamental difference between cross-sectional and longitudinal studies is that cross-sectional studies take place at a single point in time and that a longitudinal study involves a series of measurements taking over a period of time. Cross-sectional studies are used in most branches of science, in the social sciences and in other fields as well. Cross-sectional research takes a 'slice' of its target group and bases its overall finding on the views or behaviours of those targeted, assuming them to be typical of the whole group. The alternative is longitudinal studies.

Cross-Sectional Studies in Medicine

Cross-sectional studies can be thought of as providing a "snapshot" of the frequency and characteristics of a disease in a population at a particular point in time. This type of data can be used to assess the prevalence of acute or chronic conditions in a population. However, since exposure and disease status are measured at the same point in time, it may not always be possible to distinguish whether the exposure preceded or followed the disease. The cross-sectional survey—which, like a snapshot, "freezes" a specific moment in time—aims at finding the same kind of relationships that might be shown by the "moving picture" of the cohort study, but at far less cost. In a cross-sectional survey, a specific group is looked at to see if a substance or activity, say smoking, is related to the health effect being investigated—for example, lung cancer. If a significantly greater number of smokers already have lung cancer than those who don't smoke, this would support the hypothesis that lung cancer is caused by smoking.

Cross-sectional analysis studies the relationship between different variables at a point in time. For instance, the relationship between income, locality, and personal expenditure. Unlike time series, cross-sectional analysis relates to how variables affect each other at the same time.

A question commonly asked in an epidemiological investigation into the aetiology of a disease is whether some manifestation of ill-health is associated with certain personal characteristics or habits or with a particular aspect of the environment in which a person has lived or with experiences he has undergone. For example, is the risk of death from lung cancer related to the extent of cigarette smoking? Is the risk of incurring a certain illness greater for individuals who treated with a particular dose of drug during a previous illness? Sometimes, questions like these can be answered by controlling experimentation in which the presumptive personal factor can be administered or withheld at the investigator's discretion. More often, however, the experimental approach is out of question, the investigator must then be satisfied with observing whether there is an association between the presumed factor and the disease? These questions, then, will usually be studied by surveys rather than experiments. There are two main designs for aetiological surveys: Casecontrol study and Cohort study.

What is Case-Control Study?

Case control study is a non-experimental one in which subjects are enrolled contingent to the presence (cases) or absence (control) of the defined outcome. Then cases and control are compared with regard to prior exposure to the suspected causal factor(s) as shown in figure 4.1.

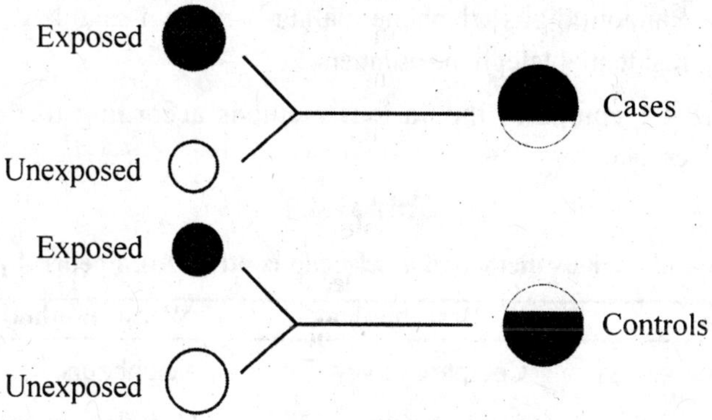

Figure 4.1

The central problems in a case-control study is the method by which the controls are chosen. Usual sources for selection of control subjects are (a) hospitalised patients and (b) the community. For these two sources, there are some advantages besides limitations, the advantages for the selection of hospital controls are that they are (a) easily accessible, (b) usually willing to co-operate and (c) tend to have socio-economic features similar to the cases in all respects expect the medical conditions under study and it is desirable to select the control subjects from the same areas i.e. community source. the advantage of selecting community control is that the prevalence of exposure is likely to be indicative of non-disease persons. However, selecting community control is (a) expensive and time consuming, (b) tends to have a low level of co-operation and (c) certain groups (examples: siblings, neighbours) may be so similar to the cases that associations are obsecured.

There are some other approaches to the selection of controls from the general population, namely:

1. A complex sample survey: A random sample drawn from census tracts with weightage proportional to the size of the population.
2. A sample of neighbour cases.
3. A random sample of names from existing rosters, for example, health care financing, administration register, town books, voters lists etc.

4. Random digits telephone dialing–a random sample drawn from residential telephone numbers.

Table 4.1 compares the various methods according to the criteria considered crucial.

Table - 4.1

Comparison of various methods for selecting controls from general population

Criterion	Best method	Worst method
Representativeness	Complex survey	Neighbours
Cost	Existing rosters	Complex survey
Speed	Existing rosters	Complex survey
Staff safety	Random	Complex survey
	Telephone dialling	

It is necessary to observe that control groups selected by either of these methods are unlikely to share the same aetiological factors experience. Further, the frequencies with which the various factors are found will usually vary with age and sex of cases and controls.

The typical sources of the identification of cases are hospitals, disease registers, vital records bureaus, outpatient clinics, diagnostic laboratories and insurance claims. Cases should be chosen in such a way that they share the same characteristics such as social and environmental conditions or ethnic features. Comparison between cases and controls must, therefore, take account of any differences there may be ın age and sex distribution of the two groups.

Such adjustments are commonly avoided by arranging that each case is paired with a control individual who is deliberately chosen to be of the same age and share any other demographic features which may be thought to be relevant.

Working Example

In a case control or retrospective inquiry, the started point is the affected person.

For example, in a person having active pulmonary tuberculosis, uncovering of features in his history which may have led to that condition, say, cigarette smoking, occupational hazards, overcrowding, malnutrition, etc. may be relevant. Does one or more of these features appear more frequently in the histories of the affected persons than in the unaffected normal population? This indeed is the classical method of epidemiology which seeks to show that of the persons infected, say, with any type of fever, most had consumed a particular type of water while of those who were not affected, relatively few had done so.

Example

A retrospective study to investigate the role of smoking in the aetiology of pulmonary tuberculosis was carried out. A consecutive group of patients who reported to a chest clinic for diagnosis were questioned regarding smoking history. Each person was interviewed on the basis of a pre-designed questionnaire. The only difference between the cases and controls was in their reported smoking habit, the aim of the study was to assess whether symptomatic patients with history of smoking were more likely to be tuberculosis than those without such a history. A total of 4,683 persons (2,410 cases and 2273 controls) were selected and interviewed.

Table - 4.2

Distribution of cases and controls according to sex

Sex	Cases	Controls
Male	1279 (53.1%)	932 (41.1%)
Female	1131 (46.9%)	1341 (58.9%)
Total	2410 (100.0%)	2273 (100.0%)

All the selected subjects were examined and their smoking histories were recorded. Table 4.2 shows the sex distribution of cases and controls according to the factor of smoking. From 2273 healthy controls, 599 were exposed to 'risk factor' smoking while of the total 2410 cases, 1005 were so exposed. The difference in the proportion of non-smokers in males and females is statistically significant (Table 4.3). As smokers and exsmokers among females were only 9.5% in the control group, only males are considered for further analysis. Since the age distribution of smokers and non-smokers was not similar, due allowance was made for this during analysis.

Table - 4.3

Distribution of cases and controls according to sex and smoking habit

Risk Factor (Smoking)	**Sex**	**Cases**	**Controls**
Exposed	Male	910 (90.5%)	520 (86.8%)
	Female	95 (9.5%)	79 (13.2%)
	Total	1005 (100.0%) 41.7%	599 (100.0%) 26.4%
Unexposed	Male	369 (26.3%)	412 (24.6%)
	Female	1036 (73.7%)	1262 (75.4%)
	Total	1405 (100.0%) 58.3%	1674 (100.0%) 73.6%
	Grand Total	2410 100.0%	2273 100.0%

Assuming the hypothesis that there is no relationship between smoking and diagnosis of tuberculosis among symptomatic patients and for testing the hypothesis, χ^2 test was applied. It was observed that smoking was highly and significantly associated with diagnosis of tuberculosis ($\chi^2 = 55.63$ for 1 d.f., $p < 0.001$).

The case control approach is commonly used to assess the risk of developing disease from environmental exposure. The parameter of interest is the estimation of the relative risk of developing a disease in the presence of a characteristic, as compared to the absence of the same characteristic. One can see that the relative risk is the proportion of diseased persons among the exposed as compared that with among those non-exposed to a certain factor(s). In this situation the ratio is 1.95. This suggests that the probability of being diagnosed tuberculosis is about two times more among smokers than in non-smokers.

For this 95% confidence interval for relative risk $RR^{|\nabla|.96/\chi}$ is (1.63, 2.32).

Table - 4.4

Age wise distribution of cases and controls according to sex and smoking habits

Age	18-30 yrs.		31-40 yrs.		41-50 yrs.		51-60 yrs.		60 & more		Total	
	Cases	Controls	Cases	Controls	Cases	Controls	Cases	Controls	Cases	Controls	Cases	Controls
Risk Factor (Smoking)												
Exposed	422	292	241	109	148	76	78	34	21	9	910	520
%	46.4	56.2	26.5	20.9	16.3	14.7	8.6	6.5	2.2	1.7	100.0	100.0
Unexposed	303	349	37	34	18	19	8	8	3	2	369	412
%	82.1	84.7	10.0	8.3	4.9	4.6	2.2	1.9	0.8.	0.5	100.0	100.0

Thus, for the study, distribution of cases and control subjects was used in the Table 4.4 to assess the association between smoking and tuberculosis in different ages. Mantel-Haenszel test was applied and χ^2 was found to be 9.59, which is significant ($p < 0.05$). Further, the relative risks for each age group were calculated as 1.66, 2.03, 2.06, 2.29 and 1.56 for 18-30 years, 31-40 years, 41-50 years, 51-60 years, and more than 60 years, respectively. It was observed that as the age increased the probability of being diagnosed tuberculosis among smokers also increased.

Example

Consider another example of a case-control study of an acute condition with uncertain aetiology, carried out by Gene Mcgrady et.al. during 1985, to investigate association with transfusion of packed red blood cells. Of 187 new-borns admitted to a 33-bed, level III, neonatal intensive care unit between January 1985 and June 1985, 33 developed necrotizing enterocolitis during their hospital stay. Twenty of the 33 newborns (61%) had onset of symptoms between April to June, suggesting clustering during this period. A case-control study, with matching on birth weight class, and approximate duration of stay failed to reveal any association of the syndrome with type or time of feeding, perinatal drypoxic events as determined by APGAR scores or specific microbial organisms. By contrast, the transfusion of packed red cells was highly and significantly associated with the syndrome (odds ratio=15.1 and 95% confidence interval 2.59-95.1). In addition, therapy with caffeine, theophyline and furosemide was moderately associated with the syndrome, although not so significantly. During this period, the incidence of necrotizing enterocolitis by birth weight was 30.6% in infants less than 1500 gm., 10.8% in infants 1500-2500 g. and 11.9% in infants 2500 g or more. These findings confirmed the importance of low birth weight as a risk factor for the development of the syndrome.

Multiple Control Groups

In some case-control studies, the exposure histories of cases are compared separately, against separate control groups. The purpose of making multiple case-control comparisons on the exposure factor of interest is to provide an internal assessment of the reproducibility and, hence, generalisibility of the relationship under study.

A case-control study involving the use of two control groups is given below.

Example

A case-control study was carried out in 1982–83 by Robert, S *et.al.* to investigate the possible influence of behavioural factors on the risk of urinary tract infection. Study participants were college women attending a student health service. Cases were 43 women with culture confirmed urinary tract infection. There were two control groups:149 women with upper respiratory tract infection and 227 women visiting the gynecology clinic. Using each set of controls, the study confirmed that sexual intercourse was the risk factor. And, there was a dose-response effect with increasing level of coital frequency.

The study also found that the use of diaphragm was significantly associated with UTI (Odds ratio 3.0, 2.3), an association which remained significant even after allowing for possible confounding by coital frequency.

Thus, case-control studies can be used for the advantages such as (a) efficient sampling of diseased persons, (b) inexpensive, and (c) rapid conclusions. Further, it has some disadvantages namely, (a) indirect estimate of risk ratio, (b) inefficient for rare exposure, and (c) occasional bias.

With these advantages and disadvantages, in certain circumstances, one might choose to make a pilot case-control inquiry before embarking upon a more arduous cohort investigation.

A **cohort study** is a form of longitudinal study used in medicine and social science. It is one type of study design and should be compared with a cross-sectional study.

A cohort is a group of people who share a common characteristic or experience within a defined period (e.g., are born, leave school, lose their job, are exposed to a drug or a vaccine, etc.). Thus a group of people who were born on a day or in a particular period, say 1948, form a birth cohort. The comparison group may be the general population from which the cohort is drawn, or it may be another cohort of persons thought to have had little or no exposure to the substance under investigation, but otherwise similar. Alternatively, subgroups within the cohort may be compared with each other.

Application

In medicine, a cohort study is often undertaken to obtain evidence to try to refute the existence of a suspected association between cause and disease; failure to refute a hypothesis strengthens confidence in it. Crucially, the cohort is identified before the appearance of the disease under investigation. The study groups, so defined, are observed over a period of time to determine the frequency of new incidence of the studied disease among them. The cohort cannot therefore be defined as a group of people who already have the disease. Distinguishing causality from mere correlation cannot usually be done with results of a cohort study alone.

Some cohort studies track groups of children from their birth, and record a wide range of information (exposures) about them. The value of a cohort study depends on the researchers' capacity to stay in touch with all members of the cohort. Some of these studies have continued for decades.

Examples

An example of an epidemiology question that can be answered by the use of a cohort study is: does exposure to X (say, smoking) correlate with outcome Y (say, lung cancer)? Such a study would recruit a group of smokers and a group of non-smokers (the unexposed group) and follow them for a set period of time and note differences in the incidence of lung cancer between the groups at the end of this time. The groups are *matched* in terms of many other variables such as economic status and other health status so that the variable being assessed, the independent variable (in this case, smoking) can be isolated as the cause of the dependent variable (in this case, lung cancer).

In this example, a statistically significant increase in the incidence of lung cancer in the smoking group as compared to the non-smoking group is evidence in favour of the hypothesis. However, rare outcomes, such as lung cancer, are generally not studied with the use of a cohort study, but are rather studied with the use of a case-control study.

Shorter term studies are commonly used in medical research as a form of clinical trial, or means to test a particular hypothesis of clinical importance. Such studies typically follow two groups of patients for a period of time and compare an endpoint or outcome measure between the two groups.

Randomized controlled trials, or RCTs are a superior methodology in the hierarchy of evidence, because they limit the potential for bias by randomly assigning one patient pool to an intervention and another patient pool to non-intervention (or placebo). This minimises the chance that the incidence of confounding variables will differ between the two groups.

Nevertheless, it is sometimes not practical or ethical to perform RCTs to answer a clinical question. To take our example, if we already had reasonable evidence that smoking causes lung cancer then persuading a pool of non-smokers to take up smoking in order to test this hypothesis would generally be considered quite unethical.

An example of a cohort study that has been going on for more than 50 years is the Framingham Heart Study.

The largest cohort study in women is the Nurses' Health Study. Started in 1976, it is tracking over 120,000 nurses and has been analyzed for many different conditions and outcomes.

Retrospective Cohort

A "prospective cohort" defines the groups before the study is done, while a "retrospective cohort" does the grouping after the data is collected.

Whereas prospective cohorts should be summarized with the relative risk, retrospective cohorts should be summarized with the odds ratio. An example of a retrospective cohort is *Long-Term Mortality after Gastric Bypass Surgery*.

4.3 SAMPLE SIZE

If done properly, the correct estimation of sample size is a significant statistical exercise. Sometimes we bypass this process (often for sensible reasons) by adopting an *ad hoc* approach of using a fixed sample proportion (such as 10% of the population size) or sample size (such as 100). In relatively large populations (say at least 2000) this will normally produce results that are no worse than those produced by a sample based on a carefully calculated sample size (provided, of course, that the sample units that make up the 10% sample are properly selected, so that they are representative of the population).

The basis for calculating the size of samples is that there is a minimum sample size required for a given population to provide estimates with an acceptable level of precision. Any sample larger than this minimum size (if chosen properly) should yield results no less precise, but not necessarily more precise, than the minimum sample. This means that, although we may choose to use a larger sample for other reasons, there is no *statistical* basis for thinking that it will provide better results. On the other hand, a sample size less than the minimum will almost certainly produce results with a lower level of precision. Again, there may be other external factors that make it necessary to use a sample *below* this minimum. If the sample is too small the estimate will be too imprecise, but if the sample is too large, there will be more work but no necessary increase in precision.

But remember that we are primarily interested in *accuracy*. Our aim in sampling is to get an accurate estimate of the population's characteristics from measuring the sample's characteristics. The main controlling factor in deciding whether the estimates will be accurate is how representative the sample is. Using a small sample increases the possibility that the sample will not be representative, but a sample that is larger than the minimum calculated sample size does not necessarily increase the probability of getting a representative sample. As with precision, a larger-than-necessary sample may be used, but is not justified on statistical grounds.

Of course, both an appropriate sample size with the proper sampling technique are required. If the sampling process is carried out correctly, using an effective sample size, the sample will be representative and the estimates it generates will be useful.

Assumptions

In estimating sample sizes we need to make the following assumptions:

- The estimates produced by a set of samples from the same population are *normally-distributed*. (This is *not* the same as saying that the values of the variable we are measuring are actually normally-distributed within the population.) A well-designed random sample is the sampling method that will most usually produce such a distribution.
- We can decide on the required *accuracy* of the sample estimate. For example, if we decide that the accuracy has to be ± 5%, the estimated value must be within five percent either way of the 'true' value, within the margin of error defined in the next assumption.
- We can decide on a *margin of error* for the estimate, usually expressed as a probability of error (5% or 0.05). This means that in an acceptably small number of cases (e.g. five out of a hundred) our sample estimate is *not* within the accuracy range of the population estimate defined in the last assumption.
- We can provide a value for the population variance (S^2) of the variable being estimated. This is a measure of how much variation there is within the population in the value of the property we are trying to estimate. In general we will require a larger sample to accurately estimate something that is very variable, whilst something that has a similar value for all members of the population will require a markedly smaller sample. As we shall discuss shortly, although we almost never have a value for the population variance (if we knew it we probably wouldn't need to do the survey...) there are various ways of obtaining an estimate for use in calculating sample sizes.

4.4 ESTIMATION OF SAMPLE SIZE

Based on these assumptions there are several formulae that have been developed for estimating minimum sample sizes. The format presented here is the simplest, and is applicable to simple random samples, but more complex versions are available for use with systematic and stratified samples (and their various combinations).

We assume that the population mean is to be estimated from the sample mean by a simple random sample of n_o units (equivalent formulae exist for estimating parameters other than the mean). If n_o is much smaller than N (say 10% of N) n_o is given by $n_o = Z^2 \sigma^2 / d^2$

σ^2 is has to be estimated and estimates of σ^2 may be available from previous or similar studies.

The values of Z and d are obtained from the assumption of normal-distribution.

Note particularly that the sample size is *not* related to N; it depends on the variability of the population and the accuracy that we wish to achieve. It may be that this 'independence' of the sample size from the population size is the origin of the widely-held use of a fixed sample proportion (such as 10%) rather than a calculated sample size.

Estimating Population Variance

Even if we don't actually know the population variance there are several methods of deriving a value for it:

- We can split the sample into two (n_1 and n_2, where n_1 is smaller than n_2) and use the results from the first sample to estimate the value of the population variance (S^2) and thus calculate the size of n_2, the 'real' sample.
- We can use a *pilot* survey (the broader significance of which we will consider in a later section) to estimate the value of S^2.
- We can use an estimate for S^2 based on previous samples of the same (or a similar) population.
- We can use 'educated guess work' based on prior experience of the same (or a similar) population.

The question of how large a sample to take arises early in the planning of any survey. This is an important question that should not be treated lightly. To take a large sample than is needed to achieve the desired results is wasteful of resources whereas very small samples often lead to that are no practical use of making good decision. The main objective is to obtain both a desirable accuracy and a desirable confidence level with minimum cost.

Pilot Sample: A pilot or preliminary sample must be drawn from the population and the statistics computed from this sample are used in determination of the sample size. Observations used in the pilot sample may be counted as part of the final sample, so that the computed sample size minus the pilot sample size is the number of observations needed to satisfy the total sample size requirement.

People sometimes ask me, what fraction of the population do you need? I answer, "It's irrelevant; accuracy is determined by sample size alone". This answer has to be modified if the sample is a sizable fraction of the population.

For an item scored 0/1 for no/yes, the standard deviation of the item scores is given by $SD = [p(1-p)/N]^{1/2}$ where p is the proportion obtaining a score of 1, and N is the sample size.

The standard error of estimate SE (the standard deviation of the range of possible p values based on the pilot sample estimate) is given by $SE = SD/N^{1/2}$. Thus, SE is at a maximum when $p = 0.5$. Thus the worst case scenario occurs when 50% agree, 50% disagree.

The sample size, N, can then be expressed as largest integer less than or equal to $0.25/SE^2$.

Thus, for SE to be 0.01 (i.e. 1%), a sample size of 2500 would be needed; 2%, 625; 3%, 278; 4%, 156, 5%, 100.

Note: incidentally, that as long as the sample is a small fraction of the total population, the actual size of the population is entirely irrelevant for the purposes of this calculation.

Sample sizes with regard to binary data:

$$n = [t^2 N p(1-p)] / [t^2 p(1-p) + \alpha^2 (N-1)]$$

with N being the size of the total number of cases, n being the sample size, α the expected error, t being the value taken from the t distribution corresponding to a certain confidence interval, and p being the probability of an event.

For a finite population of size N, the standard error of the sample mean of size n, is:

$$\sigma[(N - n)/(nN)]^{1/2}$$

There are several formulas for the sample size needed for a t-test. The simplest one is

$$n = 2(Z_\alpha + Z_\beta)^2\sigma^2/D^2$$

which underestimates the sample size, but is reasonable for large sample sizes. A less inaccurate formula replaces the Z values with t values, and requires iteration, since the df for the t distribution depends on the sample size. The accurate formula uses a non-central t distribution and it also requires iteration.

The simplest approximation is to replace the first Z value in the above formula with the value from the studentized range statistic that is used to derive Tukey's follow-up test. If you don't have sufficiently detailed tables of the studentized range, you can approximate the Tukey follow-up test using a Bonferroni correction. That is, change the first Z value to Z_α where k is the number of comparisons.

Neither of these solutions is exact and the exact solution is a bit messy. But either of the above approaches is probably close enough, especially if the resulting sample size is larger than (say) 30.

A better stopping rule for conventional statistical tests is as follows:

Test some minimum (pre-determined) number of subjects.

Stop if p-value is equal to or less than .01, or p-value equal to or greater than .36; otherwise, run more subjects.

Obviously, another option is to stop if/when the number of subjects becomes too great for the effect to be of practical interest. This procedure maintains α about 0.05.

We may categorize probability proportion to size (PPS) sampling, stratification, and ratio estimation (or any other form of model assisted estimation) as tools that protect one from the results of a very unlucky sample.

The first two (PPS sampling and stratification) do this by manipulation of the sampling plan (with PPS sampling conceptually a limiting case of stratification). Model assisted estimation methods such as ratio estimation serve the same purpose by introduction of ancillary information into the estimation procedure. Which tools are preferable depends, as others have said, on costs, availability of information that allows use of these tools, and the potential payoffs (none of these will help much if the stratification/PPS/ratio estimation variable is not well correlated with the response variable of interest).

There are also heuristic methods for determination of sample size. For example, in healthcare behaviour and process measurement sampling criteria are designed for a 95% CI of 10 percentage points around a population mean of 0.50. There is a heuristic rule: "If the number of individuals in the target population is smaller than 50 per month, systems do not use sampling procedures but, attempt to collect data from all individuals in the target population."

Sample size determination is very important in any study to be carried out keeping all the advantages in terms of cost and time saving and for better administrative convenience. Sample size determination required different information for different type of conditions. These are as follows:

Estimating a Population Proportion with Specified Absolute Precision

Required Information and Notation

1.	Anticipated population proportion	P
2.	Confidence Interval	$100(1-\alpha)\%$
3.	Absolute precision required on either side of the proportion	d

The sample size would be

$$n = Z^2_{1-\alpha/2}\ P(1-P)/d^2$$

Working Example

A local health department wishes to estimate the prevalence of tuberculosis among school children under five years of age in its locality. How many children should be included in the sample so that the prevalence may be estimated to within 5% point of true value with 95% confidence interval, if it is known that true rate is unlikely to exceed 20%?

Information available:

1.	Anticipated population proportion	20%
2.	Confidence interval	95%
3.	Absolute precision required on either size of the proportion	5%

$$n = (1.96)^2 0.20(1-0.20)/(0.05)^2$$

$$= 246 \text{ children would be needed.}$$

If it is impractical, w.r.t. time and money to study 246 children, the investigator should lower down the requirement of confidence to 90% then in that case the required sample size would be 173.

Estimating a Population Proportion with Specified Relative Precision

Required information and notation:

1.	Anticipated population proportion	P
2.	Confidence Interval	$100(1-\alpha)\%$
3.	Relative precision	€

The choice of P for the sample size estimation should be as conservative (small) as possible, since the smaller P is the greater is the minimum sample size.

Working Example

An investigator working for a national programme of immunization seeks to estimate the proportion of children in the country who are receiving appropriate childhood vaccinations. How many children must be studied if the resulting estimate is to fall within 10% of true proportions with 95% confidence? (the vaccination coverage is not expected to be below 50%).

Solution

Information given

1. Anticipated population proportion 50%

2. Confidence interval 95%

3. Relative precision 10% (of 50%)

$P = 0.50$

$\epsilon = 0.10$

$$n = Z^2_{1-\alpha/2} P(1-P)/\epsilon^2 P$$

A sample of size of 384 would be needed.

If it is impractical, w.r.t. time and money to study 384 children, the investigator should lower down the requirement of confidence to 90% then in that case the required sample size would be 271.

TWO SAMPLE SITUATIONS

Estimating the Difference Between the Population Proportion and Specified Absolute Precision

Required information and notation:

1. Anticipated population proportion P_1 and P_2
2. Confidence Interval $100(1-\alpha)\%$
3. Absolute precision required on either side of the true value of the difference between the proportions d
4. Intermediate value $v = P_1(1-P_1) + P_2(1-P_2)$

For any value of d, the sample size required will be largest when both P_1 and P_2 are equal to 50%; therefore if it is not possible to estimate either population proportion, the 'safest' choice of 0.50 should be used in both cases.

Working Example

What size sample should be selected from each of two groups of people to estimate a risk difference to within 5% points of the true difference with 95% confidence, when no reasonable estimate of P_1 and P_2 can be made?

Information given:

1. Anticipated population proportion 50% and 50%
2. Confidence Interval 95%

3.	Absolute precision	5% point
4.	Intermediate value	0.50

$$n = Z^2_{1-\alpha/2} V/d^2 \text{ where } v = P_1(1-P_1) + P_2(1-P_2)$$

A sample of size 769 would be needed in each group.

Estimating a Relative Risk with Specified Relative Precision

Required Information and Notation:

Two of the following should be known.

1. Anticipated probability of disease in people exposed to factor of interest	P_1
Anticipated probability of disease in people not exposed to factor of interest	P_2
Anticipated relative risk	RR
2. Confidence Interval	$100(1-\alpha)\%$
3. Relative precision	€

For determining sample size; when $RR \geq 1$, the value of both P_2 and RR are needed. Either of these may be calculated, if necessary, provided that P_1 is known; $RR = P_1/P_2$ and $P_2 = P_1/RR$. If $RR < 1$, the value of P_1 and $1/RR$ should be used instead.

Working Example

An epidemiologist is planning a study to investigate the possibility that a certain lung disease is linked with exposure to a recently identified air pollutant. What sample size would be needed in each of two groups, exposed and not exposed, if the epidemiologist wishes to estimate the relative risk to within 50% of the true value (which is believed to be approximately 2) with 95% confidence? The disease is present in 20% of people who are not exposed to the air pollutant.

Solution

A.	Anticipated probability of disease given 'exposure'	?
	Anticipated probability of disease given 'no exposure'	20%
	Anticipated relative risk	2

B. Confidence level 95%

C. Relative precision 50%

$$n = Z^2_{1-\alpha/2} \{ (1-P_1)/P_1 + (1-P_2)/P_2 \} / \{\log (1-€)\}^2$$

RR=2

$P_2 = 0.20$

A sample size of 44 would be needed in each group.

Estimating an Incidence Rate with Specified Relative Precision

Required information and notation

a. Confidence interval 100(1-α)%

b. Relative precision €

Working Example

How large a sample of patients should be followed up if an investigator wishes to estimate the incidence rate of a disease to within 10% of its true value with 95% confidence?

Solution

a. Confidence interval 10%

b. Relative precision 95%

$$n = (Z_{1-\alpha/2} / €)^2$$

€ =0.10

C.I. = 95% so n=385

The sample of size 385 would be needed.

Choosing a Statistical Test

This table is designed to help you to decide which statistical test or descriptive statistic is appropriate for your experiment. In order to use it, you must be able to identify all the variables in the data set and tell what kind of variables they are.

Test	*Attribute variables*	*Continuous variables*	*Rank variables*	*Purpose*	*Notes*	*Example*
Exact binomial test for goodness-of-fit	1	-	-	Test fit of observed frequencies to expected frequencies	Used for small sample sizes, binomial data (attribute variable has only two values)	Count the number of males and females in a small sample, test fit to expected 1:1 ratio
G-test for goodness-of-fit	1	-	-	Test fit of observed frequencies to expected frequencies	Used for large sample sizes (smallest expected class >=5)	Count the number of red, pink and white flowers in a genetic cross, test fit to expected 1:2:1 ratio
Chi-square test for goodness-of-fit	1	-	-	Test fit of observed frequencies to expected frequencies	Used for large sample sizes (smallest expected class >=5)	Count the number of red, pink and white flowers in a genetic cross, test fit to expected 1:2:1 ratio
Randomization test for goodness-of-fit	1	-	-	Test fit of observed frequencies to expected frequencies	Used for small sample sizes (smallest expected class <5)	Count the number of red, pink and white flowers in a genetic cross, test fit to expected 1:2:1 ratio
G-test of independence	2+	-	-	Test hypothesis that proportions are the same in different groups	Sample sizes shouldn't be too small (expected numbers greater than 5 in each cell)	Count the number of apoptotic vs. non-apoptotic cells in liver tissue of organic chemists, molecular biologists, and regular people, test the hypothesis that the proportions are the same
Chi-square test of independence	2+	-	-	Test hypothesis that proportions are the same in different groups	Sample sizes shouldn't be too small (expected numbers greater than 5 in each cell)	Count the number of apoptotic vs. non-apoptotic cells in liver tissue of organic chemists, molecular biologists, and regular people, test the hypothesis that the proportions are the same
Fisher's exact test	2	-	-	Test hypothesis that	Used for small sample sizes; for	Count the number of left-handed vs. right-handed grad students in

Contd.

contd.

				proportions are the same in different groups	2x2 tests only (each attribute variable has only two values)	Biology and Animal Science, test the hypothesis that the proportions are the same
Mantel-Haenzel test	3	-	-	Test hypothesis that proportions are the same in repeated pairings of two groups	-	Count the number of left-handed vs. right-handed grad students in Biology and Animal Science at several universities, test the hypothesis that the proportions are the same; alternate hypothesis is a consistent direction of difference
Randomization tests	1+	-	-	Test fit of observed data to complicated hypothesis	-	Classroom has hexagonal tables with 5,4,6,6 and 3 people, estimate probability that all three left-handed people sit next to each other at the same table
Arithmetic mean	-	1	-	Description of central tendency data	-	-
Median	-	1	-	Description of central tendency of data	More useful than mean for very skewed data	Median height of trees in forest, if most trees are short seedlings and the mean would be skewed by the few very tall trees
Range	-	1	-	Description of dispersion of data	Used more in everyday life than in scientific statistics	-
Variance	-	1	-	Description of dispersion of data	Forms the basis of many statistical tests; in squared units, so not very understandable	-
Standard Deviation	-	1	-	Description of dispersion of data	In same units as original data, so understandable than variance	-

contd.

contd.

Standard error of the mean	-	1	-	Description of accuracy of an estimate of a mean	-	-
Confidence limits	-	1	-	Description of accuracy of an estimate of a mean		-
Single-classification anova, model I	1	1	-	Test the hypothesis that the mean values of the continuous variable are the same in different groups	Model I: the attribute variable is meaningful, differences among groups are interesting	Compare mean heavy metal content in mussels from Nova Scotia, Maine, Massachusetts, Connecticut, NewYork and New Jersey, to see whether there is variation in the level of pollution
Single-classification anova, model II	1	1	-	Estimate the proportion of variance in the continuous variable "explained" by the attribute variable	Model II: the attribute variable is somewhat arbitrary, partitioning variance is more interesting than determining which groups are different	Compare mean heavy metal content in mussels from five different families raised under common conditions, to see if there is heritable variation in heavy metal uptake
Sequential Dunn-Sidak method	1	1	-	After a significant single-classification model I anova, test homogeneity of means of planned, non-orthogonal comparisons of groups	-	C ompare mean heavy metal content in mussels from Nova Scotia+Maine vs. Massachusetts+Connecticut, also Nova Scotia vs. Massachusetts+Connecticut+New York
Bartlett's test	1	1	-	Test the hypothesis that the variance of a continuous variable is the same in different groups	Usually used to see whether data fit one of the assumptions of an anova	-

contd.

contd.

Nested anova, mixed-model	2+	1	-	Test hypothesis that the mean values of the continous variable are the same in different groups, when each group is divided into subgroups	Top level groups are meaningful (model I), subgroups are arbitrary (model II)	Compare mean heavy metal content in mussels from Nova Scotia, Maine, Massachusetts, Connecticut, New York and New Jersey; several mussels from each location, with several metal measurements from each mussel
Nested anova, pure model II	2+	1	-	Test hypothesis that the mean values of the continuous variable are the same in different groups, when each group is divided into subgroups	Both top-level groups and subgroups are arbitrary (model II)	Compare mean heavy metal content in mussels from five different families raised under common conditions; several mussels from each family, with several metal measurements from each mussel
Two-way anova	2	1	-	Test the hypothesis that different groups, classified two ways, have the same means of the continuous variable	-	Compare cholesterol levels in blood of male vegetarians, female vegetarians, male carnivores, and female carnivores
Paired t-test	2	1	-	Test the hypothesis that the means of the continuous variable are the same in paired data	-	Compare the cholesterol level in blood of people before vs. after switching to a vegetarian diet
Linear regression	-	2	-	See whether variation in an independent variable causes some of the variation in a dependent variable; estimate the value	-	Measure chirping speed in crickets at different temperatures, test whether variation in temperature causes variation in chirping speed; or use the estimated relationship to estimate temperature from chirping speed when no thermometer is available

contd.

contd.

				of one unmeasured variable corresponding to a measured variable		
Correlation	-	2	-	See whether two variables covary	-	Measure salt intake and fat intake in different people's diets, to see if people who eat a lot of fat also eat a lot of salt
Multiple regression	-	3+	-	Fit an equation relating several X variables to a single Y variable	-	Measure air temperature, humidity, body mass, leg length, see how they relate to chirping speed in crickets
Curvilinear regression	-	2	-	Test the hypothesis that an equation with X2, X3, etc. fits the Y variable significantly better than a linear regression	-	-
Analysis of covariance	1	2	-	Test the hypothesis that different groups have the same regression lines	First step is to test the homogeneity of slopes; if they are not significantly different, the homogeneity of the Y-intercepts is tested	Measure chirping speed vs. temperature in four species of crickets, see if there is significant variation among the species in the slope or Y-intercept of the relationships
Sign test	2	-	1	Test randomness of direction of difference in paired data	Often used as a non-parametric alternative to a paired t-test	Compare the cholesterol level in blood of people before vs. after switching to a vegetarian diet, only record whether it is higher or lower after the switch

contd.

contd.

Kruskal-Walls test	1	-	1	Test the hypothesis that rankings are the same in different groups	Often used as a non-parametric alternative to single classification anova	Five members of an admissions committee rank applicants to graduate school; see whether their rankings are the same
Spearman's rank correlation	-	-	2	See whether the ranks of two variables covary	Often used as a non-parametric alternative to regression or correlation	Applicants to a graduate program are ranked based on undergraduate GPA and undergraduate research experience; see whether the rankings are correlated

CHAPTER 5	STATISTICAL INFERENCE

5.1 INTRODUCTION

Main objects of sampling theory are (i) Estimation (ii) Testing a hypothesis, which are two important parts of statistical inference.

Estimation we have discussed in the previous chapter. In this chapter we will discuss the other part of inference i.e. Testing of hypothesis. Before discussing the tesing of hypothesis we should have knowledge of Central Limit Theroem.

Central Limit Theorem

It states that 'when the size of the sample increases and becomes sufficiently large the distribution of the sample means tends to Normal Distribution'.

Now here we must take one thing in our notice that the theorem is equally valid for both normal and strongly non-normal. We restate the central limit theorem as: "Even if the population distribution is strongly non-normal, its sampling distribution of means tends to normal distribution for large sample size".

The natural question that comes to one's mind is as to what will be the size which can be taken as the large size?

The following diagrams show how sampling distribution of means approaches normal distribution even if the parent distribution is not normal.

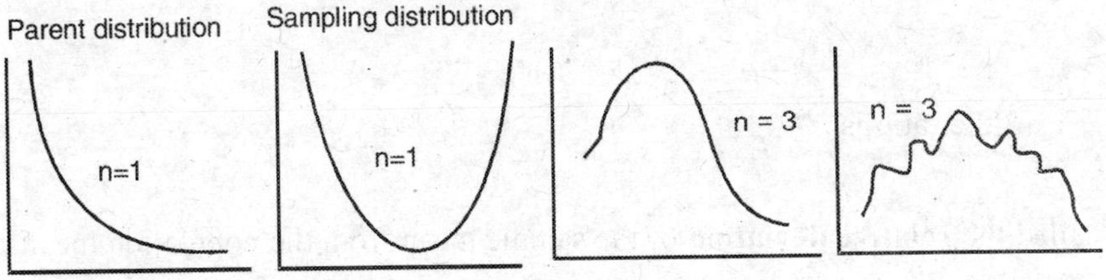

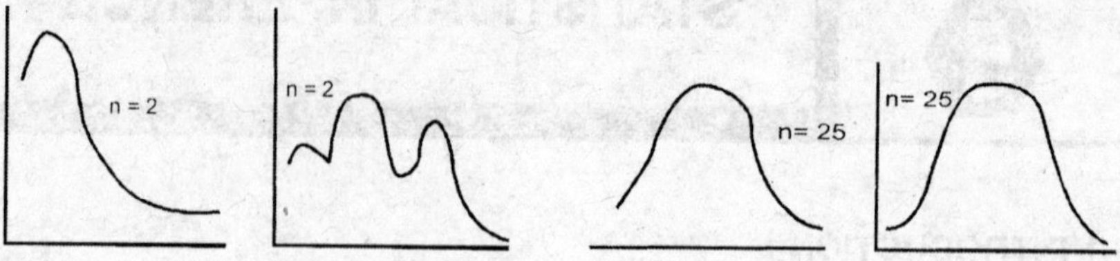

The answer to the above question is that the "large sample size" means n > 30 i.e. over 30.

We have seen that the sample mean $\overline{x}$ is distributed normally with mean m, the mean of the population which is an unbiased estimator. It can be shown that the standard deviation of the sample means, called **Standard error (S.E.)** is equal to

Thus $\mu_{\overline{x}} = \mu$ and $\sigma_{\overline{x}} = \dfrac{\sigma}{\sqrt{n}}$

If we put, $z = \dfrac{\overline{x} - \mu}{\sigma/\sqrt{n}}$

then z - score is called a standard normal variate, with the mean as zero and the standard deviation as 1. If μ is the population mean and $\overline{x}$ is the sample mean then $\overline{x}-\mu$ is the deviation of the sample mean from the population mean.

When this deviation is divided by, $\sigma/\sqrt{n}$

the ratio is $\dfrac{\overline{x} - \mu}{\sigma/\sqrt{n}}$.

called the **relative deviation** of the sample mean from the population mean.

Critical Region

Now $$z = \frac{\overline{x} - \mu}{\sigma / \sqrt{n}}$$

i. e. the relative deviation of sample is a standard normal variate from which it is extremely useful to draw statistical inference.

We know that the standard normal variate is our z - score. 95% area under the curve lies between -1.96 and +1.96, 99% lies between -2.58 and +2.58 and 99.73% lies between -3 and +3. In other words, only 5% area under the normal curve lies beyond ± 1.96, 1%, beyond ± 2.58 and 0.27% lies beyond ±3. These areas also indicate the probabilities that the z - score exceeds these values i.e. the probability that z - score will exceed 1.96 numerically is 0.05.

$\therefore$ P (z < -1.96 or z > 1.96) = 0.05

$\therefore$ P (| z | > 1.96) = 0.05

This means that the probability that z - score will lie in the shaded region is 0.05 which is very small.

Similarly P (| z | > 2.58) = 0.01 and P (| z | > 3) = 0.0027.

Return to our z - score formula $$z_1 = \frac{\overline{x}_1 - \mu_0}{\sigma / \sqrt{n}}$$

where mean of sample is for which z-score is z_1 .

Now 95 out of 100 values of z_1 will lie between -1.96 and +1.96. For $z_1 > 1.96$ or $z_1 < 1.96$, a rare event has taken place because p (| z_1 | > 1.96) = 0.05 which is very small. The z - score (z_1 of x_1) from μ_0 is so significant that it cannot due to sample fluctuations alone.

If p (| z_1 | > 2.58) = 0.01, then very unusual event has taken place because this probability is extremely small (remote). Again we can firmly say that the deviation of x_1 from μ_0 (i.e. z - score) is significant and it is not due to the sample fluctuations alone.

From this discussion we come to a strong conclusion that the levels marked by the probabilities 0.05 or 0.01 which determine the significance of an event are called **Levels of Significance** and are always expressed in percentages as 5% level of significance or 1% level of significance. The corresponding regions are called **Critical Regions.**

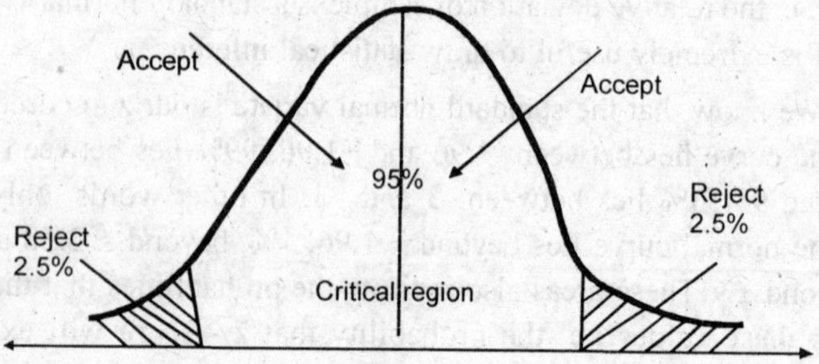

The limits within which we expect z-score lies with specified probabilities are called 'Confidence limits'. Thus $p(|z| > 1.96) = 0.05$ and the bounding values are $\pm$ 1.96 are the confidence limits or fiducial limits. It means we are confident that 95 cases out of 100, the sample mean x will be such that z lies between -1.96 and +1.96.

5.2 TESTING OF HYPOTHESIS

A **statistical hypothesis** is an assumption about a population parameter. This assumption may or may not be true.

The best way to determine whether a statistical hypothesis is true would be to examine the entire population. Since that is often impractical, researchers typically examine a random sample from the population. If sample data are consistent with the statistical hypothesis, the hypothesis is accepted; if not, it is rejected.

There are two types of statistical hypotheses :

- **Null hypothesis** : The null hypothesis, denoted by H_0, is usually the hypothesis that sample observations result purely from chance.
- **Alternative hypothesis** : The alternative hypothesis, denoted by H_1 or H_a, is the hypothesis that sample observations are influenced by some non-random cause.

For example, suppose we wanted to determine whether a coin was fair and balanced. A null hypothesis might be that half the flips would result in Heads and half, in Tails. The alternative hypothesis might be that the number of Heads and Tails would be very different. Symbolically, these hypotheses would be expressed as

$H_0: P = 0.5$

$H_a: P \neq 0.5$

Suppose we flipped the coin 50 times, resulting in 40 Heads and 10 Tails. Given this result, we would be inclined to reject the null hypothesis and accept the alternative hypothesis.

DECISION ERRORS

Two types of errors can result from a hypothesis test :

- **Type I error** : A Type I error occurs when the researcher rejects a null hypothesis when it is true. The probability of committing a Type I error is called the **significance level**. This probability is also called **alpha**, and is often denoted by α.
- **Type II error**. A Type II error occurs when the researcher accepts a null hypothesis that is false. The probability of committing a Type II error is called **beta**, and is often denoted by β. The probability of *not* committing a Type II error is called the **Power** of the test.

Errors in Testing of Hypothesis

In testing any hypothesis, we get only two results : either we accept or we reject it. We do not know whether it is true or false. Hence four possibilities may arise:

1. The hypothesis is true but test rejects it (Type I error)
2. The hypothesis is false but test accepts it (Type II error)
3. The hypothesis is true and test accepts it (correct decision)
4. The hypothesis is false and test rejects it (correct decision)

In a statistical hypothesis testing experiment, a Type I error is committed when the null hypothesis is rejected though it is true. In terms of probability, Type I error is denoted by α (alpha) where

α = probability of type I error = probability (rejecting H_o / H_α is true).

A Type II error is committed by not rejecting (i.e. accepting) the null hypothesis, when it is false. The probability of Type II error is denoted by β (beta) where

β = probability of Type - II error = probability accepting H_o / H_α is false

Now consider that the difference between two population means is actually zero i.e. $H_o : \mu_1 - \mu_2 = 0$. But our test says that the difference is significant. Here we make a Type I error.

On the other hand, suppose there is true difference between the population means i.e. $H_o : \mu_1 - \mu_2 \neq 0$, but our test says the difference is not significant. Here we commit a Type II error.

Hypothesis	**Decision**	
(H_0)	**Accept (H_0)**	**Reject (H_0)**
True	Correct decision	Type I error
False	Type II error	Correct decision

Now suppose **Suchet**, a manufacturer produces some type of articles of good quality. A purchaser by chance selects a sample randomly. It so happens that the sample contains many defective articles and it leads the purchaser to reject the whole product. Now, **Suchet** suffers a loss even though he has produced a good article of quality. Therefore, this Type I error is called "**producers risk**".

On the other hand, if we accept the entire lot on the basis of a sample and the lot is not really good, the consumers are put in loss. Therefore, this Type II error is called the "**consumers risk**".

In practical situations, still other aspects are considered while accepting or rejecting a lot. The risks involved for both producer and consumer are compared. Then Type I and Type II errors are fixed; and a decision is reached.

The measure of how well the test of hypothesis is working, is called the 'power of the test'. In hypothesis testing both α (the probability of Type I error) and β (the probability of Type II error) should be small.

Decision Rules

The analysis plan includes decision rules for accepting or rejecting the null hypothesis. In practice, statisticians describe these decision rules in two ways - with reference to a P-value or with reference to a region of acceptance.

- P-value : The strength of evidence in support of a null hypothesis is measured by the **P-value**. Suppose the test statistic is equal to *S*. The P-value is the probability of observing a test statistic as extreme as *S*, assuming the null hypothesis is true. If the P-value is less than the significance level, we reject the null hypothesis.
- Region of acceptance : The **region of acceptance** is a range of values. If the test statistic falls within the region of acceptance, the null hypothesis is accepted. The region of acceptance is defined so that the chance of making a Type I error is equal to the significance level.

The set of values outside the region of acceptance is called the **region of rejection**. If the test statistic falls within the region of rejection, the null hypothesis is rejected. In such cases, we say that the hypothesis has been rejected at the α level of significance.

These approaches are equivalent. Some statistics texts use the P-value approach; others use the region of acceptance approach.

Few points to consider before selecting the appropriate statistical test:

- Design of the study.
- Groups are unrelated/related.
- Sample size.
- Number of variables involed.
- Types of variables involved.

- Does the variable fulfill the assumptions of the test.

Many a time, we strongly believe some results to be true. but after taking a sample, we notice that one sample data does not wholly support the result. The difference is due to (i) the original belief being wrong and (ii) the sample being slightly one sided.

Tests are therefore, needed to distinguish between the two possibilities. These tests tell about the likely possibilities and reveal whether or not the difference can be due to chance elements. If the difference is not due to chance elements it is significant and therefore, these tests are called tests of significance. The whole procedure is known as Testing of Hypothesis.

A hypothesis is a statement supposed to be true till it is proved false. It may be based on previous experience or may be derived theoretically. First a statistician or the investigator forms a research hypothesis that an exception is to be tested. Then he derives a statement which is opposite the research hypothesis (noting as H_o). The approach here is to set up an assumption that there is no contraction between the **believed result** and the **sample result** and that the difference therefore can be ascribed solely to chance. Such a hypothesis is called a **null hypothesis (H_o)**. It is the null hypothesis that is actually tested, not the research hypothesis. The object of the test is to see whether the null hypothesis should be rejected or accepted.

If the null hypothesis is rejected, that is taken as evidence in favour of the research hypothesis which is called as the **alternative hypothesis (denoted by H_a)**. In usual practice we do not say that the research hypothesis has been "proved" only that it has been supported.

For example, if it is assumed that the mean of the weights of the population of a college is 110 lb, then the null hypothesis will be the mean of the population that is 110 lbs. i.e. H_o : m = 110 lbs (Null hypothesis). In terms of alternative hypothesis (i) $H_\alpha : \mu_\alpha \neq 110$ lbs (ii) $H\alpha : \mu\alpha > 110$ lbs (iii) $H\alpha : \mu\alpha < 110$ lbs.

Setting Up Levels of Significance

Once the null hypothesis is set up, the next job is to set the limits within which we expect (the null hypothesis) m lies. The idea behind it is to ensure that the difference between the sample value and the hypothesis should arise due to sampling fluctuations alone. If this difference does not exceed this limit then the sample supports the null hypothesis and the sample is accepted. If it exceeds this limit the sample does not support the hypothesis and it is rejected.

Now fixing the limits totally depends upon the accuracy desired. Generally the limits are fixed such that the probability that the difference will exceed the limits is 0.05 or 0.01. These levels are known as the 'levels of significance' and are expressed as 5% or 1% levels of significance. Rejection of null hypothesis does not mean that the hypothesis is disproved.

It simply means that the sample values does not support the hypothesis. Also, acceptance does not mean that the hypothesis is proved. It means simply it is being supported.

Confidence Limits

The limits (or range) within which the hypothesis should lie with specified probabilities are called the confidence limits or fiducial limits. It is customary to take these limits as 5% or 1% levels of significance. If sample values lies between the confidence limits, the hypothesis is accepted; if it does not, the hypothesis is rejected at the specified level of significance.

Rejecting H_0 when it is false is exactly what a good test must do. A high value of $(1 - \beta)$, mostly close to 1, means that the test is working in high gear. A low value of $(1 - \beta)$, mostly close 0, means that the test is working poorly.

Thus $(1 - \beta)$ is the measure of the power of the test. If we plot the values of $(1 - \beta)$ for each value of μ f_2 for which $H\alpha$ is true, the resulting curve is known as a **power curve.**

You can see from the figure given below that the power is simply $(1 - \beta)$. In testing of a hypothesis high power is desirable. As we know that the Type I error or a is usually set in advance by a researcher but the Type II error or b for a given test is harder to know as it requires estimation of the distribution of H_a, which is unknown in most of the cases. So like β, the power can be difficult to estimate accurately, but increasing the sample size n, we can increase the power of the test.

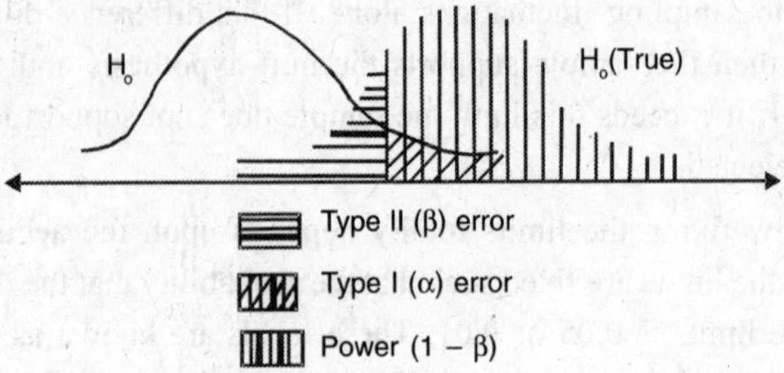

Power of a Hypothesis Test

The probability of *not* committing a Type II error is called the **power** of a hypothesis test.

Effect Size

To compute the power of the test, one offers an alternative view about the "true" value of the population parameter, assuming that the null hypothesis is false. The **effect size** is the difference between the true value and the value specified in the null hypothesis.

Effect size = True value - Hypothesized value

For example, suppose the null hypothesis states that a population mean is equal to 100. A researcher might ask: What is the probability of rejecting the null hypothesis if the true population mean is equal to 90? In this example, the effect size would be 90 - 100, which equals -10.

Factors That Affect Power

The power of a hypothesis test is affected by three factors :

- Sample size (*n*). Other things being equal, the greater the sample size, the greater the power of the test.
- Significance level (α). The higher the significance level, the higher the power of the test. If you increase the significance level, you reduce the region of acceptance. As a result, you are more likely to reject the null hypothesis. This means you are less likely to accept the null hypothesis when it is false; i.e., less likely to make a Type II error. Hence, the power of the test is increased.

The "true" value of the parameter being tested. The greater the difference between the "true" value of a parameter and the value specified in the null hypothesis, the greater the power of the test. That is, the greater the effect size, the greater the power of the test.

One-Tailed and Two-Tailed Tests

A test of a statistical hypothesis, where the region of rejection is on only one side of the sampling distribution, is called a **one-tailed test**. For example, suppose the null hypothesis states that the mean is less than or equal to 10. The alternative hypothesis would be that the mean is greater than 10. The region of rejection would consist of a range of numbers located on the right side of sampling distribution; that is, a set of numbers greater than 10.

A test of a statistical hypothesis, where the region of rejection is on both sides of the sampling distribution, is called a **two-tailed test**. For example, suppose the null hypothesis states that the mean is equal to 10. The alternative hypothesis would be that the mean is less than 10 or greater than 10. The region of rejection would consist of a range of numbers located on both sides of sampling distribution; that is, the region of rejection would consist partly of numbers that were less than 10 and partly of numbers that were greater than 10.

While testing a hypothesis, we often talk of two-tailed tests and one-tailed tests. In the previous tests the critical region lay along both the tails of the distributions. That is, we did not want sample statistic (say mean) to be away from the population parameter (say mean) in either direction. The test for such a hypothesis is non-directional or two-sided or two-tailed. A two-tailed test of hypothesis will reject the null hypothesis H_0, if the sample statistic is significantly higher than or lower than the hypothesized population parameter. Thus in two-tailed test the **rejection (critical)** region is located in both the tails.

For example, suppose you suspect that a particular 6th grader's performance on a test in Mathematics is not a true representative of the students who have appeared. The national mean score in this test was found to be 75. The alternative (or research) hypothesis is:

$H_a : \mu \neq 75$ while the null hypothesis is : $H_0 : \mu = 75$.

Now our pre-determined probability level is 95% i.e. 5% level of significance for this test. Both tests have the rejection (or critical) region of 5% i.e. 0.05. Now this rejection region is divided between both the tails of the distribution i.e. 2.5% or 0.25 in the upper tail and 2.5% or 0.25 in the upper tail and 2.5% or 0.25 in the lower tail since your hypothesis gives only a difference and not a direction. You will reject the null hypothesis on the basis that the sample mean falls into the area beyond 1.96 S.E. Otherwise if it falls into area 0.475 corresponds to 1.96 S.E. you can accept the null hypothesis.

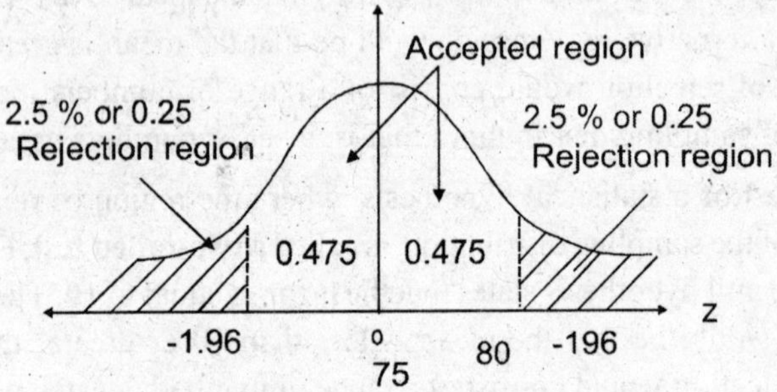

Suppose you want to reduce the risk of committing a Type I error, reduce the size of the rejection region. If the hypothesis is treated at 1% i.e. 0.01 level of significance. If we consult the table of areas under the normal curve (table - 2), we find the acceptance region of 0.495 ((one half of .99) is equal to 2.58 S.E. from μ_H i.e. z-score = 0.

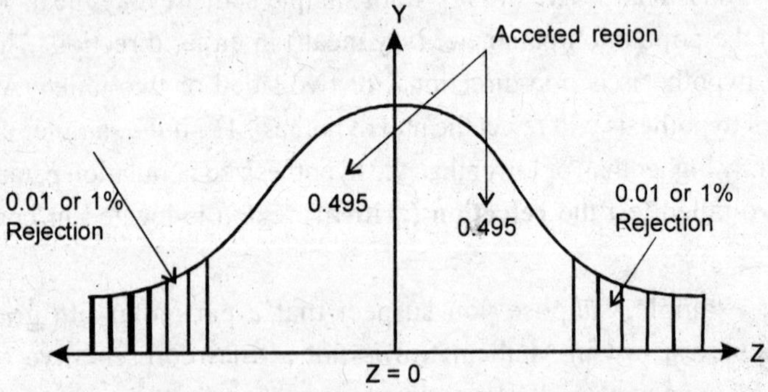

You will still reject the null hypothesis of no difference, if the class sample is either much higher or much lower than our population mean of 75.

As distinguished from the two-tailed test, we can apply a directional one sided i.e. one-tailed test also because in some cases it is necessary to guard against only small values of (i.e. sample mean). One-tailed test is socalled because the rejection region will be located in only one-tail, which may either be on the upper or the lower side of the distribution depending upon the alternative (H_a) hypothesis formula. For example, we want to test a hypothesis that the average income per household is greater than $ 5000 against the alternative hypothesis that the income is $ 1000 or more. We will place all α risk on the upper-side of the theoretical sampling distribution and the test will be one-tailed. On the other hand, if we are testing that the average income per household is $ 5000 against H_a that the income is less than $ 5000 or less, the α risk is on the lower side of the distribution and the test will be one sided.

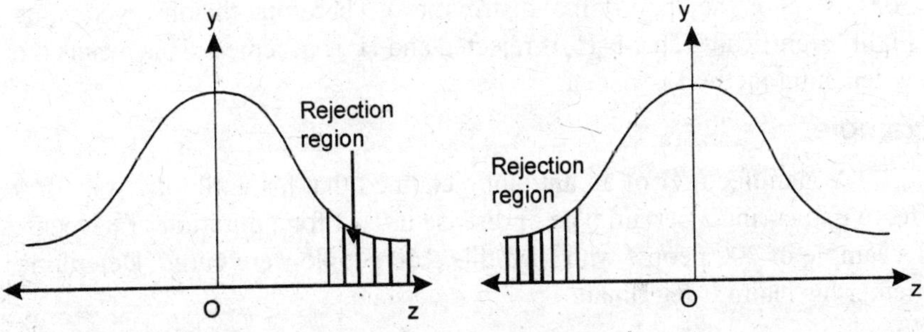

Summing up, if the population as specified mean say μo then the null hypothesis would be $H_0 : \mu = \mu_0$ and alternative (researcher's) hypothesis could be:

1. $H_a : \mu \neq \mu_0$ (i.e. $\mu > \mu_0$ or $\mu < \mu_0$)
2. $H_a : \mu > \mu_0$
3. $H_a : \mu < \mu_0$

Example

Past records show that the mean marks of students taking statistics are 60 with standard deviation of 15 marks. A new method of teaching is adopted and a random sample of 64 students is chosen. After using the new method, the sample gives the mean marks of 65. Is the new method better?

Solution

Here we are interested in knowing whether the marks increased on using the new teaching method. Therefore, we use the one-tailed method :

The null hypothesis is: $H_o : \mu = 60$

The alternative hypothesis is: $H_a : \mu > 60$.

We have $\bar{x} = 65$, $\mu = 60$, $\sigma = 16$ and $n = 64$ then

$$z = \frac{\bar{x} - \mu_0}{\sigma/\sqrt{n}} = \frac{65 - 60}{16/\sqrt{64}} = 2.5$$

Now suppose the researcher had predetermined the level of significance which is 0.01 or 1% for his decision. Then 2.5 > 2.33 (Here z-score is 2.33 for 0.01 level on the upper-tail of distribution). Therefore, the observed value is highly significant. That is H_o is rejected and H_a is accepted. This means the new teaching method is better.

Example

A manufacturer of an antibiotic claimed that his antibiotic was 90% effective in curing a certain type of disease if used for a duration of 8 weeks. In a sample of 200 people who tried this, 160 people were cured. Determine whether his claim is legitimate.

Solution

Let P = Probability for curing the disease by the use of the manufacturer's antibiotic.

Setting two types of hypothesis as :

Null hypothesis $H_o : P = 0.9 \Rightarrow$ claim is supported.

Researcher's hypothesis: $H_a : P < 0.9 \Rightarrow$ claim is rejected.

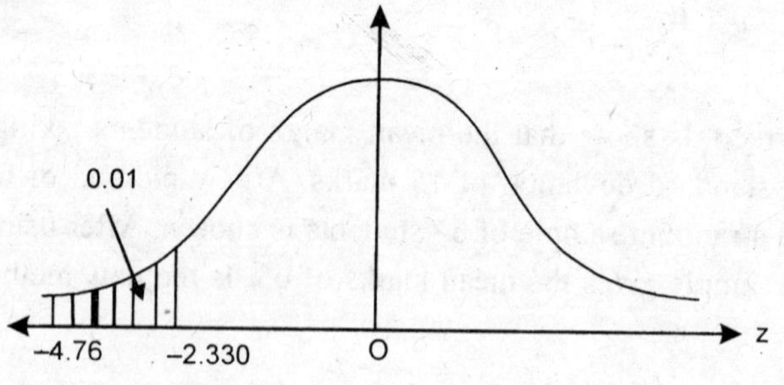

Now P′ = Proportion of success in the given sample = 160/200 = 0.8

Now P = 0.9 ⇒ q = 0.1

Therefore, $\sqrt{\frac{pq}{n}} = \sqrt{\frac{(0.9)(0.1)}{200}} = 0.021$

Thus the corresponding z-score will be

$$Z = \frac{P - P}{\sqrt{\frac{Pq}{n}}} = \frac{0.8 - 0.9}{0.021} = \frac{-0.1}{0.021} = 4.76$$

which is much less than - 2.33. Thus by our decision rule H_o is rejected and H_a is accepted stating that his claim is not legitimate and that the sample results are highly significant (at 0.01 level of significance).

Example

The breaking strengths of metal rods, produced by a certain company, have mean as 820 kg. and standard deviation as 50 kg. When a new manufacturing process is adopted, it is claimed that the breaking strength can be improved. A sample of 100 rods is tested and the results indicates that the breaking strength as 840 kg. Can we support this claim at a 1% level of significance?

Solution

Setting up the two hypotheses as:

Null hypothesis H_o : μ = 820 kg. ⇒ there is no change.

Researcher's hypothesis H_α : μ < 820 kg. ⇒ Breaking strength is improved.

A one-tailed test should be used at 0.01 level of significance for decision making rule.

Now μ = 820, = 840, n = 100 and σ = 50 then

$$Z = \frac{\bar{x} - m}{s/\sqrt{n}} = \frac{840 - 820}{50/\sqrt{100}} = \frac{20}{50/10} = 0.04$$

Now z-score 4 > 2.33 i.e. the null hypothesis H_0 is rejected and the researchers hypothesis is accepted stating that we support the claim "Breaking strength is improved by the new manufacturing process".

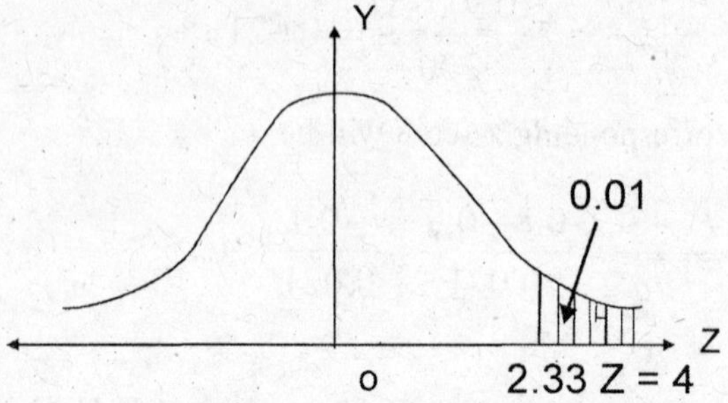

Note: In practice, one should adopt a 'one tailed test' only when he has enough reasoning to expect that the difference will be in a specified direction. A two-tailed test is conservative than a one-tailed test. Since it uses more extreme test statistic for the rejection of the null hypothesis.

Test of Significance for Small Samples

So far we have discussed problems belonging to large samples. When a small sample (size < 30) is considered, the above tests are inapplicable because the assumptions we made for large sample tests, do not hold good for small samples. In case of small samples it is not possible to assume (i) that the random sampling distribution of a statistics normal and (ii) the sample values are sufficiently close to population values to calculate the S.E. of estimate.

Thus an entirely new approach is required to deal with problems of small samples. But one should note that the methods and theory of small samples are applicable to large samples but its converse is not true.

Degree of Freedom (df)

By degree of freedom we mean the number of classes to which the value can be assigned arbitrarily or at will without voicing the restrictions or limitations placed.

For example, we are asked to choose any 4 numbers whose total is 50. Clearly we are at freedom to choose any 3 numbers say 10, 23, 7 but the fourth number, 10 is fixed since the total is 50 [50 - (10 + 23 + 7) = 10]. Thus we are given a restriction, hence the freedom of selection of number is 4 - 1 = 3.

The degree of freedom (df) is denoted by ν (nu) or df and it is given by ν = n - k, where n = number of classes and k = number of independent constiaints (or restrictions).

In general for a Binomial distribution, n = n - 1

For Poisson distribution, n = n - 2 (since we use total frequency and arithmetic mean).

For normal distribution, n = n - 3 (since we use total frequency, mean and standard deviation) etc.

Example

Other things being equal, which of the following actions will reduce the power of a hypothesis test?

I. Increasing sample size.

II. Increasing significance level.

III. Increasing beta, the probability of a Type II error.

(A) I only

(B) II only

(C) III only

(D) All of the above

(E) None of the above

Solution

The correct answer is (C). Increasing sample size makes the hypothesis test more sensitive - more likely to reject the null hypothesis when it is, in fact, false. Increasing the significance level reduces the region of acceptance, which makes the hypothesis test more likely to reject the null hypothesis, thus increasing the power of the test. Since, by definition, power is equal to one minus beta, the power of a test will get smaller as beta gets bigger.

Example

Suppose a researcher conducts an experiment to test a hypothesis. If she doubles her sample size, which of the following will increase?

I. The power of the hypothesis test.

II. The effect size of the hypothesis test.

III. The probability of making a Type II error.

(A) I only

(B) II only

(C) III only

(D) All of the above

(E) None of the above

Solution

The correct answer is (A). Increasing sample size makes the hypothesis test more sensitive M more likely to reject the null hypothesis when it is, in fact, false. Thus, it increases the power of the test. The effect size is not affected by sample size. And the probability of making a Type II error gets smaller, not bigger, as sample size increases.

5.3 HOW TO TEST SIGNIFICANCE OF TEST

This section of the chapter describes a general procedure that can be used to test statistical hypotheses.

A GENERAL PROCEDURE FOR CONDUCTING HYPOTHESIS TESTS

All hypothesis tests are conducted the same way. The researcher states a hypothesis to be tested, formulates an analysis plan, analyzes sample data according to the plan, and accepts or rejects the null hypothesis, based on results of the analysis.

- **State the hypotheses :** Every hypothesis test requires the analyst to state a **null hypothesis** and an alternative hypothesis. The hypotheses are stated in such a way that they are mutually exclusive. That is, if one is true, the other must be false; and vice versa.
- **Formulate an analysis plan** : The analysis plan describes how to use sample data to accept or reject the null hypothesis. It should specify the following elements.
- **Significance level:** Often, researchers choose significance levels equal to 0.01, 0.05, or 0.10; but any value between 0 and 1 can be used.

- **Test method :** Typically, the test method involves a test statistic and a sampling distribution. Computed from sample data, the test statistic might be a mean score, proportion, difference between means, difference between proportions, z-score, t-score, chi-square, etc. Given a test statistic and its sampling distribution, a researcher can assess probabilities associated with the test statistic. If the test statistic probability is less than the significance level, the null hypothesis is rejected.

- **Analyze sample data :** Using sample data, perform computations called for in the analysis plan.

- **Test statistic :** When the null hypothesis involves a mean or proportion, use either of the following equations to compute the test statistic.

Test statistic = (Statistic - Parameter) / (Standard deviation of statistic)

Test statistic = (Statistic - Parameter) / (Standard error of statistic)

where *Parameter* is the value appearing in the null hypothesis, and *Statistic* is the point estimate of *Parameter*. As part of the analysis, you may need to compute the standard deviation or standard error of the statistic.

When the parameter in the null hypothesis involves categorical data, you may use a chi-square statistic as the test statistic. Instructions for computing a chi-square test statistic are presented in the later chapter on the chi-square goodness of fit test.

- **P-value** : The P-value is the probability of observing a sample statistic as extreme as the test statistic, assuming the null hypotheis is true.

- **Interpret the results :** If the sample findings are unlikely, given the null hypothesis, the researcher rejects the null hypothesis. Typically, this involves comparing the P-value to the significance level, and rejecting the null hypothesis when the P-value is less than the significance level.

The next section we will see how to apply the general hypothesis testing procedure to different kinds of statistical problems.

Example

In hypothesis testing, which of the following statements are always true?

I. The P-value is greater than the significance level.

II. The P-value is computed from the significance level.

III. The P-value is the parameter in the null hypothesis.

IV. The P-value is a test statistic.

V. The P-value is a probability.

(A) I only

(B) II only

(C) III only

(D) IV only

(E) V only

Solution

The correct answer is (E). The P-value is the probability of observing a sample statistic as extreme as the test statistic. It can be greater than the significance level, but it can also be smaller than the significance level. It is not computed from the significance level, it is not the parameter in the null hypothesis, and it is not a test statistic.

Hypothesis Test for a Proportion

This lesson explains how to conduct a hypothesis test of a proportion, when the following conditions are met:

- The sampling method is simple random sampling.
- The sample includes at least 10 successes and 10 failures. (Some texts say that 5 successes and 5 failures are enough.)
- The population size is at least 10 times as big as the sample size.

This approach consists of four steps: (1) state the hypotheses, (2) formulate an analysis plan, (3) analyze sample data, and (4) interpret results.

State the Hypotheses

Every hypothesis test requires the analyst to state a null hypothesis and an alternative hypothesis. The hypotheses are stated in such a way that they are mutually exclusive. That is, if one is true, the other must be false; and vice versa.

Formulate an Analysis Plan

The analysis plan describes how to use sample data to accept or reject the null hypothesis. It should specify the following elements :

- **Significance level:** Often, researchers choose significance levels equal to 0.01, 0.05, or 0.10; but any value between 0 and 1 can be used.
- **Test method** : Use the one-sample z-test to determine whether the hypothesized population proportion differs significantly from the observed sample proportion.

Analyze Sample Data

Using sample data, find the test statistic and its associated P-value.

- **Standard deviation :** Compute the standard deviation (σ) of the sampling distribution.

  $$\sigma = \text{sqrt}[P * (1 - P) / n]$$

  where P is the hypothesized value of population proportion in the null hypothesis, and n is the sample size.
- **Test statistic :** The test statistic is a z-score (z) defined by the following equation.

  $$z = (p - P) / \sigma$$

  where P is the hypothesized value of population proportion in the null hypothesis, p is the sample proportion, and σ is the standard deviation of the sampling distribution.
- **P-value :** The P-value is the probability of observing a sample statistic as extreme as the test statistic. Since the test statistic is a z-score, use the Normal Distribution Calculator to assess the probability associated with the z-score. (See sample problems at the end of this lesson for examples of how this is done.)

Interpret Results

If the sample findings are unlikely, given the null hypothesis, the researcher rejects the null hypothesis. Typically, this involves comparing the

P-value to the significance level, and rejecting the null hypothesis when the P-value is less than the significance level.

In this section, two sample problems illustrate how to conduct a hypothesis test of a proportion. The first problem involves a two-tailed test; the second problem, a one-tailed test.

Example Two-Tailed Test

The physician of a large hospital claims that 80 percent of his 1,000,000 patients are very satisfied with the service they receive annually. To test this claim, the hospital surveyed 100 patient's , using simple random sampling. Among the sampled patients, 73 percent say they are very satisified. Based on these findings, can we reject the physicians' hypothesis that 80% of the patients are very much satisfied with the facilities given at the hospital? Use $\alpha = 0.05$ level of significance.

Solution

The solution to this problem takes four steps: (1) state the hypotheses, (2) formulate an analysis plan, (3) analyze sample data, and (4) interpret results. We work through those steps below:

- **State the hypotheses.** The first step is to state the null hypothesis and an alternative hypothesis.

  Null hypothesis: $P = 0.80$

  Alternative hypothesis: $P \neq 0.80$

  Note that these hypotheses constitute a two-tailed test. The null hypothesis will be rejected if the sample proportion is too big or if it is too small.

- **Formulate an analysis plan**. For this analysis, the significance level is 0.05. The test method, shown in the next section, is a one-sample z-test.

- **Analyze sample data**. Using sample data, we calculate the standard deviation (σ) and compute the z-score test statistic (z).

  σ = sqrt[P * (1 - P) / n] = sqrt [(0.8 * 0.2) / 100]

  = sqrt(0.0016) = 0.04

$z = (p - P) / \sigma = (.73 - .80)/0.04 = -1.75$

where P is the hypothesized value of population proportion in the null hypothesis, p is the sample proportion, and n is the sample size.

Since we have a two-tailed test, the P-value is the probability that the z-score is less than -1.75 or greater than 1.75.

We use the Normal Distribution Calculator to find $P(z < -1.75) = 0.04$, and $P(z > 1.75) = 0.04$. Thus, the P-value = 0.04 + 0.04 = 0.08.

- **Interpret results.** Since the P-value (0.08) is greater than the significance level (0.05), we cannot reject the null hypothesis.

Note: If you use this approach on an exam, you may also want to mention why this approach is appropriate. Specifically, the approach is appropriate because the sampling method was simple random sampling, the sample included at least 10 successes and 10 failures, and the population size was at least 10 times the sample size.

Example One-Tailed Test

Suppose the previous example is stated a little bit differently. Suppose the physician claims that *at least* 80 percent of the total 1,000,000 patients are very satisfied. Again, 100 patients are surveyed using simple random sampling. The result is 73 percent are very satisfied. Based on these results, should we accept or reject the physician's hypothesis? Assume a significance level of 0.05.

Solution

The solution to this problem takes four steps: (1) state the hypotheses, (2) formulate an analysis plan, (3) analyze sample data, and (4) interpret results. We work through those steps below:

- **State the hypotheses.** The first step is to state the null hypothesis and an alternative hypothesis.

  Null hypothesis: $P = 0.80$

  Alternative hypothesis: $P < 0.80$

Note that these hypotheses constitute a one-tailed test. The null hypothesis will be rejected only if the sample proportion is too small.

- **Formulate an analysis plan**. For this analysis, the significance level is 0.05. The test method, shown in the next section, is a one-sample z-test.
- **Analyze sample data**. Using sample data, we calculate the standard deviation (σ) and compute the z-score test statistic (z).

  σ = sqrt[P * (1 - P) / n] = sqrt [(0.8 * 0.2) / 100]

  = sqrt(0.0016) = 0.04

  z = (p - P) / σ = (.73 - .80)/0.04 = -1.75

  where P is the hypothesized value of population proportion in the null hypothesis, p is the sample proportion, and n is the sample size.

  Since we have a one-tailed test, the P-value is the probability that the z-score is less than -1.75. We use the Normal Distribution Calculator to find P(z < -1.75) = 0.04. Thus, the P-value = 0.04.

- **Interpret results**. Since the P-value (0.04) is less than the significance level (0.05), we cannot accept the null hypothesis.

Note: If you use this approach on an exam, you may also want to mention why this approach is appropriate. Specifically, the approach is appropriate because the sampling method was simple random sampling, the sample included at least 10 successes and 10 failures, and the population size was at least 10 times the sample size.

Hypothesis Test for Difference Between Proportions

This chapter explains how to conduct a hypothesis test to determine whether the difference between two proportions is significant. The test procedure, called the **two-proportion z-test**, is appropriate when the following conditions are met:

- The sampling method for each population is simple random sampling.
- The samples are independent.

- Each sample includes at least 10 successes and 10 failures. (Some texts say that 5 successes and 5 failures are enough)
- Each population is at least 10 times as big as its sample.

This approach consists of four steps: (1) state the hypotheses, (2) formulate an analysis plan, (3) analyze sample data, and (4) interpret results.

State the Hypotheses

Every hypothesis test requires the analyst to state a null hypothesis and an alternative hypothesis. The table below shows three sets of hypotheses. Each makes a statement about the difference *d* between two population proportions, P_1 and P_2. (In the table, the symbol '$\neq$' means " not equal to.)

Set	Null hypothesis	Alternative hypothesis	Number of tails
1	$P_1 - P_2 = 0$	$P_1 - P_2 \neq 0$	2
2	$P_1 - P_2 > 0$	$P_1 - P_2 < 0$	1
3	$P_1 - P_2 < 0$	$P_1 - P_2 > 0$	1

The first set of hypotheses (Set 1) is an example of a two-tailed test, since an extreme value on either side of the sampling distribution would cause a researcher to reject the null hypothesis. The other two sets of hypotheses (Sets 2 and 3) are one-tailed tests, since an extreme value on only one side of the sampling distribution would cause a researcher to reject the null hypothesis.

When the null hypothesis states that there is no difference between the two population proportions (i.e., d = 0), the null and alternative hypothesis for a two-tailed test are often stated in the following form:

$$H_0: P_1 = P_2$$
$$H_a: P_1 \neq P_2$$

Formulate an Analysis Plan

The analysis plan describes how to use sample data to accept or reject the null hypothesis. It should specify the following elements:

- Significance level. Often, researchers choose significance levels equal to 0.01, 0.05, or 0.10; but any value between 0 and 1 can be used.

- Test method. Use the two-proportion z-test (described in the next section) to determine whether the hypothesized difference between population proportions differs significantly from the observed sample difference.

Analyze Sample Data

Using sample data, complete the following computations to find the test statistic and its associated P-value.

- **Pooled sample proportion:** Since the null hypothesis states that $P_1 = P_2$, we use a pooled sample proportion (p) to compute the standard error of the sampling distribution.

$$p = (p_1 * n_1 + p_2 * n_2) / (n_1 + n_2)$$

  where p_1 is the sample proportion from population 1, p_2 is the sample proportion from population 2, n_1 is the size of sample 1, and n_2 is the size of sample 2.

- **Standard error:** Compute the standard error (SE) of the sampling distribution difference between two proportions.

$$SE = \text{sqrt}\{ p * (1 - p) * [(1/n_1) + (1/n_2)] \}$$

  where p is the pooled sample proportion, n_1 is the size of sample 1, and n_2 is the size of sample 2.

- **Test statistic:** The test statistic is a z-score (z) defined by the following equation.

$$z = (p_1 - p_2) / SE$$

  where p_1 is the proportion from sample 1, p_2 is the proportion from sample 2, and SE is the standard error of the sampling distribution.

- **P-value:** The P-value is the probability of observing a sample statistic as extreme as the test statistic. Since the test statistic is a z-score, use the Normal Distribution Calculator to assess the probability associated with the z-score. (See sample problems at the end of this lesson for examples of how this is done.)

The analysis described above is a two-proportion z-test.

Interpret Results

If the sample findings are unlikely, given the null hypothesis, the researcher rejects the null hypothesis. Typically, this involves comparing the P-value to the significance level, and rejecting the null hypothesis when the P-value is less than the significance level.

In this section, two sample problems illustrate how to conduct a hypothesis test for the difference between two proportions. The first problem involves a two-tailed test; the second problem, a one-tailed test.

Example Two-Tailed Test

Suppose the Acme Drug Company develops a new drug, designed to prevent colds. The company states that the drug is equally effective for men and women. To test this claim, they choose a simple random sample of 100 women and 200 men from a population of 100,000 volunteers.

At the end of the study, 38% of the women caught a cold; and 51% of the men caught a cold. Based on these findings, can we reject the company's claim that the drug is equally effective for men and women? Use a 0.05 level of significance.

Solution

The solution to this problem takes four steps: (1) state the hypotheses, (2) formulate an analysis plan, (3) analyze sample data, and (4) interpret results. We work through those steps below:

- **State the hypotheses.** The first step is to state the null hypothesis and an alternative hypothesis.

  Null hypothesis: $P_1 = P_2$

  Alternative hypothesis: $P_1 \neq P_2$

  Note that these hypotheses constitute a two-tailed test. The null hypothesis will be rejected if the proportion from population 1 is too big or if it is too small.

- **Formulate an analysis plan**. For this analysis, the significance level is 0.05. The test method is a two-proportion z-test.

- **Analyze sample data**. Using sample data, we calculate the pooled sample proportion (p) and the standard error (SE). Using those measures, we compute the z-score test statistic (z).

$p = (p_1 * n_1 + p_2 * n_2) / (n_1 + n_2) = [(0.38 * 100) + (0.51 * 200)] / (100 + 200) = 140/300 = 0.467$

$SE = sqrt\{ p * (1 - p) * [(1/n_1) + (1/n_2)] \}$

$SE = sqrt [0.467 * 0.533 * (1/100 + 1/200)] = sqrt [0.003733] = 0.061$

$z = (p_1 - p_2) / SE = (0.51 - 0.38)/0.061 = 2.13$

where p_1 is the sample proportion in sample 1, where p_2 is the sample proportion in sample 2, n_1 is the size of sample 1, and n_2 is the size of sample 2.

Since we have a two-tailed test, the P-value is the probability that the z-score is less than -2.13 or greater than 2.13.

We use the Normal Distribution Calculator to find $P(z < -2.13) = 0.017$, and $P(z > 2.13) = 0.017$. Thus, the P-value = 0.017 + 0.017 = 0.034.

- **Interpret results**. Since the P-value (0.034) is less than the significance level (0.05), we cannot accept the null hypothesis.

Note: If you use this approach on an exam, you may also want to mention why this approach is appropriate. Specifically, the approach is appropriate because the sampling method was simple random sampling, the samples were independent, each population was at least 10 times larger than its sample, and each sample included at least 10 successes and 10 failures.

Example One-Tailed Test

Suppose the previous example is stated a little bit differently. Suppose the Acme Drug Company develops a new drug, designed to prevent colds. The company states that the drug is more effective for women than for men. To test this claim, they choose a simple random sample of 100 women and 200 men from a population of 100,000 volunteers.

At the end of the study, 38% of the women caught a cold; and 51% of the men caught a cold. Based on these findings, can we conclude that the drug is more effective for women than for men? Use a 0.01 level of significance.

Solution

The solution to this problem takes four steps: (1) state the hypotheses, (2) formulate an analysis plan, (3) analyze sample data, and (4) interpret results. We work through those steps below:

- **State the hypotheses.** The first step is to state the null hypothesis and an alternative hypothesis.

  Null hypothesis: $P_1 = P_2$

  Alternative hypothesis: $P_1 < P_2$

Note that these hypotheses constitute a one-tailed test. The null hypothesis will be rejected if the proportion of women catching cold (p_1) is sufficiently smaller than the proportion of men catching cold (p_2).

- **Formulate an analysis plan**. For this analysis, the significance level is 0.01. The test method is a two-proportion z-test.

- **Analyze sample data**. Using sample data, we calculate the pooled sample proportion (p) and the standard error (SE). Using those measures, we compute the z-score test statistic (z).

  p = $(p_1 * n_1 + p_2 * n_2) / (n_1 + n_2)$ = [(0.38 * 100) + (0.51 * 200)] / (100 + 200) = 140/300 = 0.467

  SE = sqrt{ p * (1 - p) * [$(1/n_1) + (1/n_2)$] }

  SE = sqrt [0.467 * 0.533 * (1/100 + 1/200)] = sqrt [0.003733] = 0.061

  z = $(p_1 - p_2)$ / SE = (0.38 - 0.51)/0.061 = -2.13

  where p_1 is the sample proportion in sample 1, where p_2 is the sample proportion in sample 2, n_1 is the size of sample 2, and n_2 is the size of sample 2.

  Since we have a one-tailed test, the P-value is the probability that the z-score is less than -2.13. We use the Normal Distribution Calculator to find P(z < -2.13) = 0.017. Thus, the P-value = 0.017.

- **Interpret results**. Since the P-value (0.017) is greater than the significance level (0.01), we cannot reject the null hypothesis.

Note: If you use this approach on an exam, you may also want to mention why this approach is appropriate. Specifically, the approach is appropriate because the sampling method was simple random sampling, the samples were independent, each population was at least 10 times larger than its sample, and each sample included at least 10 successes and 10 failures.

Hypothesis Test of the Mean

This chapter explains how to conduct a hypothesis test of a mean, when the following conditions are met:

- The sampling method is simple random sampling.
- The sample is drawn from a normal or near-normal population.

Generally, the sampling distribution will be approximately normally distributed if any of the following conditions apply:

- The population distribution is normal.
- The sampling distribution is symmetric, unimodal, without outliers, and the sample size is 15 or less.
- The sampling distribution is moderately skewed, unimodal, without outliers, and the sample size is between 16 and 40.
- The sample size is greater than 40, without outliers.

This approach consists of four steps: (1) state the hypotheses, (2) formulate an analysis plan, (3) analyze sample data, and (4) interpret results.

State the Hypotheses

Every hypothesis test requires the analyst to state a null hypothesis and an alternative hypothesis. The hypotheses are stated in such a way that they are mutually exclusive. That is, if one is true, the other must be false; and vice versa.

The table below shows three sets of hypotheses. Each makes a statement about how the population mean μ is related to a specified value *M*. (In the table, the symbol ≠ means " not equal to".)

Set	Null hypothesis	Alternative hypothesis	Number of tails
1	$\mu = M$	$\mu \neq M$	2
2	$\mu \geqslant M$	$\mu < M$	1
3	$\mu \leqslant M$	$\mu > M$	1

The first set of hypotheses (Set 1) is an example of a two-tailed test, since an extreme value on either side of the sampling distribution would cause a researcher to reject the null hypothesis. The other two sets of hypotheses

(Sets 2 and 3) are one-tailed tests, since an extreme value on only one side of the sampling distribution would cause a researcher to reject the null hypothesis.

Formulate An Analysis Plan

The analysis plan describes how to use sample data to accept or reject the null hypothesis. It should specify the following elements:

- **Significance level.** Often, researchers choose significance levels equal to 0.01, 0.05, or 0.10; but any value between 0 and 1 can be used.
- **Test method.** Use the one-sample t-test to determine whether the hypothesized mean differs significantly from the observed sample mean.

Analyze Sample Data

Using sample data, conduct a one-sample t-test. This involves finding the standard error, degrees of freedom, test statistic, and the P-value associated with the test statistic.

- **Standard error.** Compute the standard error (SE) of the sampling distribution.

  $SE = s * sqrt\{ (1/n) * (1 - n/N) * [N / (N - 1)] \}$

  where *s* is the standard deviation of the sample, N is the population size, and *n* is the sample size. When the population size is much larger (at least 10 times larger) than the sample size, the standard error can be approximated by:

  $$SE = s / sqrt(n)$$

- **Degrees of freedom.** The degrees of freedom (DF) is equal to the sample size (n) minus one. Thus, DF = n - 1.
- **Test statistic.** The test statistic is a t-score (t) defined by the following equation:

  $$t = (\bar{x} - \mu) / SE$$

  where $\bar{x}$ is the sample mean, μ is the hypothesized population mean in the null hypothesis, and SE is the standard error.

- P-value. The P-value is the probability of observing a sample statistic as extreme as the test statistic. Since the test statistic is a t-score, use the t Distribution Calculator to assess the probability associated with the t-score, given the degrees of freedom computed above. (See sample problems at the end of this lesson for examples of how this is done).

Interpret Results

If the sample findings are unlikely, given the null hypothesis, the researcher rejects the null hypothesis. Typically, this involves comparing the P-value to the significance level, and rejecting the null hypothesis when the P-value is less than the significance level.

In this section, two sample problems illustrate how to conduct a hypothesis test of a mean score. The first problem involves a two-tailed test; the second problem, a one-tailed test.

Example Two-Tailed Test

An inventor has developed a new, energy-efficient lawn mower engine. He claims that the engine will run continuously for 5 hours (300 minutes) on a single gallon of regular gasoline. Suppose a simple random sample of 50 engines is tested. The engines run for an average of 295 minutes, with a standard deviation of 20 minutes. Test the null hypothesis that the mean run time is 300 minutes against the alternative hypothesis that the mean run time is not 300 minutes. Use a 0.05 level of significance. (Assume that run times for the population of engines are normally distributed).

Solution

The solution to this problem takes four steps: (1) state the hypotheses, (2) formulate an analysis plan, (3) analyze sample data, and (4) interpret results. We work through those steps below:

- **State the hypotheses.** The first step is to state the null hypothesis and an alternative hypothesis.

  Null hypothesis: $\mu = 300$

  Alternative hypothesis: $\mu \neq 300$

Note that these hypotheses constitute a two-tailed test. The null hypothesis will be rejected if the sample mean is too big or if it is too small.

- **Formulate an analysis plan.** For this analysis, the significance level is 0.05. The test method is a one-sample t-test.
- **Analyze sample data.** Using sample data, we compute the standard error (SE), degrees of freedom (DF), and the t-score test statistic (t).

  SE = s / sqrt(n) = 20 / sqrt(50) = 20/7.07 = 2.83

  DF = n - 1 = 50 - 1 = 49

  t = (x - μ) / SE = (295 - 300)/2.83 = 1.77

  where s is the standard deviation of the sample, x is the sample mean, μ is the hypothesized population mean, and n is the sample size.

  Since we have a two-tailed test, the P-value is the probability that the t-score having 49 degrees of freedom is less than -1.77 or greater than 1.77.

  We use the t Distribution Calculator to find P(t < -1.77) = 0.04, and P(t > 1.75) = 0.04. Thus, the P-value = 0.04 + 0.04 = 0.08.
- **Interpret results.** Since the P-value (0.08) is greater than the significance level (0.05), we cannot reject the null hypothesis.

Note: If you use this approach on an exam, you may also want to mention why this approach is appropriate. Specifically, the approach is appropriate because the sampling method was simple random sampling, and the population was normally distributed.

Example: One-Tailed Test

Bon Air Elementary School has 300 students. The principal of the school thinks that the average IQ of students at Bon Air is at least 110. To prove her point, she administers an IQ test to 20 randomly selected students. Among the sampled students, the average IQ is 108 with a standard deviation of 10. Based on these results, should the principal accept or reject her original hypothesis? Assume a significance level of 0.01.

Solution

The solution to this problem takes four steps: (1) state the hypotheses, (2) formulate an analysis plan, (3) analyze sample data, and (4) interpret results. We work through those steps below:

- **State the hypotheses.** The first step is to state the null hypothesis and an alternative hypothesis.

  Null hypothesis: $\mu = 110$

  Alternative hypothesis: $\mu < 110$

Note that these hypotheses constitute a one-tailed test. The null hypothesis will be rejected if the sample mean is too small.

- **Formulate an analysis plan.** For this analysis, the significance level is 0.01. The test method is a one-sample t-test.

- **Analyze sample data.** Using sample data, we compute the standard error (SE), degrees of freedom (DF), and the t-score test statistic (t).

  SE = s / sqrt(n) = 10 / sqrt(20) = 10/4.472 = 2.236

  DF = n - 1 = 20 - 1 = 19

  $t = (\bar{x} - \mu) / SE = (108 - 110)/2.236 = -0.894$

  where s is the standard deviation of the sample, $\bar{x}$ is the sample mean, μ is the hypothesized population mean, and n is the sample size.

  Since we have a one-tailed test, the P-value is the probability that the t-score having 19 degrees of freedom is less than -0.894.

  We use the t Distribution Calculator to find $P(t < -0.894) = 0.19$. Thus, the P-value is 0.19.

- **Interpret results.** Since the P-value (0.19) is greater than the significance level (0.01), we cannot reject the null hypothesis.

Note: If you use this approach on an exam, you may also want to mention why this approach is appropriate. Specifically, the approach is appropriate because the sampling method was simple random sampling, and the population was normally distributed.

Hypothesis Test for the Difference Between Two Means

This chapter explains how to conduct a hypothesis test for the difference between two means. The test procedure, called the **two-sample t-test**, is appropriate when the following conditions are met:

- The sampling method for each sample is simple random sampling.
- The samples are independent.
- Each population is at least 10 times larger than its respective sample.
- Each sample is drawn from a normal or near-normal population.

Generally, the sampling distribution will be approximately normal if any of the following conditions apply:

- The population distribution is normal.
- The sample data are symmetric, unimodal, without outliers, and the sample size is 15 or less.
- The sample data are slightly skewed, unimodal, without outliers, and the sample size is 16 to 40.
- The sample size is greater than 40, without outliers.

This approach consists of four steps: (1) state the hypotheses, (2) formulate an analysis plan, (3) analyze sample data, and (4) interpret results.

State the Hypotheses

Every hypothesis test requires the analyst to state a null hypothesis and an alternative hypothesis. The hypotheses are stated in such a way that they are mutually exclusive. That is, if one is true, the other must be false; and vice versa.

The table below shows three sets of null and alternative hypotheses. Each makes a statement about the difference *d* between the mean of one population μ_1 and the mean of another population μ_2. (In the table, the symbol $\neq$ means " not equal to".)

Set	Null hypothesis	Alternative hypothesis	Number of tails
1	$\mu_1 - \mu_2 = d$	$\mu_1 - \mu_2 \neq d$	2
2	$\mu_1 - \mu_2 \geqslant d$	$\mu_1 - \mu_2 < d$	1
3	$\mu_1 - \mu_2 \leqslant d$	$\mu_1 - \mu_2 > d$	1

The first set of hypotheses (Set 1) is an example of a two-tailed test, since an extreme value on either side of the sampling distribution would cause a researcher to reject the null hypothesis. The other two sets of hypotheses (Sets 2 and 3) are one-tailed tests, since an extreme value on only one side of the sampling distribution would cause a researcher to reject the null hypothesis.

When the null hypothesis states that there is no difference between the two population means (i.e., d = 0), the null and alternative hypothesis are often stated in the following form:

$H_0: \mu_1 = \mu_2$

$H_a: \mu_1 \neq \mu_2$

Formulate An Analysis Plan

The analysis plan describes how to use sample data to accept or reject the null hypothesis. It should specify the following elements:

- **Significance level:** Often, researchers choose significance levels equal to 0.01, 0.05, or 0.10; but any value between 0 and 1 can be used.
- **Test method:** Use the two-sample t-test to determine whether the difference between means found in the sample is significantly different from the hypothesized difference between means.

Analyze Sample Data

Using sample data, find the standard error, degrees of freedom, test statistic, and the P-value associated with the test statistic.

- **Standard error:** Compute the standard error (SE) of the sampling distribution.

  $$SE = sqrt[(s_1^2/n_1) + (s_2^2/n_2)]$$

  where s_1 is the standard deviation of sample 1, s_2 is the standard deviation of sample 2, n_1 is the size of sample 1, and n_2 is the size of sample 2.

- **Degrees of freedom:** The degrees of freedom (DF) is:

  $$DF = (s_1^2/n_1+s_2^2/n_2)^2 / \{[(s_1^2 / n_1)^2 / (n_1-1)]+[(s_2^2 / n_2)^2 / (n_2-1)] \}$$

  If DF does not compute to an integer, round it off to the nearest whole number. Some texts suggest that the degrees of freedom can be approximated by the smaller of n_1 - 1 and n_2 - 1; but the above formula gives better results.

- **Test statistic.** The test statistic is a t-score (t) defined by the following equation:

  $$t = [(x_1 - x_2) - d] / SE$$

  where x_1 is the mean of sample 1, x_2 is the mean of sample 2, d is the hypothesized difference between population means, and SE is the standard error.

- **P-value.** The P-value is the probability of observing a sample statistic as extreme as the test statistic. Since the test statistic is a t-score, use the t Distribution Calculator to assess the probability associated with the t-score, having the degrees of freedom computed above. (See sample problems at the end of this lesson for examples of how this is done.

Interpret Results

If the sample findings are unlikely, given the null hypothesis, the researcher rejects the null hypothesis. Typically, this involves comparing the P-value to the significance level, and rejecting the null hypothesis when the P-value is less than the significance level.

In this section, two sample problems illustrate how to conduct a hypothesis test of a difference between mean scores. The first problem involves a two-tailed test; the second problem, a one-tailed test.

Example Two-Tailed Test

Within a district hospital, patients were randomly given one of two treatments, 30 patients were chosen of treatment A and 25 patients were given treatment B.

At the end of the year, each patient took the same standardized test for diagnosis. Patient with treatment A had an average test score of 78, with a standard deviation of 10; and patients with treatment B had an average test score of 85, with a standard deviation of 15.

Test the hypothesis that treatment A and treatment B are equally effective. Use a 0.10 level of significance.

Solution

The solution to this problem takes four steps: (1) state the hypotheses, (2) formulate an analysis plan, (3) analyze sample data, and (4) interpret results. We work through those steps below:

- **State the hypotheses.** The first step is to state the null hypothesis and an alternative hypothesis.

  Null hypothesis: $\mu_1 - \mu_2 = 0$

  Alternative hypothesis: $\mu_1 - \mu_2 \neq 0$

Note that these hypotheses constitute a two-tailed test. The null hypothesis will be rejected if the difference between sample means is too big or if it is too small.

- **Formulate an analysis plan**. For this analysis, the significance level is 0.05. Using sample data, we will conduct a two-sample t-test of the null hypothesis.

- **Analyze sample data**. Using sample data, we compute the standard error (SE), degrees of freedom (DF), and the t-score test statistic (t).

  $SE = sqrt[(s_1^2/n_1) + (s_2^2/n_2)]$

  $SE = sqrt[(10^2/30) + (15^2/25] = sqrt(3.33 + 9)$

  $= sqrt(12.33) = 3.51$

  $DF = (s_1^2/n_1 + s_2^2/n_2)^2 / \{ [(s_1^2 / n_1)^2 / (n_1 - 1)] + [(s_2^2 / n_2)^2 / (n_2 - 1)] \}$

  $DF = (10^2/30 + 15^2/25)^2 / \{ [(10^2 / 30)^2 / (29)] + [(15^2 / 25)^2 / (24)] \}$

  $DF = (3.33 + 9)^2 / \{ [(3.33)^2 / (29)] + [(9)^2 / (24)] \}$

  $= 152.03 / (0.382 + 3.375) = 152.03/3.757 = 40.47$

  $t = [(x_1 - x_2) - d] / SE = [(78 - 85) - 0] / 3.51 = -7/3.51 = -1.99$

  where s_1 is the standard deviation of sample 1, s_2 is the standard deviation of sample 2, n_1 is the size of sample 1, n_2 is the size of sample 2, x_1 is the mean of sample 1, x_2 is the mean of sample 2, d is the hypothesized difference between the population means, and SE is the standard error.

  Since we have a two-tailed test, the P-value is the probability that a t-score having 40 degrees of freedom is more extreme than -1.99; that is, less than -1.99 or greater than 1.99.

We use the t Distribution Calculator to find $P(t < -1.99) = 0.027$, and $P(t > 1.99) = 0.027$. Thus, the P-value = 0.027 + 0.027 = 0.054.

- **Interpret results.** Since the P-value (0.054) is less than the significance level (0.10), we cannot accept the null hypothesis.

Note: If you use this approach on an exam, you may also want to mention why this approach is appropriate. Specifically, the approach is appropriate because the sampling method was simple random sampling, the samples were independent, the sample size was much smaller than the population size, and the samples were drawn from a normal population.

Example: One-Tailed Test

The Acme Company has developed a new drug. The researcher claims that the new drug will more effective as compare to the existing drug.

To test the claim, the company selects a simple random sample of 100 patients using new drug and 100 patients using old drug. The old drug gives the results with recovery in 190 days with a standard deviation of 20 days; the new drug, 200 days with a standard deviation of 40 days.

Test the researcher's claim that the new drug will more effective as compared to the existing drug.

Use a 0.05 level of significance. (Assume that there are no outliers in either sample.)

Solution

The solution to this problem takes four steps: (1) state the hypotheses, (2) formulate an analysis plan, (3) analyze sample data, and (4) interpret results. We work through those steps below:

- **State the hypotheses.** The first step is to state the null hypothesis and an alternative hypothesis.

  Null hypothesis: $\mu_1 - \mu_2 >= 7$

  Alternative hypothesis: $\mu_1 - \mu_2 < 7$

Note that these hypotheses constitute a one-tailed test. The null hypothesis will be rejected if the mean difference between sample means is too small.

- **Formulate an analysis plan**. For this analysis, the significance level is 0.05. Using sample data, we will conduct a two-sample t-test of the null hypothesis.
- **Analyze sample data**. Using sample data, we compute the standard error (SE), degrees of freedom (DF), and the t-score test statistic (t).

  $SE = sqrt[(s_1^2/n_1) + (s_2^2/n_2)]$

  $SE = sqrt[(40^2/100) + (20^2/100] = sqrt(16 + 4) = 4.472$

  $DF = (s_1^2/n_1 + s_2^2/n_2)^2 / \{ [(s_1^2 / n_1)^2 / (n_1 - 1)] + [(s_2^2 / n_2)^2 / (n_2 - 1)] \}$

  $DF = (40^2/100 + 20^2/100)^2 / \{[(40^2 / 100)^2 / (99)]+[(20^2 / 100)^2 / (99)]\}$

  $DF = (20)^2 / \{[(16)^2 / (99)] + [(2)^2/(99)]\}= 400 / (2.586 + 0.162) = 145.56$

  $t = [(x_1 - x_2) - d] / SE = [(200 - 190) - 7] / 4.472 = 3/4.472 = 0.67$

  where s_1 is the standard deviation of sample 1, s_2 is the standard deviation of sample 2, n_1 is the size of sample 1, n_2 is the size of sample 2, x_1 is the mean of sample 1, x_2 is the mean of sample 2, d is the hypothesized difference between population means, and SE is the standard error.

  For this one-tailed test, the region of rejection is on the positive end of the sampling distribution. Thus, the P-value is the probability that a t-score having 146 degrees of freedom is greater than 0.67.

  We use the t Distribution Calculator to find $P(t > 0.67) = 0.25$. Thus, the P-value = 0.25.

- **Interpret results**. Since the P-value (0.25) is greater than the significance level (0.05), we cannot reject the null hypothesis.

Note: If you use this approach on an exam, you may also want to mention why this approach is appropriate. Specifically, the approach is appropriate because the sampling method was simple random sampling, the samples were independent, the sample size was much smaller than the population size, and the sample size was large without outliers.

Hypothesis Test for Difference Between Matched Pairs

This chapter explains how to conduct a hypothesis test for the difference between paired means. The test procedure, called the **matched-pairs t-test**, is appropriate when the following conditions are met:

- The sampling method for each sample is simple random sampling.
- The test is conducted on paired data. As a result, the data sets are *not* independent.
- Each sample is drawn from a normal or near-normal population.

Generally, the sampling distribution will be approximately normal if any of the following conditions apply:

- The population distribution is normal.
- The sample data are symmetric, unimodal, without outliers, and the sample size is 15 or less.
- The sample data are slightly skewed, unimodal, without outliers, and the sample size is 16 to 40.
- The sample size is greater than 40, without outliers.

This approach consists of four steps: (1) state the hypotheses, (2) formulate an analysis plan, (3) analyze sample data, and (4) interpret results.

State the Hypotheses

Every hypothesis test requires the analyst to state a null hypothesis and an alternative hypothesis. The hypotheses are stated in such a way that they are mutually exclusive. That is, if one is true, the other must be false; and vice versa.

The hypotheses concern a new variable d, which is based on the difference between paired values from two data sets.

$d = x_1 - x_2$

where x_1 is the value of variable x in the first data set, and x_2 is the value of the variable from the second data set that is paired with x_1.

The table below shows three sets of null and alternative hypotheses. Each makes a statement about how the true difference in population values μ_d is related to some hypothesized value D. (In the table, the symbol $\neq$ means " not equal to".)

Set	Null hypothesis	Alternative hypothesis	Number of tails
1	$\mu_d = D$	$\mu_d \neq D$	2
2	$\mu_d \geqslant D$	$\mu_d < D$	1
3	$\mu_d \leqslant D$	$\mu_d > D$	1

The first set of hypotheses (Set 1) is an example of a two-tailed test, since an extreme value on either side of the sampling distribution would cause a researcher to reject the null hypothesis. The other two sets of hypotheses (Sets 2 and 3) are one-tailed tests, since an extreme value on only one side of the sampling distribution would cause a researcher to reject the null hypothesis.

Formulate an Analysis Plan

The analysis plan describes how to use sample data to accept or reject the null hypothesis. It should specify the following elements:

- **Significance level.** Often, researchers choose significance levels equal to 0.01, 0.05, or 0.10; but any value between 0 and 1 can be used.
- **Test method.** Use the matched-pairs t-test to determine whether the difference between sample means for paired data is significantly different from the hypothesized difference between population means.

Analyze Sample Data

Using sample data, find the standard deviation, standard error, degrees of freedom, test statistic, and the P-value associated with the test statistic.

- **Standard deviation.** Compute the standard deviation (s_d) of the differences computed from n matched pairs.

  s_d = sqrt [($\sum$(d_i - d)^2 / (n - 1)]

  where d_i is the difference for pair *i*, d is the sample mean of the differences, and n is the number of paired values.

- **Standard error.** Compute the standard error (SE) of the sampling distribution of d.

  SE = s_d * sqrt{ (1/n) * (1 - n/N) * [N / (N - 1)] }

  where s_d is the standard deviation of the sample difference, *N* is the population size, and *n* is the sample size. When the population size is much larger (at least 10 times larger) than the sample size, the standard error can be approximated by:

  SE = s_d / sqrt(n)

- **Degrees of freedom.** The degrees of freedom (DF) is: DF = n - 1
- **Test statistic.** The test statistic is a t-score (t) defined by the following equation:

$$t = [(x_1 - x_2) - D] / SE = (d - D) / SE$$

where x_1 is the mean of sample 1, x_2 is the mean of sample 2, d is the mean difference between paired values in the sample, D is the hypothesized difference between population means, and SE is the standard error.

- **P-value.** The P-value is the probability of observing a sample statistic as extreme as the test statistic. Since the test statistic is a t-score, use the t Distribution Calculator to assess the probability associated with the t-score, having the degrees of freedom computed above. (See the sample problem at the end of this lesson for guidance on how this is done.)

Interpret Results

If the sample findings are unlikely, given the null hypothesis, the researcher rejects the null hypothesis. Typically, this involves comparing the P-value to the significance level, and rejecting the null hypothesis when the P-value is less than the significance level.

Example

Forty-four sixth graders were randomly selected from a school district. Then, they were divided into 22 matched pairs, each pair having equal IQ's. One member of each pair was randomly selected to receive special training. Then, all of the students were given an IQ test. Test results are summarized below:

Pair	Training	No training	Difference, d	$(d - d)^2$
1	95	90	5	16
2	89	85	4	9
3	76	73	3	4
4	92	90	2	1
5	91	90	1	0
6	53	53	0	1
7	67	68	-1	4

contd..

contd..

8	88	90	-2	9
9	75	78	-3	16
10	85	89	-4	25
11	90	95	-5	36
12	85	83	2	1
13	87	83	4	9
14	85	83	2	1
15	85	82	3	4
16	68	65	3	4
17	81	79	2	1
18	84	83	1	0
19	71	60	11	100
20	46	47	-1	4
21	75	77	-2	9
22	80	83	-3	16

$$\sum (d - d)^2 = 270$$

$$d = 1$$

Do these results provide evidence that the special training helped or hurt student performance? Use an 0.05 level of significance. Assume that the mean differences are approximately normally distributed.

Solution

The solution to this problem takes four steps: (1) state the hypotheses, (2) formulate an analysis plan, (3) analyze sample data, and (4) interpret results. We work through those steps below:

- **State the hypotheses.** The first step is to state the null hypothesis and an alternative hypothesis.

  Null hypothesis: $\mu_d = 0$

  Alternative hypothesis: $\mu_d \neq 0$

Note that these hypotheses constitute a two-tailed test. The null hypothesis will be rejected if the difference between sample means is too big or if it is too small.

- **Formulate an analysis plan.** For this analysis, the significance level is 0.05. Using sample data, we will conduct a matched-pairs t-test of the null hypothesis.

- **Analyze sample data.** Using sample data, we compute the standard deviation of the differences (s), the standard error (SE) of the mean difference, the degrees of freedom (DF), and the t-score test statistic (t).

  s = sqrt [($\sum$ (d_i - d)^2 / (n - 1)] = sqrt[270/(22-1)] = sqrt(12.857) = 3.586

  SE = s / sqrt(n) = 3.586 / [sqrt(22)] = 3.586/4.69 = 0.765

  DF = n - 1 = 22 -1 = 21

  t = [(x_1 - x_2) - D] / SE = (d - D)/ SE = (1 - 0)/0.765 = 1.307

  where d_i is the observed difference for pair *i*, d is mean difference between sample pairs, D is the hypothesized mean difference between population pairs, and n is the number of pairs.

  Since we have a two-tailed test, the P-value is the probability that a t-score having 21 degrees of freedom is more extreme than 1.307; that is, less than -1.307 or greater than 1.307.

  We use the t Distribution Calculator to find P(t < -1.307) = 0.103, and P(t > 1.307) = 0.103. Thus, the P-value = 0.103 + 0.103 = 0.206.

- **Interpret results.** Since the P-value (0.206) is greater than the significance level (0.05), we cannot reject the null hypothesis.

Note: If you use this approach on an exam, you may also want to mention why this approach is appropriate. Specifically, the approach is appropriate because the sampling method was simple random sampling, the samples consisted of paired data, and the mean differences were normally distributed. In addition, we used to approximation formula to compute the standard error, since the sample size was small relative to the population size.

Chi-Square Goodness of Fit Test

This chapter explains how to conduct a **chi-square goodness of fit test**. The test is applied when you have one categorical variable from a single population. It is used to determine whether sample data are consistent with a hypothesized distribution.

For example, suppose a company printed baseball cards. It claimed that 30% of its cards were rookies; 60%, veterans; and 10%, All-Stars. We could gather a random sample of baseball cards and use a chi-square goodness of fit test to see whether our sample distribution differed significantly from the distribution claimed by the company. The sample problem at the end of the lesson considers this example.

The test procedure described in this lesson is appropriate when the following conditions are met:

- The sampling method is simple random sampling.
- The population is at least 10 times as large as the sample.
- The variable under study is categorical.
- The expected value for each level of the variable is at least 5.

This approach consists of four steps: (1) state the hypotheses, (2) formulate an analysis plan, (3) analyze sample data, and (4) interpret results.

State the Hypotheses

Every hypothesis test requires the analyst to state a null hypothesis and an alternative hypothesis. The hypotheses are stated in such a way that they are mutually exclusive. That is, if one is true, the other must be false; and vice versa.

For a chi-square goodness of fit test, the hypotheses take the following form:

H_0: The data are consistent with a specified distribution.

H_a: The data are *not* consistent with a specified distribution.

Typically, the null hypothesis specifies the proportion of observations at each level of the categorical variable. The alternative hypothesis is that *at least* one of the specified proportions is not true.

Formulate An Analysis Plan

The analysis plan describes how to use sample data to accept or reject the null hypothesis. The plan should specify the following elements:

- **Significance level.** Often, researchers choose significance levels equal to 0.01, 0.05, or 0.10; but any value between 0 and 1 can be used.
- **Test method.** Use the chi-square goodness of fit test to determine whether observed sample frequencies differ significantly from expected frequencies specified in the null hypothesis. The chi-square goodness of fit test is described in the next section, and demonstrated in the sample problem at the end of this lesson.

Analyze Sample Data

Using sample data, find the degrees of freedom, expected frequency counts, test statistic, and the P-value associated with the test statistic.

- **Degrees of freedom.** The degrees of freedom (DF) is equal to one minus the number of levels (k) of the categorical variable: DF = k - 1
- **Expected frequency counts.** The expected frequency counts at each level of the categorical variable are equal to the sample size times the hypothesized proportion from the null hypothesis:

  $$E_i = np_i$$

  where E_i is the expected frequency count for the *i*th level of the categorical variable, n is the total sample size, and p_i is the hypothesized proportion of observations in level *i*.
- **Test statistic.** The test statistic is a chi-square random variable (χ^2) defined by the following equation:

  $$\chi^2 = \Sigma [(O_i - E_i)^2 / E_i]$$

  where O_i is the observed frequency count for the *i*th level of the categorical variable, and E_i is the expected frequency count for the *i*th level of the categorical variable.
- **P-value.** The P-value is the probability of observing a sample statistic as extreme as the test statistic. Since the test statistic is a chi-square, use the Chi-Square Distribution Calculator to assess the probability associated with the test statistic. Use the degrees of freedom computed above.

Interpret Results

If the sample findings are unlikely, given the null hypothesis, the researcher rejects the null hypothesis. Typically, this involves comparing the P-value to the significance level, and rejecting the null hypothesis when the P-value is less than the significance level.

Example

Acme Toy Company prints baseball cards. The company claims that 30% of the cards are rookies, 60% veterans, and 10% are All-Stars. The cards are sold in packages of 100.

Suppose a randomly-selected package of cards has 50 rookies, 45 veterans, and 5 All-Stars. Is this consistent with Acme's claim? Use a 0.05 level of significance.

Solution

The solution to this problem takes four steps: (1) state the hypotheses, (2) formulate an analysis plan, (3) analyze sample data, and (4) interpret results. We work through those steps below:

- **State the hypotheses.** The first step is to state the null hypothesis and an alternative hypothesis.

  Null hypothesis: The proportion of rookies, veterans, and All-Stars is 30%, 60% and 10%, respectively.

  Alternative hypothesis: At least one of the proportions in the null hypothesis is false.

- **Formulate an analysis plan**. For this analysis, the significance level is 0.05. Using sample data, we will conduct a chi-square goodness of fit test of the null hypothesis.

- **Analyze sample data**. Applying the chi-square goodness of fit test to sample data, we compute the degrees of freedom, the expected frequency counts, and the chi-square test statistic. Based on the chi-square statistic and the degrees of freedom, we determine the P-value.

  $DF = k - 1 = 3 - 1 = 2$

  $(E_i) = n * p_i$

$(E_1) = 100 * 0.30 = 30$

$(E_2) = 100 * 0.60 = 60$

$(E_3) = 100 * 0.10 = 10$

$\chi^2 = \Sigma\ [(O_i - E_i)^2 / E_i]$

$\chi^2 = [(50 - 30)^2 / 30] + [(45 - 60)^2 / 60] + [(5 - 10)^2 / 10]$

$\chi^2 = (400 / 30) + (225 / 60) + (25 / 10) = 13.33 + 3.75 + 2.50 = 19.58$

where DF is the degrees of freedom, k is the number of levels of the categorical variable, n is the number of observations in the sample, E_i is the expected frequency count for level i, O_i is the hypothesized frequency count for level i, and χ^2 is the chi-square test statistic.

The P-value is the probability that a chi-square statistic having 2 degrees of freedom is more extreme than 19.58.

We use the Chi-Square Distribution Calculator to find $P(\chi^2 > 19.58) = 0.0001$.

- **Interpret results**. Since the P-value (0.0001) is less than the significance level (0.05), we cannot accept the null hypothesis.

Note: If you use this approach on an exam, you may also want to mention why this approach is appropriate. Specifically, the approach is appropriate because the sampling method was simple random sampling, the population was more than 10 times larger than the sample, the variable under study was categorical, and each level of the categorical variable had an expected frequency count of at least 5.

Chi-Square Test for Homogeneity

This chapter explains how to conduct a **chi-square test of homogeneity**. The test is applied to a single categorical variable from two different populations. It is used to determine whether frequency counts are distributed identically across different populations.

For example, in a survey of TV viewing preferences, we might ask respondents to identify their favourite program. We might ask the same question of two different populations, such as males and females. We could use a chi-square test for homogeneity to determine whether male viewing preferences differed significantly from female viewing preference. The sample problem at the end of the lesson considers this example.

The test procedure described in this lesson is appropriate when the following conditions are met:

- For each population, the sampling method is simple random sampling.
- Each population is at least 10 times as large as its respective sample.
- The variable under study is categorical.
- If sample data are displayed in a contingency table (Populations multiply Category levels), the expected frequency count for each cell of the table is at least 5.

This approach consists of four steps: (1) state the hypotheses, (2) formulate an analysis plan, (3) analyze sample data, and (4) interpret results.

State the Hypotheses

Every hypothesis test requires the analyst to state a null hypothesis and an alternative hypothesis. The hypotheses are stated in such a way that they are mutually exclusive. That is, if one is true, the other must be false; and vice versa.

Suppose that data were sampled from *r* populations, and assume that the categorical variable had *c* levels. At any specified level of the categorical variable, the null hypothesis states that each population has the same proportion of observations. Thus,

$$H_0: P_{\text{level 1 of population 1}} = P_{\text{level 1 of population 2}} = \ldots = P_{\text{level 1 of population r}}$$

$$H_0: P_{\text{level 2 of population 1}} = P_{\text{level 2 of population 2}} = \ldots = P_{\text{level 2 of population r}}$$

$$H_0: P_{\text{level c of population 1}} = P_{\text{level c of population 2}} = \ldots = P_{\text{level c of population r}}$$

The alternative hypothesis (H_a) is that *at least* one of the null hypothesis statements is false.

Formulate An Analysis Plan

The analysis plan describes how to use sample data to accept or reject the null hypothesis. The plan should specify the following elements:

- **Significance level.** Often, researchers choose significance levels equal to 0.01, 0.05, or 0.10; but any value between 0 and 1 can be used.
- **Test method**. Use the chi-square test for homogeneity to determine whether observed sample frequencies differ significantly from expected frequencies specified in the null hypothesis. The chi-square test for homogeneity is described in the next section.

Analyze Sample Data

Using sample data from the contingency tables, find the degrees of freedom, expected frequency counts, test statistic, and the P-value associated with the test statistic. The analysis described in this section is illustrated in the sample problem at the end of this lesson.

- **Degrees of freedom**. The degrees of freedom (DF) is equal to:

  $DF = (r - 1) * (c - 1)$

  where r is the number of populations, and c is the number of levels for the categorical variable.

- **Expected frequency counts**. The expected frequency counts are computed separately for each population at each level of the categorical variable, according to the following formula:

  $$E_{r,c} = (n_r * n_c) / n$$

  where $E_{r,c}$ is the expected frequency count for population r at level *c* of the categorical variable, n_r is the total number of observations from population r, n_c is the total number of observations at treatment level *c*, and n is the total sample size.

- **Test statistic.** The test statistic is a chi-square random variable (x^2) defined by the following equation:

  $$x^2 = \Sigma [(O_{r,c} - E_{r,c})^2 / E_{r,c}]$$

  where $O_{r,c}$ is the observed frequency count in population *r* for level *c* of the categorical variable, and $E_{r,c}$ is the expected frequency count in population *r* for level *c* of the categorical variable.

- **P-value.** The P-value is the probability of observing a sample statistic as extreme as the test statistic. Since the test statistic is a chi-square, use the Chi-Square Distribution Calculator to assess the probability associated with the test statistic. Use the degrees of freedom computed above.

Interpret Results

If the sample findings are unlikely, given the null hypothesis, the researcher rejects the null hypothesis. Typically, this involves comparing the P-value to the significance level, and rejecting the null hypothesis when the P-value is less than the significance level.

Example

In a study of the television viewing habits of children, a developmental psychologist selects a random sample of 300 first graders - 100 boys and 200 girls. Each child is asked which of the following TV programs they like best: The Lone Ranger, Sesame Street, or The Simpsons. Results are shown in the contingency table below.

Viewing Preferences

	Lone Ranger	Sesame Street	The Simpsons	Row total
Boys	50	30	20	100
Girls	50	80	70	200
Column total	100	110	90	300

Do the boys' preferences for these TV programs differ significantly from the girls' preferences? Use a 0.05 level of significance.

Solution

The solution to this problem takes four steps: (1) state the hypotheses, (2) formulate an analysis plan, (3) analyze sample data, and (4) interpret results. We work through those steps below:

- **State the hypotheses.** The first step is to state the null hypothesis and an alternative hypothesis.
- **Null hypothesis:** The null hypothesis states that the proportion of boys who prefer the Lone Ranger is identical to the proportion of girls. Similarly, for the other programs. Thus,

$$H_0: P_{\text{boys who prefer Lone Ranger}} = P_{\text{girls who prefer Lone Ranger}}$$

H_0: $P_{\text{boys who prefer Sesame Street}} = P_{\text{girls who prefer Sesame Street}}$

H_0: $P_{\text{boys who prefer The Simpsons}} = P_{\text{girls who prefer The Simpsons}}$

Alternative hypothesis: At least one of the null hypothesis statements is false.

- **Formulate an analysis plan**. For this analysis, the significance level is 0.05. Using sample data, we will conduct a chi-square test for homogeneity.
- **Analyze sample data**. Applying the chi-square test for homogeneity to sample data, we compute the degrees of freedom, the expected frequency counts, and the chi-square test statistic. Based on the chi-square statistic and the degrees of freedom, we determine the P-value.

$$DF = (r - 1) * (c - 1) = (2 - 1) * (3 - 1) = 2$$

$$E_{r,c} = (n_r * n_c) / n$$

$$E_{1,1} = (100 * 100) / 300 = 10000/300 = 33.3$$

$$E_{1,2} = (100 * 110) / 300 = 11000/300 = 36.7$$

$$E_{1,3} = (100 * 90) / 300 = 9000/300 = 30.0$$

$$E_{2,1} = (200 * 100) / 300 = 20000/300 = 66.7$$

$$E_{2,2} = (200 * 110) / 300 = 22000/300 = 73.3$$

$$E_{2,3} = (200 * 90) / 300 = 18000/300 = 60.0$$

$$\chi^2 \Sigma [(O_{r,c} - E_{r,c})^2 / E_{r,c}]$$

$$\chi^2 = (50 - 33.3)^2/33.3 + (30 - 36.7)^2/36.7 + (20 - 30)^2/30 + (50 - 66.7)^2/66.7 + (80 - 73.3)^2/73.3 + (70 - 60)^2/60$$

$$\chi^2 = (16.7)^2/33.3 + (-6.7)^2/36.7 + (-10.0)^2/30 + (-17.7)^2/66.7 + (3.3)^2/73.3 + (10)^2/60$$

$$\chi^2 = 8.38 + 1.22 + 3.33 + 4.70 + 0.61 + 1.67 = 19.91$$

where DF is the degrees of freedom, r is the number of populations, c is the number of levels of the categorical variable, n_r is the number of observations from population *r*, n_c is the number of observations from level *c* of the categorical variable, n is the number of observations in the sample, $E_{r,c}$ is the expected frequency count in population r for level c, and $O_{r,c}$ is the observed frequency count in population r for level c.

The P-value is the probability that a chi-square statistic having 2 degrees of freedom is more extreme than 19.91.

We use the Chi-Square Distribution Calculator to find $P(\chi^2 > 19.91) = 0.0000$. (The actual P-value, of course, is not exactly zero. If the Chi-Square Distribution Calculator reported more than four decimal places, we would find that the actual P-value is a very small number that is less than 0.00005 and greater than zero.

- **Interpret results**. Since the P-value (0.0000) is less than the significance level (0.05), we cannot accept the null hypothesis.

Note: If you use this approach on an exam, you may also want to mention why this approach is appropriate. Specifically, the approach is appropriate because the sampling method was simple random sampling, each population was more than 10 times larger than its respective sample, the variable under study was categorical, and the expected frequency count was at least 5 in each population at each level of the categorical variable.

Chi-Square Test for Independence

This chapter explains how to conduct a **chi-square test for independence**. The test is applied when you have two categorical variables from a single population. It is used to determine whether there is a significant association between the two variables.

For example, in an election survey, voters might be classified by gender (male or female) and voting preference (Democrat, Republican, or Independent). We could use a chi-square test for independence to determine whether gender is related to voting preference. The sample problem at the end of the lesson considers this example.

The test procedure described in this lesson is appropriate when the following conditions are met:

- The sampling method is simple random sampling.
- Each population is at least 10 times as large as its respective sample.
- The variables under study are each categorical.
- If sample data are displayed in a contingency table, the expected frequency count for each cell of the table is at least 5.

This approach consists of four steps: (1) state the hypotheses, (2) formulate an analysis plan, (3) analyze sample data, and (4) interpret results.

State the Hypotheses

Suppose that Variable A has *r* levels, and Variable B has *c* levels. The null hypothesis states that knowing the level of Variable A does not help you predict the level of Variable B. That is, the variables are independent.

H_0 : Variable A and Variable B are independent.

H_a : Variable A and Variable B are not independent.

The alternative hypothesis is that knowing the level of Variable A *can* help you predict the level of Variable B.

Note: Support for the alternative hypothesis suggests that the variables are related; but the relationship is not necessarily causal, in the sense that one variable "causes" the other.

Formulate An Analysis Plan

The analysis plan describes how to use sample data to accept or reject the null hypothesis. The plan should specify the following elements:

- **Significance level.** Often, researchers choose significance levels equal to 0.01, 0.05, or 0.10; but any value between 0 and 1 can be used.
- **Test method.** Use the chi-square test for independence to determine whether there is a significant relationship between two categorical variables.

Analyze Sample Data

Using sample data, find the degrees of freedom, expected frequencies, test statistic, and the P-value associated with the test statistic. The approach described in this section is illustrated in the sample problem at the end of this lesson.

- **Degrees of freedom.** The degrees of freedom (DF) is equal to:

$$DF = (r - 1) * (c - 1)$$

where r is the number of levels for one categorical variable, and c is the number of levels for the other categorical variable.

- **Expected frequencies**. The expected frequency counts are computed separately for each level of one categorical variable at each level of the other categorical variable. Compute r * c expected frequencies, according to the following formula.

$$E_{r,c} = (n_r * n_c) / n$$

where $E_{r,c}$ is the expected frequency count for level *r* of Variable A and level *c* of Variable B, n_r is the total number of sample observations at level r of Variable A, n_c is the total number of sample observations at level *c* of Variable B, and n is the total sample size.

- **Test statistic.** The test statistic is a chi-square random variable (χ^2) defined by the following equation:

$$\chi^2 = \Sigma [(O_{r,c} - E_{r,c})^2 / E_{r,c}]$$

where $O_{r,c}$ is the observed frequency count at level *r* of Variable A and level *c* of Variable B, and $E_{r,c}$ is the expected frequency count at level *r* of Variable A and level *c* of Variable B.

- **P-value.** The P-value is the probability of observing a sample statistic as extreme as the test statistic. Since the test statistic is a chi-square, use the Chi-Square Distribution Calculator to assess the probability associated with the test statistic. Use the degrees of freedom computed above.

Interpret Results

If the sample findings are unlikely, given the null hypothesis, the researcher rejects the null hypothesis. Typically, this involves comparing the P-value to the significance level, and rejecting the null hypothesis when the P-value is less than the significance level.

Example

A public opinion poll surveyed a simple random sample of 1000 voters. Respondents were classified by gender (male or female) and by voting preference (Republican, Democrat, or Independent). Results are shown in the contingency table below:

Voting Preferences

	Republican	**Democrat**	**Independent**	**Row total**
Male	200	150	50	400
Female	250	300	50	600
Column total	450	450	100	1000

Is there a gender gap? Do the men's voting preferences differ significantly from the women's preferences? Use a 0.05 level of significance.

Solution

The solution to this problem takes four steps: (1) state the hypotheses, (2) formulate an analysis plan, (3) analyze sample data, and (4) interpret results. We work through those steps below:

- **State the hypotheses.** The first step is to state the null hypothesis and an alternative hypothesis.

  H_0: Gender and voting preferences are independent.

  H_a: Gender and voting preferences are not independent.

- **Formulate an analysis plan.** For this analysis, the significance level is 0.05. Using sample data, we will conduct a chi-square test for independence.

- **Analyze sample data.** Applying the chi-square test for independence to sample data, we compute the degrees of freedom, the expected frequency counts, and the chi-square test statistic. Based on the chi-square statistic and the degrees of freedom, we determine the P-value.

  $DF = (r - 1) * (c - 1) = (2 - 1) * (3 - 1) = 2$

  $E_{r,c} = (n_r * n_c) / n$

  $E_{1,1} = (400 * 450) / 1000 = 180000/1000 = 180$

  $E_{1,2} = (400 * 450) / 1000 = 180000/1000 = 180$

  $E_{1,3} = (400 * 100) / 1000 = 40000/1000 = 40$

  $E_{2,1} = (600 * 450) / 1000 = 270000/1000 = 270$

$E_{2,2} = (600 * 450) / 1000 = 270000/1000 = 270$

$E_{2,3} = (600 * 100) / 1000 = 60000/1000 = 60$

$\chi^2 = \Sigma [(O_{r,c} - E_{r,c})^2 / E_{r,c}]$

$\chi^2 = (200 - 180)^2/180 + (150 - 180)^2/180 + (50 - 40)^2/40$

$+ (250 - 270)^2/270 + (300 - 270)^2/270 + (50 - 60)^2/40$

$\chi^2 = 400/180 + 900/180 + 100/40 + 400/270 + 900/270 + 100/60$

$\chi^2 = 2.22 + 5.00 + 2.50 + 1.48 + 3.33 + 1.67 = 16.2$

where DF is the degrees of freedom, r is the number of levels of gender, c is the number of levels of the voting preference, n_r is the number of observations from level *r* of gender, n_c is the number of observations from level *c* of voting preference, n is the number of observations in the sample, $E_{r,c}$ is the expected frequency count when gender is level *r* and voting preference is level *c*, and $O_{r,c}$ is the observed frequency count when gender is level *r* voting preference is level *c*.

The P-value is the probability that a chi-square statistic having 2 degrees of freedom is more extreme than 16.2.

We use the Chi-Square Distribution Calculator to find $P(\chi^2 > 16.2) = 0.0003$.

- **Interpret results.** Since the P-value (0.0003) is less than the significance level (0.05), we cannot accept the null hypothesis. Thus, we conclude that there is a relationship between gender and voting preference.

Note: If you use this approach on an exam, you may also want to mention why this approach is appropriate. Specifically, the approach is appropriate because the sampling method was simple random sampling, each population was more than 10 times larger than its respective sample, the variables under study were categorical, and the expected frequency count was at least 5 in each cell of the contingency table.

Hypothesis Test for Slope of Regression Line

This chapter describes how to conduct a hypothesis test to determine whether there is a significant linear relationship between an independent variable

X and a dependent variable *Y*. The test focuses on the slope of the regression line

$$Y = B_0 + B_1 X$$

where B_0 is a constant, B_1 is the slope (also called the regression coefficient), X is the value of the independent variable, and Y is the value of the dependent variable.

Test Requirements

The approach described in this lesson is valid whenever the standard requirements for simple linear regression are met.

- The dependent variable *Y* has a linear relationship to the independent variable *X*.
- For each value of X, the probability distribution of Y has the same standard deviation σ.
- For any given value of X:

  The Y values are independent.

  The Y values are roughly normally distributed (i.e.; symmetric and unimodal). A little skewness is ok if the sample size is large.

Previously, we described how to verify that regression requirements are met.

The test procedure consists of four steps: (1) state the hypotheses, (2) formulate an analysis plan, (3) analyze sample data, and (4) interpret results.

State the Hypotheses

If there is a significant linear relationship between the independent variable *X* and the dependent variable *Y*, the slope will *not* equal zero.

$H_0: B_1 = 0$

$H_a: B_1 \neq 0$

The null hypothesis states that the slope is equal to zero, and the alternative hypothesis states that the slope is not equal to zero.

Formulate An Analysis Plan

The analysis plan describes how to use sample data to accept or reject the null hypothesis. The plan should specify the following elements:

- **Significance level.** Often, researchers choose significance levels equal to 0.01, 0.05, or 0.10; but any value between 0 and 1 can be used.

- **Test method.** Use a linear regression t-test (described in the next section) to determine whether the slope of the regression line differs significantly from zero.

Analyze Sample Data

Using sample data, find the standard error of the slope, the slope of the regression line, the degrees of freedom, the test statistic, and the P-value associated with the test statistic. The approach described in this section is illustrated in the sample problem at the end of this lesson.

- **Standard error.** Many statistical software packages and some graphing calculators provide the standard error of the slope as a regression analysis output. The table below shows hypothetical output for the following regression equation: y = 76 + 35x .

Predictor	Coef	SE Coef	T	P
Constant	76	30	2.53	0.01
X	.35	20	1.75	0.04

- In the output above, the standard error of the slope (shaded in gray) is equal to 20. In this example, the standard error is referred to as "SE Coeff". However, other software packages might use a different label for the standard error. It might be "St Dev", "SE", "Std Dev", or something else.

- If you need to calculate the standard error of the slope (SE) by hand, use the following formula:

  $SE = s_{b1} = \text{sqrt} [\sum (y_i - y_i)^2 / (n - 2)] / \text{sqrt} [\sum (x_i - x)^2]$

  where y_i is the value of the dependent variable for observation *i*, y_i is estimated value of the dependent variable for observation *i*, x_i is the observed value of the independent variable for observation *i*, x is the mean of the independent variable, and n is the number of observations.

- **Slope.** Like the standard error, the slope of the regression line will be provided by most statistics software packages. In the hypothetical output above, the slope is equal to 35.
- **Degrees of freedom.** The degrees of freedom (DF) is equal to:

  $$DF = n - 2$$

  where n is the number of observations in the sample.
- **Test statistic.** The test statistic is a t-score (t) defined by the following equation.

  $$t = b_1 / SE$$

  where b_1 is the slope of the sample regression line, and SE is the standard error of the slope.
- **P-value.** The P-value is the probability of observing a sample statistic as extreme as the test statistic. Since the test statistic is a t-score, use the t Distribution Calculator to assess the probability associated with the test statistic. Use the degrees of freedom computed above.

Interpret Results

If the sample findings are unlikely, given the null hypothesis, the researcher rejects the null hypothesis. Typically, this involves comparing the P-value to the significance level, and rejecting the null hypothesis when the P-value is less than the significance level.

Example

The local utility company surveys 101 randomly selected customers. For each survey participant, the company collects the following: annual electric bill (in dollars) and home size (in square feet). Output from a regression analysis appears below:

Regression equation: Annual bill = 0.55 * Home size + 15

Predictor	**Coef**	**SE Coef**	**T**	**P**
Constant	15	3	5.0	0.00
Home size	0.55	0.24	2.29	0.01

Is there a significant linear relationship between annual bill and home size? Use a 0.05 level of significance.

Solution

The solution to this problem takes four steps: (1) state the hypotheses, (2) formulate an analysis plan, (3) analyze sample data, and (4) interpret results. We work through those steps below:

- **State the hypotheses.** The first step is to state the null hypothesis and an alternative hypothesis.

  H_0: The slope of the regression line is equal to zero.

  H_a: The slope of the regression line is *not* equal to zero.

  If the relationship between home size and electric bill is significant, the slope will *not* equal zero.

- **Formulate an analysis plan**. For this analysis, the significance level is 0.05. Using sample data, we will conduct a linear regression t-test to determine whether the slope of the regression line differs significantly from zero.

- **Analyze sample data**. To apply the linear regression t-test to sample data, we require the standard error of the slope, the slope of the regression line, the degrees of freedom, the t-score test statistic, and the P-value of the test statistic.

  We get the slope (b_1) and the standard error (SE) from the regression output:

  $b_1 = 0.55 \quad SE = 0.24$

  We compute the degrees of freedom and the t-score test statistic, using the following equations:

  $DF = n - 2 = 101 - 2 = 99$

  $t = b_1/SE = 0.55/0.24 = 2.29$

  where DF is the degrees of freedom, n is the number of observations in the sample, b_1 is the slope of the regression line, and SE is the standard error of the slope.

  Based on the t-score test statistic and the degrees of freedom, we determine the P-value. The P-value is the probability that a t-score having 99 degrees of freedom is more extreme than 2.29. Since this is a two-tailed test, "more extreme" means greater than 2.29 or less than -2.29. We use the t Distribution Calculator to find P(t > 2.29) = 0.0121 and P(t < 2.29) = 0.0121. Therefore, the P-value is 0.0121 + 0.0121 or 0.0242.

- **Interpret results.** Since the P-value (0.0242) is less than the significance level (0.05), we cannot accept the null hypothesis.

Example

A certain stimulus administered to each of 12 patients resulted in the following increments in 'Blood pressure' 5, 2, 8, -1, 3, 0, 6, -2, 1, 5, 0, 4. Can it be concluded that the stimulus will in general be accompanied by an increase in blood pressure, given that for all df the value of t (.05) = 2.201?

Solution

$$\bar{x} = \frac{\Sigma X_i}{n} = \frac{31}{12} = 2.583 \approx 2.6$$

$$\text{Also } S = \sqrt{\frac{\Sigma(x_i - \bar{X})^2}{n-1}} = \sqrt{\frac{104.92}{12-1}} = 3.08$$

The null hypothesis $H_0 : \mu = 0$ i.e. assuming that the stimulus will not be accompanied by an increase in blood pressure (or the mean increase in blood pressure for the population is zero).

$$\text{Now } t = \frac{\bar{x} - \mu}{s}\sqrt{n} = \frac{2.6 - 0}{3.08}\sqrt{12} = 2.924$$

The table value, $t_{0.05}$, n = 11 = 2.201

Therefore, 2.924 > 2.201

Thus the null hypothesis H_0 is rejected i.e. we find that our assumption is wrong and we say that as a result of the stimulus the blood pressure will increase.

Distribution of 't' for Comparison of Two Samples Means Independent Samples

Let X_{1i} (i = 1, 2, 3, ..., n_1) and X_{2i} (i = 1, 2, 3, ..., n_2) be two random independent samples drawn from two normal populations with mean

m_1 and m_2 respectively but with same variance s^2. Let $\bar{x}_1$ and $\bar{x}_2$ be sample means and let

$$s^2_1 = \frac{1}{n_1-1}\sum_1^{n_1}(x_i - \bar{x}_1)^2 \text{and } s^2_2 = \frac{1}{n_2-1}\sum_1^{n2}(x_i - \bar{x}_1)^2$$

Then the static t is given by

$$t = \frac{(\bar{x}_1 - \bar{x}_2) - (\mu_1 - \mu_2)}{\sqrt{s^2{}_p(\frac{1}{n_1} + \frac{1}{n_2})}}$$

Where $s^2{}_p = \frac{(n_1 - 1)s^2{}_1 + (n_2 - 1)s^2{}_2}{n_1 + n_2 - 2}$ is called the **pooled estimate** of the population variance.

Example

Two types of drugs were used on 5 and 7 patients for reducing their weights in Jerry's 'slim-beauty' health club. Drug A was allopathic and drug B was Herbal. The decrease in the weight after using drugs for six months was as follows :

Drug A : 10 12 13 11 14

Drug B : 8 9 12 14 15 10 9

Is there a significant difference in the efficiency of the two drug ? If not which drug should you buy ?

Solution:

Let the null hypothesis $H_0 : \mu_1 = \mu_2$ or $H_0 : \mu_1 - \mu_2 = 0$

Alternative hypothesis $H_\alpha : \mu_1 \neq \mu_2$ or $H_\alpha : \mu_1 - \mu_2 \neq 0$

x_{1i}	$(x_1-\bar{x}_1)$	$(x_1-\bar{x}_1)^2$	x_{2i}	$(x_2-\bar{x}_2)$	$(x_2-\bar{x}_2)^2$
10	-2	4	8	-3	9
12	0	0	9	-2	4
13	1	1	12	1	1
11	-1	1	1	3	9
14	2	4	15	4	16
			10	-1	1
			9	-2	4
$x_{1i}=60$	$(x_1-\bar{x}_1)^2=10$		$x_{2i}=77$	$(x_2-\bar{x}_2)^2=44$	

Now $\bar{x}_1 = \dfrac{\Sigma x_{1i}}{n} = \dfrac{60}{5} = 12$ and $\bar{x}_2 = \dfrac{\Sigma x_{2i}}{n} = \dfrac{77}{7} = 11$

$$\text{Also } S^2_p = \frac{(n_1-1)S^2_1+(n_2-1)S^2_2}{n_1+n_2-2}$$

$$\text{Where } S^2_1 = \frac{\Sigma(x_1-\bar{x}_1)^2}{n_1-1} = \frac{10}{5-1} = 25\text{and}$$

$$S^2_2 = \frac{\Sigma(x_2-\bar{x}_2)^2}{n_2-1} = \frac{44}{7-1} = 7.3$$

$$\text{Therefore } S^2_p = \frac{(5-1)2.5+(7-1)7.3}{5+7-2}$$

$$= \frac{4\times 2.5+6\times 7.3}{10} = 5.38$$

Using the formulae

$$t = \frac{(\bar{x}_1-\bar{x}_2)-(\mu_1-\mu_2)}{\sqrt{s^2{}_p\left(\frac{1}{n_1}+\frac{1}{n_2}\right)}} \quad \text{Where } \mu_1-\mu_2=0$$

We get

$$t = \frac{12-11}{\sqrt{5.38(\frac{1}{5}+\frac{1}{7})}} = \frac{1}{\sqrt{5.38\times\frac{12}{35}}} = \frac{1}{\sqrt{5.38\times 0.342}} = 0.735$$

Now $\nu\,(df) = n_1 + n_2 - 2 = 10$

For $\nu = 10.\ t_{0.05} = 2.228$

Therefore $0.735 < 2.228$

Thus the null hypothesis is accepted. Hence there is no significance in the efficiency of the two drugs. Since drug B is Herbal and there is no difference in efficiency between the two with no side effects, we should buy the Herbal drug.

Testing Difference Between Means of Two Samples Dependent Samples or Matched Paired Observations

Two samples are said to be dependent on each other when the elements of one are related to those of the other in any significant or meaningful manner. In fact the two samples consist of observations made of the same objects, individuals or more generally, on the same selected population elements. The 't' test is often used to compare 'before' and 'after' scores in experiments for the determination of the significant change that has occurred. We may carry out some experiment,. say, to find the training effect on some students, to find out the efficacy of coaching class, efficacy of two drugs. Often the use of dependent or paired samples will enable us to perform a more precise analysis.

The 't' test is defined by the formula :

$$t = \frac{\bar{x}-\Delta}{s}\sqrt{n}$$ where $\Delta = 0$ (for testing equal means)

and $s = \sqrt{\frac{\Sigma d^2}{n-1}}$ Where d = Deviation from mean or the 'm'

where m = mean of the differences.

Example

Two laboratories carry out independent estimates of fat content in the ice-cream of a certain company. A sample is taken from each batch, halved and the separate halves were tested in the two laboratories. They obtain the following results:

% of fat content in ice-cream

Batch No.	1	2	3	4	5	6	7	8	9	10
Lab A	7	8	7	3	8	6	9	4	7	8
Lab B	9	8	8	4	7	7	9	6	6	6

Is the testing reliable?

Solution

The null hypothesis $H_0 : \mu_1 - \mu_2$ or $H_0 : \mu_1 - \mu_2 = 0$ i.e. If the testing is reliable the mean of the difference in the results should not be significantly differ from 0.

Difference of result (Lab A - Lab B)	Deviation from Mean (m), (d)	d^2
+2	+1.7	2.89
0	-0.3	0.09
+1	+0.7	0.49
+1	+0.7	0.49
-1	-1.3	1.69
+1	+0.7	0.49
0	-0.3	0.09
+2	-1.7	2.89
-1	-1.3	1.69
-2	-2.3	5.29
$\sum m = +3$		$Sd^2 = 16.10$

Mean of the difference $\bar{x} = \frac{\sum m}{n} = \frac{3}{10} = 0.3$

Standard deviation of the differences

$$S = \sqrt{\frac{\Sigma d^2}{n-1}} = \sqrt{\frac{16.1}{10-1}} = 1.33$$

Using the formula

$$t = \frac{\bar{x} - \Delta}{s}\sqrt{n} \text{ where } \Delta = 0 \text{ (for testing equal means)}$$

$$\text{We get} = \frac{0.3 - 0}{1.33}\sqrt{10} = 0.71$$

For $\nu = 10 - 1 = 9$, $t\ 0.05 = 2.57$. Therefore , $0.71 < 2.57$.

The null hypothesis is accepted i.e. the testing is reliable.

Example

A dietitian decided to try out a new type of diet program on 10 boys. Before applying this program, he recorded their weights. Three months later, he recorded their weights again. The weight would have grown by an average of 6 kgs. during this period even without this special diet program. Did this special diet program help? Use 0.05 level of significance.

Boys	1	2	3	4	5	6	7	8	9	10
Before weight	36	32	31	36	23	28	25	26	35	28
After weight	45	37	39	45	31	34	29	36	42	35

Solution

The null hypothesis $H_0 : \mu_1 \neq \mu_2$ or $H_0 : \mu_1 - \mu_2 \neq 0$

or more clearly $H_0 : \mu_1 - \mu_2 \text{i.e.} \Delta \leq 6$

alternative hypothesis $H_\alpha : \Delta > 6$

Boys	Difference of weight	Deviation from 'm' (d)	d^2
1	+9	+1.5	2.25
2	+5	-2.5	6.25
3	+8	+0.5	0.25
4	+9	+1.5	2.25
5	+8	+0.5	0.25
6	+8	+0.5	0.25
7	+4	-2.5	6.25
8	+10	+2.5	6.25
9	+7	-0.5	0.25
10	+7	-0.5	0.25
n = 10	$\sum m = 75$		$\sum d^2 = 24.50$

Mean of difference $\bar{x} = \frac{\sum m}{n} = \frac{75}{10} = 7.5$

Standard deviation of the difference $S = \sqrt{\frac{\sum d^2}{n-1}} = \sqrt{\frac{24.50}{10-1}} = 1.65$

$$\text{Therefore, } t = \frac{\bar{x} - \Delta}{S}\sqrt{n} = \frac{7.5 - 6}{1.65}\sqrt{10} = 2.87$$

The degree of freedom ν (df) = 10 - 1 = 9. The test is one-tailed because we are asked only whether the new diet program increases the weight and not whether it reduces it.

Now $t_{0.05}$, ν = 9 = 2.26 (i,e. $t_{0.025}$, ν = 9 = 2.25 for one tailed test) Because 2.87 > 2.26. The null hypothesis can be rejected. Thus the test has provided evidence that the new diet program caused the weight increase in boys. Though the amount of actual increase was not large (1.6 kgs over normal weight) but it was statistically significant.

Chi-Square

Tests like z-score, t, F are based on the assumption that the samples were drawn from normally distributed populations or more accurately that the sample means were normally distributed. As these tests require assumption about the type of population or parameters, these tests are known as 'parametric tests;

If the calculated value of χ^2 is very small, compared to table value then expected frequencies are very little and the fit is good.

If the calculated value of χ^2 is very large as compared to table value then divergence between the expected and the observed frequencies is very big and the fit is poor.

We know that the degree of freedom r (df) is the number of independent constraints in a set of data.

Suppose there is a 2 × 2 association table and actual frequencies of the various classes are as follows:

	A	a	
B	AB	aB	
	22	38	60
b	Ab	ab	
	8	32	40
	30	70	100

Now the formula for calculating expected frequency of any class (cell)

$$= \frac{\text{Row total for row containing the cell multiply column total for column containing the cell}}{\text{The total number of observations}}$$

In notations : Expected frequemcy $= \dfrac{R \times C}{N}$

For example, if we have two attributes A and B that are independent then the expected frequency

of the class (cell) AB would be $\dfrac{30 \times 60}{100} = 18$

Once the expected frequency of cell (AB) is decided the expected frequencies of remaining three classes are automatically fixed.

Thus for class (aB) it would be 60 - 18 = 42

for class (Ab) it would be 30 - 18 = 12

for class (ab) it would be 70 – 42 = 28

This means that so far as 2 × 2 association (contingency). Table is concerned, there is 1 degree of freedom.

In such tables the degrees of freedom are given by a formula n = (c - 1) (r - 1)

where c = Number of columns, r = Number of rows

Thus in 2 ´ 2 table df = (2 - 1) (2 - 1) = 1

3 ´ 3 table df = (3 - 1) (3 - 1) = 4

4 ´ 4 table df = (4 - 1) (4 - 1) = 9 etc.

If the data is not in the form of contingency tables but as a series of individual observations or discrete or continuous series then it is calculated by n = n - 1 where n is the number of frequencies or values of number of independent individuals.

$$\chi^2 = \Sigma\left[\frac{(\text{Observe frequency - Expected frequency})^2}{\text{Expected frequency}}\right]$$

$$\chi^2 = \Sigma\left[\frac{(O - E)^2}{E}\right]$$

where O = observed frequency and E = expected frequency.

Example

The following table shows the age groups of people interviewed according to their age-group and the number in each group estimated to have T.B.:

Age group	Nos. interviewed	T.B. cases
15-20	199	1
20-25	300	8
25-30	1128	38
35-45	1375	96
45-55	1089	105
55-65	625	56
65-75	155	12
Total	4871	316

Do these figures justify the hypothesis that T. B. is equally popular in all age groups?

Solution

If T.B. equally popular in all groups then in each age group

$$\left[\frac{316}{4871}\times 100 = 65\% \text{ of the people suffer from it}\right]$$

On this basis the observed and expected frequencies would be as:

Age group	Observed Cases	Expected cases
15 - 20	1	13
20 - 25	8	19.5
25 - 35	38	73
35 - 45	96	89
45 - 55	105	71
55 - 65	56	40.5
65 - 75	12	10

Using formula a we get

$$\chi^2 = \frac{(1-13)^2}{13} + \frac{(8-19.5)^2}{19.5} + \frac{(38-73)^2}{73} + \frac{(96-89)^2}{89}$$

$$+ \frac{(105-71)^2}{71} + \frac{(56-40.5)^2}{40.5} + \frac{(12-10)^2}{10}$$

Therefore $\chi^2 = 57.6$

Also n (df) = (c - 1) (n - 1) = (7 - 1) (2 - 1) = 6

From the χ^2 - table, χ^2 0.05, n = 6, χ^2 = 12.59

Since 57.6 > 12.59 at 0.05 level of significance for 6 degree of freedom, the difference is significant and the hypothesis is not justified.

Example

In a certain town 100 persons were randomly chosen and interviewed for their educational stature. The results are as:

Education

		Middle	HighSchool	College	Total
	Male	10	15	25	50
Sex	Female	25	10	15	50
	Total	35	25	40	100

Can you say that education depends on the sex of the individual?

Solution

The null hypothesis: That there is no association between education and sex. On this hypothesis the expected frequencies are as below:

	Middle	HighSchool	College	Total
Male	17.5	12.5	20	50
Female	17.5	12.5	20	50
Total	35	25	40	100

$$\chi^2 = \frac{(10-17.5)^2}{17.5} + \frac{(15-12.5)^2}{12.5} + \frac{(25-20)^2}{20}$$

$$+ \frac{(25-17.5)^2}{17.5} + \frac{(10-12.5)^2}{12.5} + \frac{(15-20)^2}{20}$$

The numbers degree of freedom $\nu = (c-1)(r-1)$

$$\chi^2 = 9.93(\text{approx.}) = (3-1)(2-1) = 2$$

From the table $\chi^2 0.05$, $\nu = 2 = 5.99$ and $\chi^2\ 0.01$, $\nu = 2 = 9.21$

Thus the calculated value of χ^2 is highly significant and the null hypothesis which stated that, education does not depend on sex is, discredited.

Example

The following table is published in a memoir written by 'Karl Pearsons':

		Eye color in sons		
		not light	light	Total
Eye color of fathers	not light	230	148	378
	light	151	471	622
Total		381	619	1000

Test whether the color of son's eyes is associated with that of fathers.

Solution

The null hypothesis : The eye color of sons and eye color of fathers are independent. If this is true the expected frequencies are

		Eye color in sons	
		not light	light
Eye color of fathers	not light	144	234
	light	237	385

$$\chi^2 = \frac{(230-144)^2}{144} + \frac{(184-234)^2}{234} + \frac{(151-237)^2}{237} + \frac{(471-385)^2}{385}$$

$$\chi^2 = 133.37$$

The nos. of degree of freedom $v = (c - 1)(r - 1)$

$= (2 - 1)(2 - 1) = 1$

The table value of χ^2 at 0.05 level of significance for df = 1 is 3.841 which is extremely poor compared to the calculated 133.37. Thus we reject the null hypothesis saying that there is high association between the sons' eyes and that of the father.

Example

In an experiment on the immunization of goats from anthrax, the following results were obtained. Derive the inference on the efficacy of the vaccine.

	Died of anthrax	**Survived**	**Total**
Inoculated	2	10	12
Non-inoculated	6	6	12
Total	8	16	24

Solution

The null hypothesis: Inoculation of vaccine and survival are independent attributes. The expected frequencies would be:

	Died of anthrax	Survived	Total
Inoculated	4	8	12
Non-inoculated	4	8	12
Total	8	16	24

Therefore by formula $\chi^2 = \frac{(2-4)^2}{4} + \frac{(10-8)^2}{8} + \frac{(6-4)^2}{4} + \frac{(6-8)^2}{8}$

$\chi^2 = 3$

The nos. of degree of freedom n $= (c - 1)(r - 1)$

$= (2 - 1)(2 - 1)$

$= 1$

From the table χ^2 0.05, $\nu = 1 = 3.841$.

Thus the calculated value is less than table value. Hence the hypothesis is accepted.

Note : Brandt and Snedecor gave a simple formula for 2×2 contingency table, in order to calculate χ^2. Representing the (2×2) fold contingency table as:

b_1	b_2	T_b
c_1	c_2	T_c
T_1	T_2	T

$$\chi_1 = \frac{(b_1c_2 - c_1b_2)^2}{T_1 \times T_2 \times T_b \times T_c}$$

We multiply diagonal frequencies and find the difference between the two products $(b_1c_2 - c_1b_2)$

Square this i.e. $(b_1c_2 - c_1b_2)^2$

Multiply by the grand total i.e. $(b_1c_2 - c_1b_2)^2 \times T$

Divide the above result by the product of all the sub totals i.e. $T_1 \times T_2 \times T_b \times T_c$

2	10	12
6	6	12
8	16	24

Therefore $\chi^2 = \frac{[(2 \times 6) - (6 \times 10)^2] \times 24}{8 \times 16 \times 12 \times 12} = 3$

Sampling Theory of Correlation

By using the sampling correlation coefficient, you often have to estimate the population correlation coefficient. To do so one must know the sampling distribution of the coefficient of correlation. If the population coefficient of correlation = 0, this distribution is symmetric and the statistic having student's 't' - distribution can be used. Otherwise the distribution is skewed. For such a case a transformation, given by Fisher, which produces a statistic which is nearly normally distributed is used.

(1) In case of large sample (> 30) the standard error of coefficient of correlation 'r'

is calculated by $\frac{\sqrt{1-r^2}}{\sqrt{n}}$

(2) In case of small samples the S. E. of the coefficient of correlation is calculated in the way as in the large samples, with the difference of $1 - r^2$, is used. Instead of is used because in the calculation of coefficient of correlation, 2 degree of freedom are lost and therefore ν (df) = n - 2. Thus the S. E. of the coefficient of correlation in small samples is given by $\frac{\sqrt{1-r^2}}{\sqrt{n-2}}$

The value of 't' is calculated by finding out the ratio between the coefficient of correlation and its S. E.

Thus $t = \frac{r\sqrt{n-2}}{\sqrt{1-r^2}}$

Example

Use 't' test to find whether a correlation coefficient of 0.5 is significant if n = 51.

Solution

$$r = 0.5 \text{ and } n = 51 \text{ then } t = \frac{\sqrt{n-2}}{\sqrt{1-r^2}} \text{ will be}$$

$$t = \frac{0.5\sqrt{51-2}}{\sqrt{1-(0.5)^2}} = 4.07$$

From the table t = 0.05, r = 49 t = 2.01

Thus the calculated value is much higher than table value of 't', so the correlation is significant.

Example

A random sample of 15 from a normal population given the cocfficient of correlation of 0.5. is this significant of the existence of correlation of the population?

Solution

r = 0.5 and n = 15

$$\text{Inserting it} = \frac{r\sqrt{n-2}}{\sqrt{1-r^2}} \text{ we get } t = \frac{0.5\sqrt{15-2}}{\sqrt{1-(-0.5)^2}} = -2.07$$

The df = n - 2 = 15 - 2 = 13

From the table t = 0.05, r = 13 = 2.16.

Thus t = - 2.07 < 2.16. Hence correlation of is not significant to warrant an existence of correlation in the population.

Example

To study the correlation between stature of father and the stature of son, a sample of size 1600, is taken from the population of fathers and sons. The sample study gives the correlation between the two to be 0.80. Within what limits does it hold true for the population?

Solution

The $SE_r = \frac{1-(r)^2}{\sqrt{n}}$

r = 0.8 n = 1600

$$SE_r = \frac{1-(0.8)^2}{\sqrt{1600}} = \frac{1-0.64}{40} = 0.009$$

The correlation in the population probability lies between = r ± 3 S. E. (when the sample is random and simple)

R = S ± S. E.

= 0.8 ± 3 × (0.009)

= (0.8 - 0.027, 0.8 + 0.027)

= (0.773, 0.827)

Sampling Theory of Regression

The regression equation of a normally distributed population is y = a + bx.

Let the regression equation of a sample drawn from it be

y = c + dx.

All you have done is, replaced the intercept (a) by c and the slope (b) by d.

To find S. E. of regression coefficient of y on x i.e. $S.E_{byx}$ use

$$\frac{\sigma \times \sqrt{1-r^2}}{\sigma \times \sqrt{n}}$$

To find S. E. of regressiojn coefficient of x on y i.e. $S.E_{bxy}$ use

$$\frac{\sigma \times \sqrt{1-r^2}}{\sigma \times \sqrt{n}}$$

Also S. E. of regression estimate of y on x or $S.E_{xy} = \sigma \times \sqrt{1-r^2}$

S. E. of regression estimate of x on y or $S.E_{yx} = \sigma y \sqrt{1-r^2}$

To test b = c use t = σ_x with df = n-2

This can be used to find confidence intervals for population regression coefficient from sample values.

Example

Find the regression coefficient of the prices of city A over the prices of city B given that:

	A	B
Average price per kg	120	130
Standard deviation	4	5
Coefficient of correlation	0.6	

n = 100

Solution

Now regression coefficient of prices of city A (x) over the prices of city B.

$$b_{xy} = r.\frac{\sigma_x}{\sigma_y} = 0.6\left(\frac{4}{5}\right) = 0.48$$

The standard error of regression coefficient is:

$$\text{S.E.}(b_{yx}) = \frac{\sigma_x\sqrt{1-r^2}}{\sigma_y\sqrt{n}} = \frac{4\sqrt{1-(0.6)^2}}{5\sqrt{100}} = 0.064$$

Thus the regression coefficient of prices of the city A over the prices of city B is 0.48 and its S.E. is 0.064.

Example

For a certain group of adults, the coefficient of correlation between height and weight is 0.7. Standard deviations of height and weights are 2 inches and 10 lb respectively and the means of heights and weights for the entire group are 70 inches and 130 lbs respectively. Find out the best estimate of weight of a member who is 65 inches tall. Assign limits to this estimate, within which all probability has actual weight would lie.

Solution

Weight (y) and height (x)

Regression of y on x is given by $y-\overline{y}=r.\frac{\sigma y}{\sigma x}\left(x-\overline{x}\right)$

$\overline{y} = 130$, $\overline{x} = 70$, $\sigma y = 10$, $\sigma x = 2$, $r = 0.7$

$$y-130 = 0.7\left(\frac{10}{2}\right)(x-70)$$

y - 130 = 3.5x - 245 or y = 3.5x - 115

When x = 65, y = 3.5 (65) - 115

y = 112.51b

The standard estimate of y on x or S.Eyx is given by

$$S.Eyx = \sigma\sqrt{1-r^2} = 10\sqrt{1-(0.7)^2} = 7.41\,lb$$

Thus the best estimate of weight of an member whose weight is 112.5 lb and height 65 inches cannot deviate from the actual weight by more than 3 S. E.

∴ The estimate of all probabilities of his weight lies between

= 112.5 ± 3 (7.41)

= (112.5 - 22.23, 112.5 + 22.23)

= (90. 27 lb, 134.73 lb)

In brief, we have been in which situations what types of tests have to be applied. Table below gives a comprehensive facts of the tests to be used for different sample sizes.

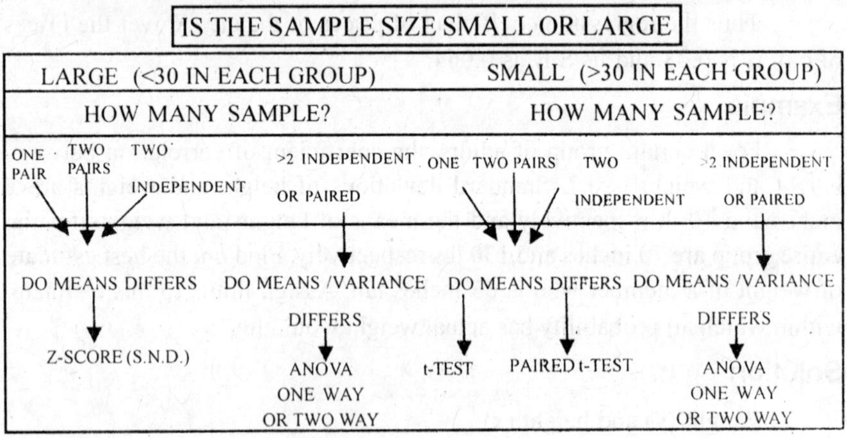

5.4 NON-PARAMETRIC TEST OR DISTRIBUTION FREE TESTS

Some of the statistical methods described above for the qualitative data involved rather simple assumptions: for example, the data is following a normal distribution or while doing simple χ^2 testing a hypothesis about the probabilities for various categories that they are equal is made. But the method used for quantitative data, by contrast have relied on relatively complex assumptions about distribution forms that the random variation is normal. These assumptions are often likely to be clearly untrue. There are methods which avoided unnecessary distributional assumptions. Such methods are called distribution-free methods and are widely used by some statisticians.

In distribution free methods there is little emphasis on population parameters, since the whole object is to avoid a particular functional form for a population distribution. The hypothesis to be tested usually relates to the nature of the distribution as a whole rather than to the values assumed by some of its parameters. For this reason they are often called non-parametric hypothesis and the appropriate techniques are often called non-parametric tests or methods. The use of non-parametric methods will require:

1. There may be obvious non-normality.
2. There may be possible non-normality perhaps to a very marked extent, but the sample size may be too small to establish whether or not this is so.
3. A rapid statistical technique, perhaps involving little or simple calculations.

The methods described in the following sections are a few of the most useful distribution free techniques. They are mainly significance tests.

One Sample Test for Location

We consider tests of the null hypothesis that the distribution of a random variable x is symmetric about zero.

The normal theory test for this hypothesis is, of course, the one sample t-test.

Working Example

In a small clinical trial to assess the value of a new tranquillizer on psycho-neurotic patients was given a week's treatment with drug and a week's treatment with placebo, the order in which the two sets of treatments were given being determined at random. At the end of each week the patient had to complete a questionnaire, on the basis of which he was given an 'anxiety score' (with possible values from 0 to 30), high scores corresponding to states of anxiety. The results are shown in the following table.

Anxiety scores recorded for ten patients receiving a new drug and a placebo in random order

Patient	Anxiety scores Drug	Placebo	Differences
1	19	22	-3
2	11	18	-7
3	14	17	-3
4	17	19	- 2
5	23	22	1
6	11	12	-1
7	15	14	1
8	19	11	8
9	11	19	-8
10	8	7	1
			-13

The last column of table shows the difference, d_i, between the anxiety scores for the ith subject on drug and on the placebo, t-test on the 10 values of d_i gives

$$\Sigma d_i = -13$$

$$\Sigma d_i^2 = 203$$

$$\Sigma(d_i - d)^2 = -186.1$$

Where d = -1.30

s^2= 186.1/9=20.68

$\sqrt{s^2/n}$ = $\sqrt{20.68/10}$ =1.438

And, to test the null hypothesis that $E(d_i)=0$,

t = - 1.30/1.438= -.90 on 9 d.f.

the difference is clearly not significant. 95% confidence interval limit for the mean difference are:

-1.30 ± 2.262x 1.438= -4.55 and 1.95

Sign Test

In a sample of size n; x_1, x_2, x_3,....,xn are n number of observations and out of these, r are positives and s are negatives. Some values of x are equally likely. Both r and s; both follows a binomial distribution with parameter n'. excessively high or low values of r can be tested exactly from the tables of binomial distribution. For large enough sample.

$$\chi^2 = (\alpha\delta - \beta\chi)^2 / \rho$$

Here n'= n= 10 (since there are no zero values)

r = 4 s = 6

for a two sided significance test the probability level is twice the probability of $r \leq 4$ which from the table of the binomial distribution is 0.75. The normal approximation with continuity correction would give

χ^2 = 0.10 (p=0.75)

So, there is no evidence that difference in anxiety score tend to be positive more or less often than they are negative.

Two Sample Tests for Location : The Mann-Whitney U Test

The observations are ranked together in order of increasing magnitude. There are n_1 n_2 pairs (xi,yj); of these.

Uxy is the number of pairs for which xi< yj,

And Uyx is the number of pairs for which xi>yj.

Any pair of which xi= yj count ½ a unit towards both Uxy and Uyx., either of these statistics may be used for a test, with exactly equivalently results. Using Uyx, for instance, the statistic must lie between 0 and n_1n_2. On the null hypothesis its expectation is ½ n_1n_2. High values will suggest a difference between the distributions, with x tending to take higher values than y. Conversely, low values of Uyx suggest x tends to be less than y.

5.5 POINTS TO BE REMEMBERED FOR TESTING OF HYPOTHESIS

You should check the normality of data distribution. The purpose of diagnosis of non-normality is:

1. To warn that mean and SD may not be proper representatives,
2. To help identify out liers.
3. To suggest transformation.

Methods to check non-normality. The following are the methods to check non-normality:

1. Mean vs. SD

   If SD> 25% of the mean i.e. non-normal or highly dispersed.

2 Mean vs. mean range

   Compare mean with (min + max.)/2.

Few Points to be Remembered Before Selecting an Appropriate Statistical Test

- Design of the study
- Groups are related/unrelated
- Sample size
- Number of variables involved
- Types of variables involved
- Does the variables fulfill the assumptions of the test

A Brief Summary of Statistical Test

Parametric Tests	Non-Parametric Tests
χ^2 Test	Wilcoxcon Rank Sum Test
t-test	Wilcoxcon Sign Rank Test
Paired t-test	Kruskal Wallis Test
ANOVA	Freedman's test Mann-Whitney U- Test
Co-effieient of correlation	Spearman's Rank Test

CHAPTER 6	CORRELATION AND REGRESSION

6.1 INTRODUCTION

When dealing with the applied problems in Medicine, Education, Psychology, Sociology etc., one might be interested in determining whether a relationship exists between two or more variables. The correlation coefficient is a useful measure of the degree of association between two characteristics, but only when their relationship is adequately described by a straight line. The equation to this line, the regression equation, allow the value of one characteristics to be estimated when the value of the other characteristics is known. The error of this estimation may be very large even when the correlation is very high.

A problem with which the scientific worker is frequently faced is measurement of the degree of relationship between two or more characteristics of a population.

6.2 CORRELATION

Correlation is a measure of linear association. We say that two variables arc positively correlated if the scatterplot slopes upwards; they are negatively correlated if the scatterplot slopes downward. Note that linear association is not the only kind of association: some variables are nonlinearly associated. For example, the average monthly rainfall in Delhi is associated with the month of the year, but that association is nonlinear: it is a seasonal variation that runs in cycles. Correlation does not measure nonlinear association, only linear association. Correlation is a measure of association, not causation. For example, the average age of people in the India has been increasing. Similarly, there is evidence that the number of plant species is decreasing with time. These two variables have a negative correlation, but there is no (straight forward) causal connection between them. The correlation coefficient r is close to 1 if the data cluster tightly around a straight line that slopes up from left to right. The correlation coefficient is close to -1 if the data cluster tightly around a straight line that slopes down from left to right. If the data do not cluster around a straight line, the correlation coefficient *r* is close to zero, even if the variables have a strong nonlinear association.

Karl Pearson Co-efficient of Correlation for r.v. X and Y

$$r(X,Y)=\frac{Cov(X,Y)}{\sigma_X\sigma_Y}=\frac{E(XY)-E(X)E(Y)}{\sigma_X\sigma_Y}=\frac{n\sum xy-\sum x\sum y}{\sqrt{n\sum x^2-\sum(x)^2}\sqrt{n\sum y^2-\sum(y)^2}}$$

Different Type of Scatter Diagram and Their Significance

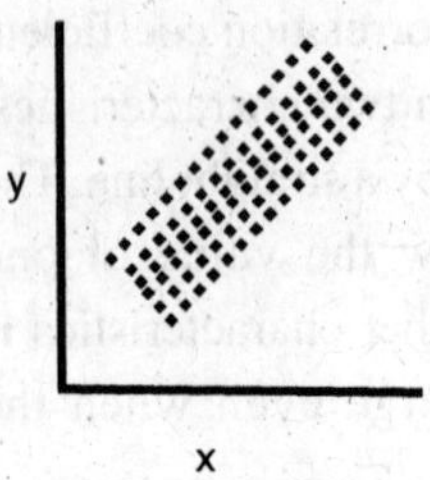

A Liner relationship

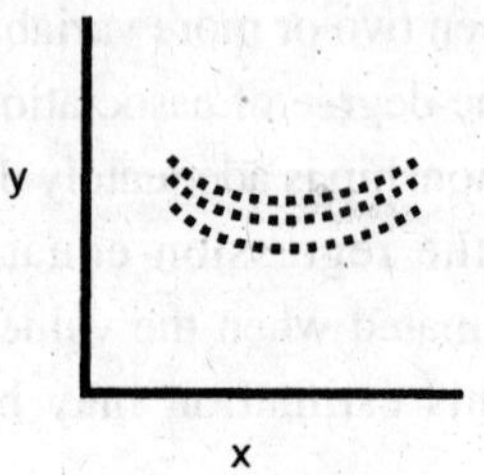

Curvilinear relationship

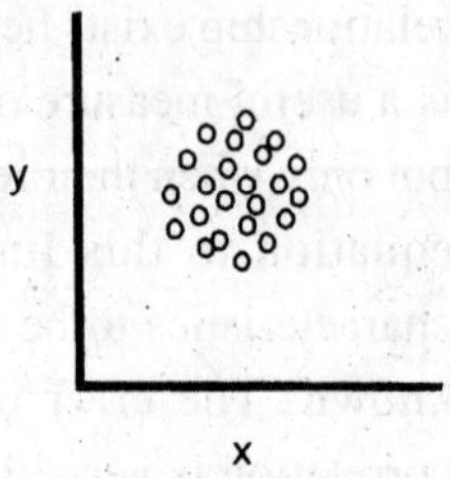

No relationship

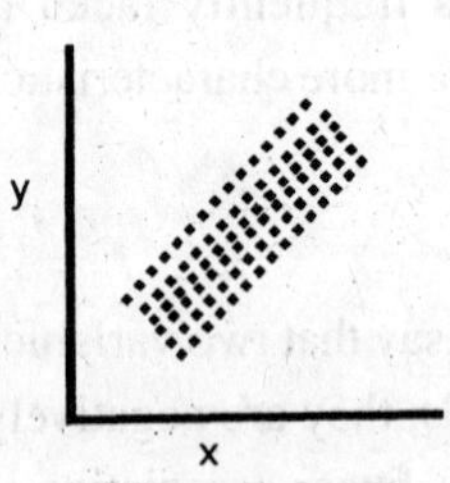

Positive Correlation

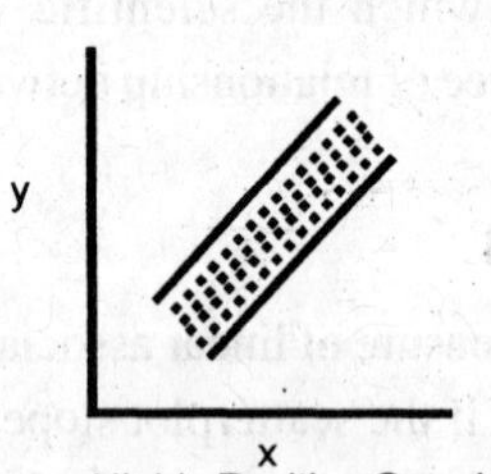

Highly Positive Correlation

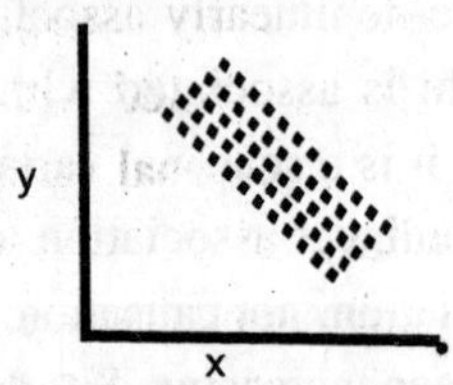

Negative Correlation

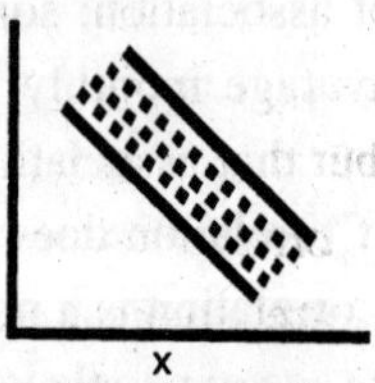

Highly Negative

SOME RESULTS

- $-1 \le r \le 1$, r = 0 implies No Correlation, r = 1 or –1 implies perfect correlation.
- Two independent variables are uncorrelated but not vice versa

- Correlation is independent of change of origin and scale
- If X & Y are r.v.'s and a, b, c, d are constants provided that $a \neq 0$, $c \neq 0$ then $r(aX + b, cY+d) = \frac{ac}{|ac|} r(X,Y)$
- If the randum variables X & Y are connected by the equation $aX + bY + c = 0$. Then the correlation between them is –1 if the sign of a and b are all alike and +1 if they are different

Example

A local health departmental store is interested in knowing whether a strong correlation exists between the amounts of money it spends on advertising and the total sales. It has the following data:

Advertising Expenditure (Rs. in 000)	Sales (Rs.)
0.75	70
0.85	83
0.92	83
1.03	84
1.55	86

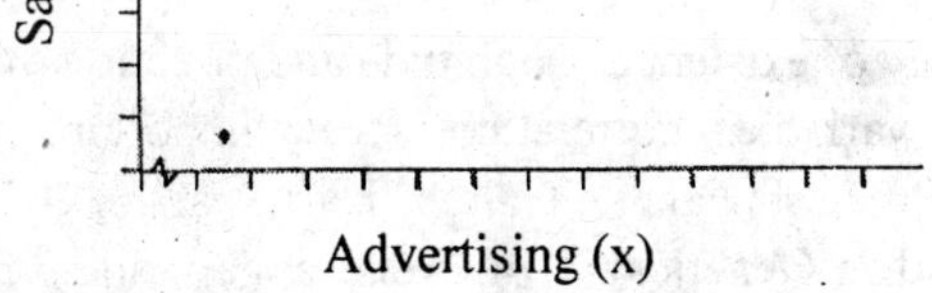

Plot of the Advertising Expenditure Vs Sales

Solution

X	Y	X	Y	XY
0.75	70	0.56	4900	52.5
0.85	83	0.72	6889	70.55
0.92	83	0.85	6889	76.36
1.03	84	1.06	7056	86.52
1.55	86	2.40	7396	133.3
5.1	406	5.59	33130	419.23

n = 5

$$r = \frac{5 \times 5{,}41.23 - 5.1 \times 406}{\sqrt{5 \times 5.59 - (5.1)^2}\ \sqrt{5 \times 33130 - (406)^2}} = 0.41$$

So far we have considered only univariate distributions. By the averages, dispersion and skewness of distribution, we get a complete idea about the structure of the distribution. Many a time, we come across problems which involve two or more variables. If we carefully study the figures of rain fall and production of paddy, figures of accidents and motor cars in a city, of demand and supply of a commodity, of sales and profit, we may find that there is some relationship between the two variables. On the other hand, if we compare the figures of rainfall in America and the production of cars in Japan, we may find that there is no relationship between the two variables. If there is any relation between two variables i.e. when one variable changes the other also changes in the same or in the opposite direction, we say that the two variables are correlated.

W. J. King: If it is proved that in a large number of instances two variables, trend always to fluctuate in the same or in the opposite direction then it is established that a relationship exists between the variables. This is called a "Correlation".

It means the study of existence, magnitude and direction of the relation between two or more variables, correlation is very important. The famous astronomist Bravais, Prof. Sir Fanci's Galton, Karl Pearson (who used this concept in Biology and in Genetics). Prof. Neiswanger and so many others have contributed to this great subject.

Types of Correlation

1. Positive and negative correlation.
2. Linear and non-linear correlation.

(A) If two variables change in the same direction (i.e. if one increases the other also increases, or if one decreases, the other also decreases), then this is called a positive correlation. For example. Advertising and sales.

(B) If two variables change in the opposite direction (i.e. if one increases, the other decreases and vice versa), then the correlation is called a negative correlation. For example: T.V. registrations and cinema attendance.

The nature of the graph gives us the idea of the linear type of correlation between two variables. If the graph is in a straight line, the correlation is called a "linear correlation" and if the graph is not in a straight line, the correlation is **non-linear** or **curvi-linear.**

For example, if variable x changes by a constant quantity, say 20 then y also changes by a constant quantity, say 4. The ratio between the two always remains the same (1/5 in this case). In case of a curvi-linear correlation this ratio does not remain constant.

Degrees of Correlation

Through the coefficient of correlation, we can measure the degree or extent of the correlation between two variables. On the basis of the coefficient of correlation we can also determine whether the correlation is positive or negative and also its degree or extent.

1. Perfect Correlation

If two variables changes in the same direction and in the same proportion, the correlation between the two is **perfect positive**. According to Karl Pearson the coefficient of correlation in this case is +1. On the other hand if the variables change in the opposite direction and in the same proportion, the correlation is **perfect negative**. Its coefficient of correlation is -1. In practice we rarely come across these types of correlations.

2. Absence of Correlation

If two series of two variables exhibit no relations between them or change in variable does not lead to a change in the other variable, then we can firmly say that there is **no correlation** or **absurd correlation** between the two variables. In such a case the coefficient of correlation is 0.

3. Limited Degrees of Correlation

If two variables are not perfectly correlated or is there a perfect absence of correlation, then we term the correlation as Limited correlation. It may be positive, negative or zero but lies with the limits ± 1.

High degree, moderate degree or low degree are the three categories of this kind of correlation. The following table reveals the effect (or degree) of coefficient or correlation.

Degrees	**Positive**	**Negative**
Absence of correlation ®	Zero	0
Perfect correlation ®	+ 1	-1
High degree ®	+ 0.75 to + 1	- 0.75 to -1
Moderate degree ®	+ 0.25 to + 0.75	- 0.25 to - 0.75
Low degree ®	0 to 0.25	0 to - 0.25

Methods of Determining Correlation

We shall consider the following most commonly used methods. (1) Scatter Plot (2) Karrl Pearson's coefficient of correlation (3) Spearman's Rank-correlation coefficient.

1. Scatter Plot (Scatter Diagram or Dot Diagram)

In this method the values of the two variables are plotted on a graph paper. One is taken along the horizontal (x-axis) and the other along the vertical (y-axis). By plotting the data, we get points (dots) on the graph which are generally scattered and hence the name 'Scatter Plot'.

The manner in which these points are scattered, suggest the degree and the direction of correlation. The degree of correlation is denoted by 'r' and its direction is given by the signs positive and negative.

(1) 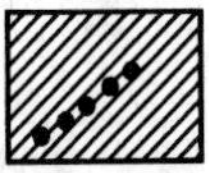 r = +1

i) If all points lie on a rising straight line the correlation is perfectly positive and r = +1 (Fig.1).

(2) 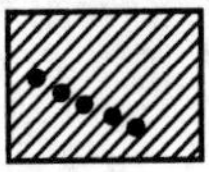 r = −1

ii) If all points lie on a falling straight line the correlation is perfectly negative and r = -1 (Fig.2).

(3) 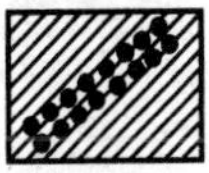 r = +↑High

iii) If the points lie in narrow strip, rising upwards, the correlation is high degree of positive (Fig.3).

(4) 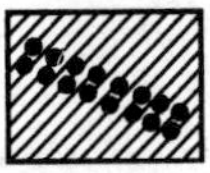 r = -↓High

iv) If the points lie in a narrow strip, falling downwards, the correlation is high degree of negative (Fig.4).

(5) 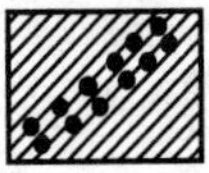 r = +↑Low

v) If the points are spread widely over a broad strip, rising upwards, the correlation is low degree positive (Fig.5).

(6) 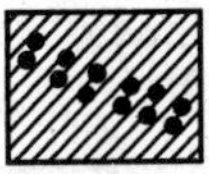 r = - ↓Low

vi) If the points are spread widely over a broad strip, falling downward, the correlation is low degree negative (Fig.6).

(7) 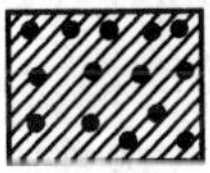 r = 0

vii) If the points are spread (scattered) without any specific pattern, the correlation is absent i.e. r = 0. (Fig.7).

Though this method is simple and is a rough idea about the existence and the degree of correlation, it is not reliable. As it is not a mathematical method, it cannot measure the degree of correlation.

2. Karl Pearson's Coefficient of Correlation

It gives the numerical expression for the measure of correlation. It is noted by 'r'. The value of 'r' gives the magnitude of correlation and sign denotes its direction. It is defined as:

$$r = \frac{\Sigma xy}{\sigma_x \sigma_y}$$

$x = (x_i - \bar{x})$, $y = (y_i - \bar{y})$, σx = s.d.of x and σy = s.d.of y where

N = Number of pairs of observation

Note : r is also known as product-moment coefficient of correlation.

$$\frac{\sum xy}{\sqrt{\sum x^2} \times \sqrt{\sum y^2}} \text{ Since } \sigma_x = \sqrt{\frac{\sum x^2}{n}} \text{ and } \sigma_y = \sqrt{\frac{\sum y^2}{n}}$$

$$\text{OR } r = \frac{\sum xy - \left(\frac{\sum x \sum y}{n}\right)}{\sqrt{\sum x^2 - \frac{\sum x^2}{n}} \cdot \sqrt{\sum y^2 - \frac{\sum y^2}{n}}}$$

Now covariance of x and y is defined as

$$\text{cov}(X,\ Y) = \frac{\sum (x_i - \bar{x})(y_i - \bar{y})}{n} \therefore r = \frac{\text{Cov}(X,\ Y)}{\sigma_x \sigma_y}$$

Example

Calculate the coefficient of correlation between the heights of father and his son for the following data:

Height of father (cm.)	165	166	167	168	167	169	170	172
Height of Son (cm.)	167	168	165	172	168	172	169	171

Solution

Height of father (cm.)	**Height of Son (cm.)**	$x = x_i - x$	$y = y_i - y$	**xy**	x^2	y^2
165	167	-3	-2	6	9	4
166	168	-2	-1	2	4	1

167	165	-1	-4	4	1	16
167	168	-1	-1	1	1	1
168	172	0	3	0	0	9
169	172	1	3	3	1	9
170	169	2	0	0	4	0
172	171	4	2	8	16	4
$\Sigma x_i = 1344$	$\Sigma y_i = 1352$	0	0	$\Sigma xy=24$	$\Sigma x^2=36$	$\Sigma y^2=44$

Calculation

$$\bar{x} = \frac{\Sigma x_i}{n} = \frac{1344}{8} = 168\text{cm} \quad \text{and} \quad \sigma_x = \sqrt{\frac{\Sigma x^2}{n}} = \sqrt{\frac{36}{8}}$$

$$\bar{y} = \frac{\Sigma y_i}{n} = \frac{1352}{8} = 169\text{cm} \quad \text{and} \quad \sigma_y = \sqrt{\frac{\Sigma y^2}{n}} = \sqrt{\frac{44}{8}}$$

Now,

$$r = \frac{\Sigma xy}{n\sigma_x\sigma_y} = \frac{24}{8\sqrt{\frac{36}{8}} \times \sqrt{\frac{44}{8}}} = \frac{24}{\sqrt{36 \times 44}}$$

$$= +0.6029$$

Since r is positive and 0.6. This shows that the correlation is positive and moderate (i.e. direct and reasonably good).

Example

From the following data compute the coefficient of correlation between x and y.

		x	y
No. of items	→	15	15
Arithmetic mean	→	25	18
$\Sigma(x_i - \bar{x}).\Sigma(y_1 - \bar{y})^2$	→	136	138
$\Sigma(x_i - \bar{x}).\Sigma(y_1.\bar{y})$	→	122	

Solution

Given $n = 15,\ \bar{x} = 25, \bar{Y} = 18$

$\Sigma(x_i - \bar{x})^2$.i.e $\Sigma x^2 = 136,\ \Sigma(y_i - \bar{y})^2$

i.e. $\Sigma y^2 = 138$

and $\Sigma(x_i - \bar{x}).\Sigma(y_i - \bar{y}) = \Sigma xy = 122$

using $r = \dfrac{\Sigma xy}{\sqrt{\Sigma x^2}.\sqrt{\Sigma y^2}}$ we get

$$= \frac{122}{\sqrt{136}.\sqrt{138}} = \frac{122}{136.9} = 0.891$$

Example

Find the number of pair of observations from the following data.

$r = 0.25$, $\Sigma (x_i - x)(y_i - y) = 60$, $\sigma_y = 4$, $\Sigma (x_i - x)2 = 90$.

Solution

Given $r = 0.25$

$\Sigma(x_i - \bar{x}).\Sigma(y_i - \bar{y}) = \Sigma xy = 60$

$$\sigma_x = \sqrt{\frac{\Sigma x^2}{n}} = \sqrt{\frac{\Sigma(x_i - \bar{x})^2}{n}} = \sqrt{\frac{90}{n}} \qquad \sigma_y = 4 = \sqrt{\frac{\Sigma y^2}{n}}$$

New, $r = \dfrac{\Sigma xy}{n\sigma_x.\sigma_y} = \dfrac{60}{n\sqrt{\dfrac{20}{n}} \times 4} = \dfrac{15}{\sqrt{90n}}$

$\therefore 0.25 = \dfrac{15}{\sqrt{90n}}$

$\therefore 0.25 \times \sqrt{90n} = 15$

on squaring

$\therefore 0.25 \times 90n = 225 \quad \therefore 90n = \dfrac{225}{0.0625}$

$\therefore 90n = 3600 \quad \therefore n = 40$

Therefore the number of pairs of obsevations = 40

If the values of x and y are very big, the calculation becomes very tedious and if we change the variable x to u = $\frac{x_1 - x_0}{c}$ and v = $\frac{y_1 - y_0}{d}$ to where x_0 and y_0 are the assumed means for variable x and y respectively, then r_{xy} = ruv

The formula for r can be simplified as

$$r_{xy} = r_{uv} = \frac{\Sigma uv - \left(\frac{(\Sigma u)(\Sigma v)}{n}\right)}{\sqrt{\Sigma u^2 - \frac{(\Sigma u^2)}{n}} \times \sqrt{\Sigma v^2 - \frac{(\Sigma v)^2}{n}}}$$

Example

Marks obtained by two brothers FRED and TED in 10 tests are as follows:

Fred:	44	80	76	48	52	72	68	56	60	64
Ted:	48	75	54	60	63	69	72	51	57	66

Find the coefficient of correlation between the two.

Solution

Here $x_0 = 60$, $c = 4$, $y_0 = 60$ and $d = 3$

Fred	Ted	$u = \frac{(x_i - x_0)}{c}$	$v = \frac{(y_i - y_0)}{c}$	uv	u^2	v^2
44	48	-4	-4	16	16	16
80	75	5	5	25	25	25
76	54	4	-2	-8	16	4
48	60	-3	0	0	9	0
52	63	-2	1	-2	4	1
72	69	3	3	9	9	9
68	72	2	4	8	4	16
56	51	-1	-3	3	1	9
60	57	0	-1	0	0	1
64	66	1	2	2	4	4
Total		$\Sigma u = 5$	$\Sigma v = 5$	$\Sigma uv = 53$	$\Sigma u^2=85$	$\Sigma v^2=85$

Calculation

$$r_{xy} = r_{uv} = \frac{\sum uv - \left(\frac{(\sum u)(\sum v)}{n}\right)}{\sqrt{\sum u^2 - \frac{(\sum u^2)}{n}} \times \sqrt{\sum v^2 - \frac{(\sum v)^2}{n}}}$$

$$= \frac{53 - \left(\frac{(5)(5)}{10}\right)}{\sqrt{85 - \frac{(5)^2}{10}} \times \sqrt{85 - \frac{(5)^2}{10}}}$$

$$= \frac{53 - 2.5}{\sqrt{82.5} \times \sqrt{82.5}}$$

$$= \frac{50.5}{82.5}$$

$$= 0.61$$

Coefficient of Correlation For Bivariate Grouped Data

When the number of observations is very large, we need to arrange the data into different classes, which are either discrete or continuous. Items having values falling in a particular class are placed together and those having values falling in another class are placed together. Due to this the whole data is divided into horizontal rows and vertical columns, with one variable placed horizontally and the other placed vertically. The table so obtained is a two-way frequency distribution table and is called the correlation table or Bi-variate frequency distribution table. The formula for calculating and for bi-variate distribution is given by

$$r_{xy} = r_{uv} = \frac{\Sigma fuv - \left(\frac{(\Sigma fu)(\Sigma fv)}{n}\right)}{\sqrt{\Sigma fu^2 - \frac{(\Sigma fu^2)}{n}} \times \sqrt{\Sigma fv^2 - \frac{(\Sigma fv)^2}{n}}}$$

Steps

First write down the mid-points of x along a horizontal raw and those of y along a vertical column.

1. Find $u = \frac{x_1 - x_0}{c}$ & $v = \frac{y_1 - y_0}{d}$

2. Multiply each frequency by the corresponding value of u then by corresponding value of v to get fuv. Write these numbers in the same box at the top.

3. Add the frequencies horizontally, and write down the total. Similarly add the frequencies vertically and write down its total.

4. Multiply this addition of x by u to get f u.

5. Multiply this addition of y by v to get f v.

6. Multiply these frequencies by the square of u to get $f\,u^2$.

7. Multiply these frequencies by the square of v to get $f\,v^2$.

8. Add horizontally (or vertically) the top numbers denoting f u v written in each box (or cell).

9. Write down $\Sigma\, f u$, $\Sigma\, f u^2$, $\Sigma\, f v$, $\Sigma\, f v^2$ and $\Sigma\, f u v$ and then use the above formula.

Example

Calculate the coefficient of correlation for the following data:

Age (years)	Age (years) of wife					Total
of husband	10 -20	20 -30	30 -40	40 -50	50 -60	
10 - 25	5	3	11	7	3	8
25 - 35	3	15	14	12	6	29
35 - 45		11	7	3		32
45 - 55						22
55 - 65						9
Total	8	29	32	22	9	100

Inserting, Σ fuv = 94, n = 100, Σ fu = -5, Σ fv = -5, Σ fu2 = 119 and Σ fv2 = 119 in

y		v	x: 10-20	20-30	30-40	40-50	50-60			
		m	15	25	35	45	55			
		u	-2	-1	0	1	2	f	fu²	fv²
10-25	20	-2	[20] 5	[6] 3				8	-16	32
25-35	30	-1		[15] 15				29	-29	29
35-45	40	0	[6] 3	[0] 11	[0] 11	[0] 7		32	0	0
45-55	50	1			[0] 14	[12] 12	[6] 3	22	+22	+22
55-65	60	2			[0] 7	[6] 3	[24] 6	9	+18	+36
		f	8	29	32	22	9	N =100	Σfv=-5	Σfv²=119
		fu	-16	-25	0	+22	+18			
		fu²	32	-29	0	+22	36	Σfuv=95		
		fuv	26	21	0	18	30			

$$r = \frac{\Sigma fuv - \dfrac{(\Sigma fu)(\Sigma fv)}{n}}{\sqrt{\Sigma fu^2 - \dfrac{(\Sigma fu)^2}{n}}\sqrt{\Sigma fv^2 - \dfrac{(\Sigma fv)^2}{n}}}$$

$$= \frac{95 - \dfrac{25}{100}}{\sqrt{119 - \dfrac{(-5)^{2'}}{100}} \times \sqrt{119 - \dfrac{(-5)^2}{100}}}$$

$$= \frac{95 - 0.25}{\sqrt{119 - 0.25} \times \sqrt{119 - 0.25}}$$

$$= \frac{94.75}{119 - 0.25}$$

$$= \frac{94.75}{118.75} = 0.7913$$

Probable Error

It is used to help in the determination of the Karl Pearson's coefficient of correlation 'r'. Due to this 'r' is corrected to a great extent but note that 'r' depends on the random sampling and its conditions. It is given by

$$\text{P. E.} = 0.6745 \left[\frac{1-r^2}{\sqrt{n}}\right]$$

i. If the value of r is less than P. E., then there is no evidence of correlation i.e. r is not significant.

ii. If r is more than 6 times the P.E. 'r' is practically certain i.e. significant.

iii. By adding or subtracting P.E. to 'r', we get the upper and lower limits within which 'r' of the population can be expected to lie.

Symbolically e = r ± P. E.

P = Correlation (coefficient) of the population.

Spearman's Rank Correlation Coefficient

This method is based on the ranks of the items rather than on their actual values. The advantage of this method over the others is that it can be used even when the actual values of items are unknown. For example if you want to know the correlation between honesty and wisdom of the boys of your class, you can use this method by giving ranks to the boys. It can also be used to find the degree of agreements between the judgements of two examiners or two judges. The formula is:

$$R = 1 - \frac{6 \Sigma D^2}{N(N^2 - 1)}$$

where R = Rank correlation coefficient

D = Difference between the ranks of two items.

N = The number of observations.

Note: $-1 \leq R \leq 1$.

i. When R = +1 ⇒ Perfect positive correlation or complete agreement in the same direction.

ii. When R = -1 ⇒ Perfect negative correlation or complete agreement in the opposite direction.

iii. When R = 0 ⇒ No correlation.

Computation

i. Give ranks to the values of items. Generally the item with the highest value is ranked 1 and then the others are given ranks 2, 3, 4, ... according to their values in the decreasing order.

ii. Find the difference $D = R_1 - R_2$

where R_1 = Rank of x and R_2 = Rank of y

Note that $\Sigma D = 0$ (always).

iii. Calculate D^2 and then find ΣD^2.

iv. Apply the formula.

★ **Note :** In some cases, there is a tie between two or more items. In such a case each items have ranks 4th and 5th respectively then they are given = (4 +5)/2 = 4.5th rank. If three items are of equal rank say 4th then they are given = (4 +5 +6)/3 = 5th rank each. If m be the number of items of equal ranks, the factor $[(m^3 - m)]\ 1/12$ is added to S. D^2. If there are more than one of such cases then this factor added as many times as the number of such cases, then

$$R = 1 - \frac{6\left\{\Sigma D^2 + \left(\frac{1}{12}(m_1^3 - m_1\right)\right\} + \frac{1}{12}\left(\frac{1}{12}(m_1^3 - m_1\right) + \cdots}{N(n^2 - 1)}$$

Example

Calculate 'R' from the following data.

Student No.:	1	2	3	4	5	6	7	8	9	10
Rank in Maths :	1	3	7	5	4	6	2	10	9	8
Rank in Stats:	3	1	4	5	6	9	7	8	10	2

Solution

Student No.	Rank in Maths (R_1)	Rank in Stats (R_2)	$R_1 - R_2$ = D	$(R_1 - R_2)^2$ = D^2
1	1	3	-2	4
2	3	1	2	4
3	7	4	3	9
4	5	5	0	0
5	4	6	-2	4
6	6	9	-3	9
7	2	7	-5	25
8	10	8	2	4
9	9	10	-1	1
10	8	2	6	36
N = 10			$\Sigma D = 0$	$\Sigma D^2 = 96$

Calculation of R:

$$R = 1 - \frac{6\sum D^2}{N(n^2 - 1)} = 1 - \frac{6(96)}{10(100 - 1)}$$

$$= 1 - \frac{6 \times (96)}{10 \times 99} = 0.4181$$

Example

Calculate 'R' of 6 students from the following data:

Marks in Stats :	40	42	45	35	36	39
Marks in English :	46	43	44	39	40	43

Solution

Marks in Stats	R_1	Marks in English	R_2	$R_1 - R_2$	$(R_1 - R_2)^2 = D^2$
40	3	46	1	2	4
42	2	43	3.5	-1.5	2.25
45	1	44	2	-1	1
35	6	39	6	0	0
36	5	40	5	0	0
39	4	43	3.5	0.5	0.25
N = 6				$\Sigma D = 0$	$\Sigma D^2 = 7.50$

Here m = 2 since in series of marks in English of items of values 43 repeated twice.

$$R = 1 - \frac{6\{\Sigma D^2 + \frac{1}{12}(2^3 - 2)\}}{N(n^2 - 1)} = 1 - \frac{6\{7.5 + \frac{1}{12}(8 - 2)\}}{6(36 - 6)}$$

$$R = 1 - \frac{6(7.5 + 0.5)}{210} = 0.771$$

6.3 REGRESSION

Correlation coefficient merely determines whether two variables are related, but does not specify how. Thus, correlation coefficient cannot be used to solve prediction problems. When a prediction problem is given, we first locate all the dots on a scatter plot and then try to fit a straight line to the data in such a way that it best represents the relationship between the two variables. Such a line is called an **estimated regression line.**

Regression is the measure of average relationship between two or more variables in terms of original units of data. Regression analysis is done for estimating or predicting the unknown values of one variable from the known values of other variables. Suppose that economic variable x causes economic variable y. Given x, one can express y as $y = a + bx$. Interpret $= a + bx$ as the best forecast of y based on x. The forecast error is e, and the intercept a and the slope b are fixed coefficients. The terminology is that x is the *independent variable* and y is the *dependent variable*; y depends on x. The intuitive concept is that an observation of x and y lies near the line $y = a + bx$. The error e is the vertical distance between the forecast (x) and the observation (x, y). The error may be either positive or negative, but on average the error is zero. (One also refers to the error as the *residual*, the component of the dependent variable not explained by the independent variable).

Correlation gives us the idea of the measure of magnitude and direction between correlated variables. Now it is natural to think of a method that helps us in estimating the value of one variable when the other is known. Also correlation does not imply causation. The fact that the variables x and y are correlated does not necessarily mean that x causes y or vice versa. For example, you would find that the number of schools in a town is correlated to the number of accidents in the town. The reason for these accidents is not the school attendance; but these two increases what is known as **population**. A statistical procedure called **regression** is concerned with causation in a relationship among variables. It assesses the contribution of one or more variable called **causing variable** or **independent variable** or one which is being **caused (dependent variable)**. When there is only one independent variable then the relationship is expressed by a straight line. This procedure is called **simple linear regression**.

Regression can be defined as a method that estimates the value of one variable when that of other variable is known, provided the variables are correlated. The dictionary meaning of regression is "to go backward". It was used for the first time by Sir Francis Galton in his research paper "Regression towards mediocrity in hereditary stature".

METHOD OF LEAST SQUARES

Fitting of a Straight Line

Whenever we draw an estimated regression line, not all points will lie on the regression line. Some will be above it and some will be below. The difference between any point and the corresponding point on the regression line is called the deviation from the line. It represents the difference between the predicted value and the actual value. The least square method fits the regression line in such a way that the sum of squares of these deviations as small as possible.

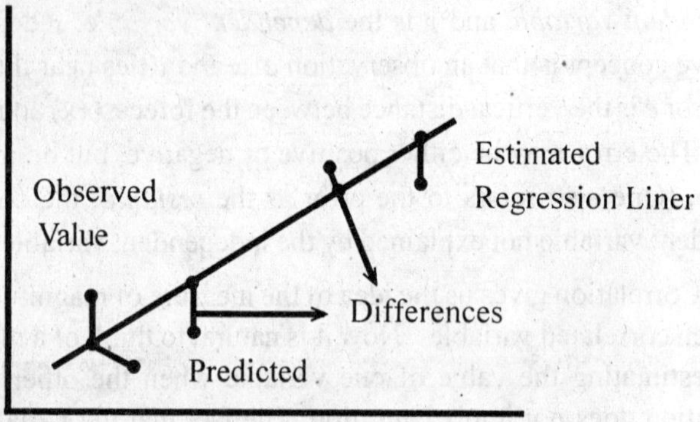

Differences Between y Values and the Estimated Regression Lines

Let us suppose that in the bivariate distribution (xi, yi); i = 1...... n, y is dependent and x is the independent variable

Let the line of regression of y on x be

$y = a + bx$

so the estimated line would be,

$\mathbf{y} = \boldsymbol{a} + \boldsymbol{b}\,\boldsymbol{x}$

we have to minimize the sum of squared error i.e. min Σdi^2 or min $\Sigma(y_i - a - bx_1)^2$ we get the following normal equations:

$$\begin{cases} \dfrac{\partial}{\partial a}\Sigma(y_i - a - bx_i)^2 = 0 \\ \dfrac{\partial}{\partial b}\Sigma(y_i - a - bx_i)^2 = 0 \end{cases}$$

or

$$\begin{cases} \Sigma(y_i - an - b\Sigma x_i)^2 = 0 \\ \Sigma(x_i y_i - a\Sigma x_i - b\Sigma x_i^2 = 0 \end{cases}$$

Solving them, we get

the slope is $\hat{b}$ = Cov(y, x) /Var (x). The estimate of the intercept is $\hat{a}$ = E (y) - $\hat{b}$ E (x) Line of regression of Y on X.

$$Y - \overline{Y} = r\frac{\sigma_y}{\sigma_x}(X - \overline{X}) = b_{YX}(X - \overline{X})$$

Line of regression of X on Y is

$$X - \overline{X} = r\frac{\sigma_x}{\sigma_y}(Y - \overline{Y}) = b_{XY}(Y - \overline{Y})$$

Where, b_{YX} and b_{XY} are coefficient of regression. If X and Y are r.v.'s, then line of regression are represented as:

$$E(Y/X) - \overline{Y} = \frac{r\sigma_y}{\sigma_x}(X - \overline{X}) = b_{XY}(X - \overline{X})$$

$$E(X/Y) - \overline{Y} = \frac{r\sigma_x}{\sigma_Y}(Y - \overline{Y}) = bxy(Y - \overline{Y})$$

SOME RESULTS

- Line of regression is the line of best fit.
- Both the lines of regression pass through (x, y).
- Correlation co-efficient is the geometric mean between the regression co-efficient i.e. $r = \pm\sqrt{b_{YX}b_{XY}}$.
- If one of the regression coefficient is greater than unity other must be less than unity.
- Arithmetic mean of the regression co-efficient is greater than the correlation coefficient i.e. $\frac{1}{2}(b_{YX} + b_{XY}) \geq r$
- Regression Coefficient are independent of change of origin but not of scale.

- Angle between the two lines of regression

$$\theta = \tan^{-1}\left\{\left(\frac{r^2-1}{r}\right)\left(\frac{\sigma_x\sigma_y}{\sigma_x^2+\sigma_y^2}\right)\right\}$$

- If r = 0, then the two lines of regression are perpendicular to each other. If, then the two lines coincides. These result leads to the conclusion that for higher degree of correlation lines of regression are nearer to each other.

Coefficient of Determination

The coefficient of determination is r^2. This represents the percent of the variation that can be explained by the regression equation. Every sample has some variation in it (unless all the values are identical, and that's unlikely to happen). The total variation is made up of two parts, the part that can be explained by the regression equation and the part that can't be explained by the regression equation. The ratio of the explained variation to the total variation is a measure of how good the regression line is. If the regression line passed through every point on the scatter plot exactly, it would be able to explain all of the variation. The further the line is from the points, the less it is able to explain.

Example

A survey was conducted to relate the performance of the student with the grades he received. The following table shows the matched data:

a. Find the regression equation that will predict a student score if we know how many hours the student studied.

b. If a student studies 0.85 hours, what is the student's predicted grade?

Hours x	0.5	0.75	1.00	1.25	1.50	1.75	2.00
Score	57	64	59	68	74	76	79

Solution

We will arrange the data in the form of a chart to enable us to perform the computations.

x	y	x^2	xy
0.50	57	0.25	28.5
0.75	64	0.56	48
1.00	59	1.00	59
1.25	68	1.56	85
1.50	74	2.25	111
1.75	76	3.06	133
2.00	79	4.00	158
2.25	83	5.06	186.75
2.50	85	6.25	212.5
2.75	86	7.56	236.5
3.00	88	9.00	246
3.25	89	10.56	289.25
3.50	90	12.25	315
3.75	94	14.06	352.5
4.00	96	16.00	384
33.75	**1188**	**93.44**	**2863**

n=15 $\hat{b}$= Cov(y, x) /Var (x) = 15(2863) – (33.75) (1188) / 15 (93.44) - $(33.75)^2$ = 10.86

$\hat{a} = E(y) - \hat{b}\,E(x) = 54.77$

Equation of predicted regression line is
Thus, y = 54.772 + 10.857 x

(b) For x = 0.85, we get

$$y = 54.772 + 10.857\ (0.85)$$
$$= 57.772 + 9.22845 = 64.00$$

Thus, the predicted score of a student who study 0.85 hrs is approximately 64.

Lines of Regression

In scatter plot, we have seen that if the variables are highly correlated then the points (dots) lie in a narrow strip. If the strip is nearly straight, we can draw a straight line, such that all points are close to it from both sides. Such a line can be taken as an ideal representation of variation. This line is called the line of best fit if it minimizes the distances of all data points from it.

This line is called **the line of regression.** Now prediction is easy because now all we need to do is to extend the line and read the value. Thus to obtain a line of regression, we need to have a line of best fit. But statisticians don't measure the distances by dropping perpendiculars from points on to the line. They measure **deviations** (or **errors** or **residuals** as they are called) (i) vertically and (ii) horizontally. Thus we get two lines of regressions as

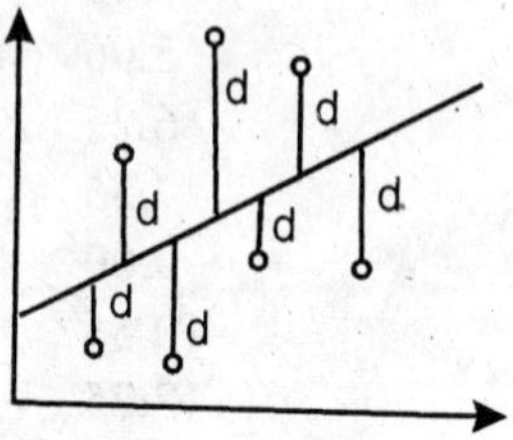

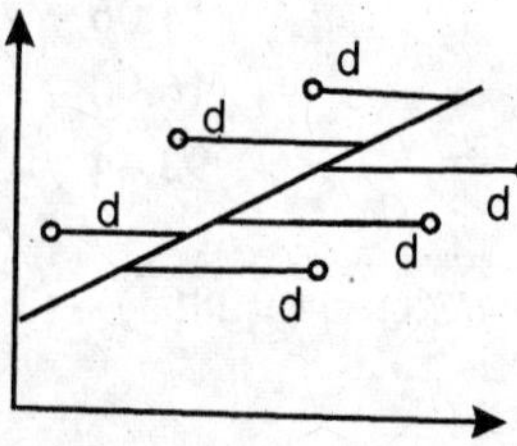

Shown in the following figures (1) and (2).

(1) Line of regression of y on x. Its form is y = a + b x. It is used to estimate y when x is given

(2) Line of regression of x on y. Its form is x = a + b y. It is used to estimate x when y is given.

They are obtained by (i) graphically– by Scatter plot (ii) Mathematically - by the method of least squares.

(ii.) Let y = a + b y .... (1)

where a and b are given by the normal equations

$$\Sigma y = n a + b \Sigma x \quad .... (2)$$

$$\Sigma xy = a \Sigma x + b \Sigma x^2 \quad .... (3)$$

where 'n' be the number of pairs of values of x and y.

Equation (1) is the equation of the **line of regression of y on x.**

$$b_{xy} = r.\frac{\sigma_X}{\sigma_Y} \quad ...(4)$$

is called the coefficient of regression of y on x which is obviously the slope of this line. Interchanging x and y in equation (1), the equation of the line of regression of x and y is given by

$$x - \bar{x} = r\frac{\sigma_x}{\sigma_y}(y - \bar{y})$$

$$\text{i.e. } x - \bar{x} = b_{xy}(y - \bar{y}) \text{ .... (5)}$$

Naturally b_{xy} is the slope of this line.

Example

A panel of two judges A and B graded dramatic performance by independently awarding marks as follows:

Performance No.:	1	2	3	4	5	6	7	8
Marks by A :	36	32	34	31	32	32	35	38
Marks by B :	35	33	31	30	34	32	36	?

Solution

Sr. No.	x_i	$x_i - \bar{x} = x$	x^2	y_i	$y_i - \bar{y} = y$	y^2	xy
1	36	+3	9	35	+2	4	6
2	32	-1	1	33	0	0	0
3	34	1	1	31	-2	4	2
4	31	-2	4	30	-3	9	6
5	32	-1	1	34	1	1	1
6	32	-1	1	32	-1	1	1
7	35	2	4	36	3	9	6
n=7	Σx_i=135		Σx^2 = 21	Σy_i=31		Σy^2 = 28	Σxy=16

$$\therefore \bar{x} = \frac{\Sigma xy}{n} = \frac{232}{7} = 33 \text{ and } \bar{y} = \frac{\Sigma y}{n} = \frac{231}{7} = 33$$

$$\text{Now } r = \frac{\Sigma xy}{\sqrt{x^2} \times \sqrt{y^2}} = \frac{16}{\sqrt{21} \times \sqrt{18}}$$

$$= \frac{16}{\sqrt{588}} = \frac{16}{24.22} = 0.65$$

$$\text{Also } \sigma_x = \sqrt{\frac{\Sigma x^2}{n}} = \sqrt{\frac{21}{7}} = \sqrt{3} = 1.73$$

$$\sigma_y = \sqrt{\frac{\Sigma y^2}{n}} = \sqrt{\frac{28}{7}} = 2$$

The equation of the line of regression of y on x

$$y - \bar{y} = r.\frac{\sigma_y}{\sigma_x}(x - \bar{x})$$

Inserting x = 38, we get

$$y - 33 = 0.74\ (38 - 33)$$

$$y - 33 = 0.74 \times 5$$

$$y - 33 = 3.7$$

$$y = 3.7 + 33$$

$$y = 36.7 = 37 \text{ (approximately)}$$

Therefore, the Judge B would have given 37 marks to 8th performance.

Example

The two regression equations of the variables x and are

$$x = 19.13 - 0.87\,y \text{ and } y = 11.64 - 0.50\,x$$

Find (1) Mean of x's

(2) Mean of y's

(3) Correlation coefficient between x and y

Solution

1. Calculation of mean.

Since lines of regression pass through means i.e. $(\bar{x} - \bar{y})$

$\bar{x} + 0.87\ \bar{y} = 19.13$............(1)

$50\,\bar{x} + \bar{y} = 11.64$

i.e $\bar{x} + 2\bar{y} = 23.28$ .... (2)

Subtracting (1) from (2) we get

$1.13\bar{y} = 4.15$ or $\bar{y} = 3.67$

Inserting $\bar{y} = 3.67$ in (2) we get $\bar{x} = 15.94$

Mean of x's = 15.94 and Mean of y's = 3.67

2. Calculation of 'r'

x = 19.93 - 0.87 y

Therefore, $b_{xy} = r.\dfrac{\sigma_x}{\sigma_y} = -0.87$.............(3)

and y = 11.64 - 0.50 x

Therefore, $b_{yx} = r.\dfrac{\sigma_y}{\sigma_x} = -0.50$.............(4)

From (3) and (4)

$r^2 = \pm\sqrt{b_{xy} \times b_{yx}} = \pm\sqrt{-0.87 \times -0.5}$

$= \pm\sqrt{0.435}$

$r = \pm 0.66$

But regression coefficient are negative

r = - 0.66

Example

In a partially destroyed laboratory record of an analysis of correlation data, the following results are legible:

Variance of x = 9

Regression equations: $8x - 10y + 66 = 6$

$40x - 18y = 214$

What are (1) Means of x's and y's (2) the coefficient of correlation between x and y (3) the standard deviation of y?

Solution

1. Means:

$8x - 10y = -66$ ------------------------- (1)

$40x - 18y = 214$ ------------------------- (2)

Solving (1) and (2) as

$40x - 50y = -330$ ------------------------- (1)

$40x - 18y = 214$ ------------------------- (2)

$-32y = -544$

$y = 17$

$\therefore$ Mean of y's ($\bar{y}$) =17

Substituting $\bar{y} = 17$ in (1) we get $8x - 10 \times 17 = -66$

or $8x = 104 \therefore x = 13$

$\therefore$ Mean of x's ($\bar{x}$) = 13

2. Coefficient of correlation between x and y

$40x = 18y + 214$

$$x = \frac{18}{40}y + \frac{214}{40}$$

$$\therefore b_{xy} = \frac{18}{40} = 0.45$$

Also $-10y = -8x - 66$

$$y = \frac{8}{10}x + \frac{66}{10}$$

$$\therefore b_{xy} = \frac{8}{10} = 0.8$$

Therefore, $r = \sqrt{b_{xy} \times b_{yx}} = \sqrt{.45 \times .8} = 0.6$

3. Standard deviation of y

$\therefore$ Variance of x i.e. $\sigma x^2 = 9 \therefore \sigma x = 3$

Now byx = $b_{yx} = r.\frac{\sigma_y}{\sigma_x}$ or $0.8 = 6 \times \frac{\sigma_y}{3} = 2\sigma_y$ $\therefore \sigma y = 0.4$

CHAPTER 7 STATISTICAL METHODS FOR VALIDITY AND RELIABILITY OF DATA

7.1 INTRODUCTION

Relative risk is used frequently in the statistical analysis of binary outcomes where the outcome of interest has relatively low probability. It is thus often suited to clinical trial data, where it is used to compare the risk of developing a disease, in people not receiving the new medical treatment (or receiving a placebo) versus people who are receiving an established (standard of care) treatment. Alternatively, it is used to compare the risk of developing a side effect in people receiving a drug as compared to the people who are not receiving the treatment (or receiving a placebo). It is particularly attractive because it can be calculated by hand in the simple case, but is also susceptible to regression modelling, typically in a Poisson regression framework.

7.2 RELATIVE RISK

In statistics and mathematical epidemiology, **relative risk (RR)** is the risk of an event (or of developing a disease) relative to exposure. Relative risk is a ratio of the probability of the event occurring in the exposed group versus the control (non-exposed) group.

$$RR = \frac{P_{exposed}}{P_{control}}$$

For example, if the probability of developing lung cancer among smokers was 20% and among non-smokers 1%, then the relative risk of cancer associated with smoking would be 20. Smokers would be twenty times as likely as non-smokers to develop lung cancer.

In a simple comparison between an experimental group and a control group:

- A relative risk of 1 means there is no difference in risk between the two groups.

- A RR of ≤ 1 means the event is less likely to occur in the experimental group than in the control group.
- A RR of > 1 means the event is more likely to occur in the experimental group than in the control group.

The log of relative risk is usually taken to have a sampling distribution that has an approximately normal distribution. This permits the construction of a confidence interval (CI) which is symmetric around log(*RR*), i.e.

$$CI = \log(RR) \pm SE \times Z_{\alpha}$$

where z_{α} is the standard score for the chosen level of significance and SE the standard error. The antilog can be taken of the two bounds of the log-CI, giving the high and low bounds for an asymmetric confidence interval around the relative risk.

In regression models, the treatment is typically included as a dummy variable along with other factors that may affect risk. The relative risk is normally reported as calculated for the mean of the sample values of the explanatory variables.

Association with Odds Ratio

Relative risk is different from the odds ratio, although it asymptotically approaches it for small probabilities. In fact, the odds ratio has much wider use in statistics, since logistic regression, often associated with clinical trials, works with the log of the odds ratio, not relative risk. Because the log of the odds ratio is estimated as a linear function of the explanatory variables, the estimated odds ratio for 70-year-olds and 60-year-olds associated with type of treatment would be the same in a logistic regression models where the outcome is associated with drug and age, although the relative risk might be significantly different. In cases like this, statistical models of the odds ratio often reflect the underlying mechanisms more effectively.

Since relative risk is a more intuitive measure of effectiveness, the distinction is important especially in cases of medium to high probabilities. If action A carries a risk of 99.9% and action B a risk of 99.0% then the relative risk is just over 1, while the odds associated with action A are almost 10 times higher than the odds with B.

In medical research, the odds ratio is favoured for case-control studies and retrospective studies. Relative risk is used in randomized controlled trials and cohort studies.

In statistical modelling, approaches like poisson regression (for counts of events per unit exposure) have relative risk interpretations: the estimated effect of an explanatory variable is multiplicative on the rate, and thus leads to a risk ratio or relative risk. Logistic regression (for binary outcomes, or counts of successes out of a number of trials) must be interpreted in odds-ratio terms: the effect of an explanatory variable is multiplicative on the odds and thus leads to an odds ratio.

Size of Relative Risk and Relevance

In the standard or classical hypothesis testing framework, the null hypothesis is that RR=1 (the putative risk factor has no effect). The null hypothesis can be rejected in favour of the alternative hypothesis of that the factor in question does affect risk if the confidence interval for RR excludes 1.

Critics of the standard approach, notably including John Brignell and Steven Milloy, believe published studies suffer from unduly high type I error rates, and have argued for an additional requirement that the point estimate of RR should exceed 2 (or, if risks are reduced, be below 0.5) and have cited a variety of statements by statisticians and others supporting this view. The issue has arisen particularly in relation to debates about the effects of passive smoking, where the effect size appears to be small (relative to smoking), and exposure levels are difficult to quantify in the affected population.

In support of this claim, it may be observed that, if the base level of risk is low, a small proportionate increase in risk may be of little practical significance. (In the case of lung cancer, however, the base risk is substantial).

In addition, if estimates are biased by the exclusion of relevant factors, the likelihood of a spurious finding of significance is greater if the estimated RR is close to 1. In his paper "Why Most Published Research Findings Are False" John Ioannidis writes, "The smaller the effect sizes in a scientific field, the less likely the research findings are to be true. Research findings are more likely true in scientific fields with relative risks 3–20, than in scientific fields where postulated effects are small (relative risks 1.1–1.5). "If the majority of true genetic or nutritional determinants of complex diseases confer relative risks less than 1.05, genetic or nutritional epidemiology would be largely utopian endeavours."

In assessing results claiming an increase of relative risk arising from exposure to a hazard, statisticians and epidemiologists consider a range of factors including the size of the effect, the level of statistical significance, whether the results arise from a clinical trial or observation of a population, the significance of possible confounding factors, the extent to which results have been replicated, and the presence or absence of a biomedical model for the claimed effect. Important confounding factors for observational studies of health risks include tobacco smoking and social class.

While few statisticians accept the general claim that a relative risk level greater than 2 is required before a finding of increased risk can be accepted, most agree with this view in relation to findings from single studies without biomedical support. Marcia Angell of the New England Journal of Medicine has stated:

"As a general rule of thumb we are looking for a relative risk of three or more [before accepting a paper for publication], particularly if it is biologically implausible or if it's a brand-new finding".

Statistical Significance (Confidence) and Relative Risk

Whether a given relative risk can be considered statistically significant is dependent on the relative difference between the conditions compared, the amount of measurement and the noise associated with the measurement (of the events considered). In other words, the confidence one has, in a given relative risk being non-random (i.e. it is not a consequence of chance), depends on the signal-to-noise ratio and the sample size.

Expressed mathematically, the confidence that a result is not by random chance is given by the following formula by Sackett:

$$\text{Confidence} = \frac{\text{Signal}}{\text{Noise}} . \sqrt{\text{Sample Size.}}$$

For clarity, the above formula is presented in tabular form below:

Dependence of Confidence with Noise, Signal and Sample Size (Tabular Form)

Parameter	Parameter increases	Parameter decreases
Noise	Confidence decreases	Confidence increases
Signal	Confidence increases	Confidence decreases
Sample size	Confidence increases	Confidence decreases

In words, the confidence is higher if the noise is lower and/or the sample size is larger and/or the effect size (signal) is increased. The confidence of a relative risk value (and its associated confidence interval) is *not* dependent on effect size alone. If the sample size is large and the noise is low a small effect size can be measured with great confidence. Whether a small effect size is considered important is dependent on the context of the events compared.

In medicine, small effect sizes (reflected by small relative risk values) are usually considered clinically relevant (if there is great confidence in them) and are frequently used to guide treatment decisions. A relative risk of 1.10 may seem very small, but over a large number of patients will make a noticeable differencc. Whcther a given treatment is considered a worthy endeavour is dependent on the risks, benefits and costs.

Thc **numbcr needed to treat** (NNT) is an epidemiological measure that indicates how many patients would require treatment with a form of medication to reduce the expected number of cases of a defined endpoint by one. It is defined as the inverse of the absolute risk reduction. It was described in 1988.

For example, consider a hypothetical drug which reduces the risk of colon cancer by 50%. Even without the drug, colon cancer is fairly rare, may be 1 in 3,000 in every 5year period. The NNT for a 5-year treatment with the drug is therefore 6,000: by treating 6,000 people with the drug, one can expect to reduce the number of colon cancer cases from 2 to 1.

In general, NNT is always computed with respect to two treatments *A* and *B*, with *A* typically a drug and *B* a placebo (in our example above, *A* is a 5-year treatment with the hypothetical drug, and *B* is no treatment). A defined endpoint has to be specified (in our example: the appearance of colon cancer in the 5year period). If the probabilities p_A and p_B of this endpoint under treatments *A* and *B*, respectively, are known, then the NNT is computed as

$$1/(P_B - P_A).$$

The NNT is an important measure in pharmacoeconomics. If a clinical endpoint is devastating enough (*e.g.* death, heart attack), drugs with a high NNT may still be indicated in particular situations. If the endpoint is minor, health insurers may decline to reimburse drugs with a high NNT.

Abbreviation	Variable	Equation	Value
-	subjects in control group	-	250
-	subjects in experimental group	-	150
-	events in control group	-	100
-	events in experimental group	-	15
CER	control event rate	=event /subjects in control group	0.4, or 40%
EER	experimental event rate	=events/subjects in experimental group	0.1, or 10%
ARR	absolute risk reduction (or increase)	= CER - EER	0.3, or 30%
RRR	relative risk reduction (or increase)	= (CER - EER) / CER	0.75
NNT	**number needed to treat/** number needed to harm	= 1 / ARR	3.33
OR, RR	odds ratio, relative risk (not really identical, but similar)	= CER / EER	4

Odds Ratio

The **odds ratio** is a measure of effect size particularly important in Bayesian statistics and logistic regression.

It is defined as the ratio of the odds of an event occurring in one group to the odds of it occurring in another group, or to a sample-based estimate of that ratio. These groups might be men and women, an experimental group and a control group, or any other dichotomous classification. If the probabilities of the event in each of the groups are p (first group) and q (second group), then the odds ratio is:

$$\frac{\frac{p}{(1-p)}}{\frac{q}{(1-q)}} = \frac{P(1-q)}{q(1-p)}$$

An odds ratio of 1 indicates that the condition or event under study is equally likely in both groups. An odds ratio greater than 1 indicates that the condition or event is more likely in the first group. And an odds ratio less than 1 indicates that the condition or event is less likely in the first group. The odds ratio must be greater than or equal to zero. As the odds of the first group approaches zero, the odds ratio approaches zero. As the odds of the second group approaches zero, the odds ratio approaches positive infinity.

For example, suppose that in a sample of 100 men, 90 have drunk wine in the previous week, while in a sample of 100 women only 20 have drunk wine in the same period. The odds of a man drinking wine are 90 to 10, or 9:1, while the odds of a woman drinking wine are only 20 to 80, or 1:4 = 0.25:1. Now, 9/0.25 = 36, so the odds ratio is 36, showing that men are much more likely to drink wine than women. Using the above formula for the calculation yields:

$$\frac{0.9/0.1}{0.2/0.8} = \frac{0.9 \times 0.8}{0.1 \times 0.2} = \frac{0.72}{0.02} = 36$$

This example also shows how odds ratios can sometimes seem to overstate relative positions: in this sample men are 4.5 times more likely to have drunk wine than women, but have 36 times the odds.

Taking the logarithm of the odds ratio ameliorates this effect, and also improves symmetry. For example, using natural logarithms, an odds ratio of 36 maps to 3.584, an odds ratio of one maps to zero, and an odds ratio of 1/36 maps to -3.584.

The logarithm of the odds ratio is the difference of the logistics of the probabilities.

The increased use of logistic regression in medical and social science research means that the odds ratio is commonly used as a means of expressing the results in some forms of clinical trials, in survey research, and in epidemiology, such as in case-control studies. It is often abbreviated "OR" in reports. When data from multiple surveys is combined, it will often be expressed as "Pooled OR".

Calculating and Interpreting Odds Ratios

The Odds Ratio is a widely used statistic to compare the frequency of exposure to risk factors in epidemiological studies. Most people will be familiar with odds from betting, and odds ratios are simply comparing the retrospective/ posterior odds of exposure to a given risk factor in two groups of individuals (there are special methods that allow you to calculate multiple levels of odds ratio, these are mentioned briefly at the end.

Calculating Odds Ratios

Calculating the odds-ratio for a set of data is fairly straight-forward, you need to construct a contingency table in the same manner as you do for χ^2 calculations, although in this instance you should *always* have the cases in the first row and the risk factor in the first column.

Working Example

Suppose you have a cohort of cases and controls, for a particular disease (choose your disease of preference, it really makes no difference, you will still divide individuals into cases or controls dependent upon their disease status). You have collected 248 cases with the disease, and 246 controls who are matched on age and sex to help avoid confounding factors. You have decided to screen for mutations in candidate gene X which is involved in some biological aspect of the disease, and you have identified ten polymorphic loci within the gene, three are in the promoter region, three are within exons but are synonymous, two are intronic, and one is exonic and causes a non-synonymous amino-acid substitution.

For each SNP you should construct the contingency table shown below:

	Allele 1	Allele 2	Total
Cases	A = 332	B = 164	496
Controls	C = 230	D = 262	492
Total	562	426	988

In order to calculate your odds-Ratio you need to calculate the odds of exposure to the risk factor (in this case allele 1) in the cases and the controls independently. The odds in the cases and controls are calculated as shown below, along with a few simple algebraic simplifications to aid in the calculation.

Odds of Exposure in Cases = A x (A + B)/ B x (A + B) = A / B

= 332 / 164 = 2.0244

Odds of Exposure in Controls = C x (C + D) / D x (C + D)

= C / D = 230 / 262 = 0.8779

You then calculate the Odds Ratio by dividing the odds in the cases by the odds in the controls which is shown below:

Odds Ratio = 2.0244 / 0.8779 = 2.306

The same simplification of inverting the numerator and denominator of the fraction you are dividing by and multiplying the two fractions together can be used to give one simple formula for the calculation of the odds ratio as shown below:

Odds Ratio $= {}^{(A/B)}/_{(C/D)} = (A \times D)/(B \times C) = (332 \times 262)/(164 \times 230) = 2.306$
and it is this formula that you should use to calculate your Odds Ratio.

Calculating the Odds Ratio for exposure to a risk factor is fine, as it is only based on the sample you have made from a population, it is essentially only an estimate. The accuracy of this estimate is in part determined by the size of your sample, and in general the larger the sample size the better (although you should be cautious of over-interpreting Odds Ratios from studies with huge sample sizes). For this reason it is conventional to calculate the 95% Confidence Interval (CI) for the Odds Ratio.

There are several different ways of calculating a CI for the odds ratio, however one method provided by Woolf will suffice, and is shown below:

95% CI of ln(OR) $= \ln(OR) \pm 1.96(^1/_A + ^1/_B + ^1/_C + ^1/_D)^{0.5}$

For the above example this works out as being:

95% CI of ln(OR) $= \ln(OR) \pm 1.96(^1/_{332} + ^1/_{164} + ^1/_{230} + ^1/_{262})^{0.5}$

$= \ln(OR) \pm 1.96(0.0030125 + 0.00609756 + 0.00434783 + 0.00381679)^{0.5}$

$= \ln(OR) \pm 1.96(0.01727423)^{0.5}$

$= \ln(OR) \pm 1.96 \times 0.13143146$

$= \ln(OR) \pm 0.25760567$

$= 0.83551442 \pm 0.2576056$

95% CI of ln(OR) = 0.57790875 to 1.0931201

95% CI of OR = $e^{0.57790875}$ to $e^{0.25760567}$

95% CI of OR = 1.7823073 to 2.9835686

The above example is to calculate a 95% Confidence Interval, if you wished to calculate an alternative width confidence interval then you would simply replace the 1.96 in the above equation with the appropriate value from the standard normal distribution.

Interpreting Odds Ratio

In order to interprete the odds ratio you need to have calculated a confidence interval as shown above. You can say that a proposed risk factor acts as a significant risk to disease if the odds ratio is greater than one **and** the lower bound of the confidence interval does **not** go below 1.

Getting Computers to Do the Work For You

To sit down and calculate odds ratio statistics for each and every SNP that you are testing would take you maybe an hour or so, however there is a much easier solution, and that is to use a computer program to do this for you. The use of stata to calculate allelic and genotypic associations can be found from the software available in market nowadays.

7.3 DIAGNOSTIC TESTS

Correct diagnosis forms an important and indispensible part of clinical practice. Much of the medical research is carried out to improve the method of diagnosis.

Assessment of validity and reliability of a diagnostic and screening test is essential not only for medical research but also to provide appropriate and effective health care. This is important issue both in clinical practice as well as, in the Planning of Public Health intervention programmes.

Working Example

Sputum sample of a total of 5776 pulmonary TB patients were examined by direct Smear and culture examination. The DS examination of sputum was carried out by Z N staining technique which is the only cost effective tool for diagnosis of patients with infection 2-4 tuberculosis, the technique consists of making a Smear and drying it for 15-30 minutes, fixing it over the flame and staining with steaming hot carbol fuchsin for 5 minutes, decolorisation with 25% sulphuric acid for 2-4 minutes and counterstaining with 0.1 % methylene blue for half a minute and examining under oil immersion lens of microscope. the detection limit with this method is 5x103 bacilli/ml. of sputum. Increasing concentration of sputum sample has been found to increase the sensitivity. The culture of M tuberculosis from the sputum sample is taken as gold standard for diagnosis of tuberculosis.

Out of 5776 sputum samples examined by ZN staining, 1169 were found positive for A F B as 1889 were positive by culture. 720 samples found negative by DS examination were observed by culture.

Relationship Between DS Culture for Diagnosis of Pulmonary TB (n = 5776)

DS	Culture on LJ Medium (PTB)		Total
	Positive	Negative	
Positive	1169	44	1213
Negative	720	3843	4563
Total	1889	3887	5776

Sensitivity of DS (i.e. proportion of true positive identified Correctly) in the above study is:

$$\text{Sensitivity} = \frac{TP}{TP + FN} = \frac{1169}{1169+720} = 0.62 = 62\%$$

Specificity of DS (i.e. proportion of true negative identified correctly) in the above study is:

$$\text{Sepecificity} = \frac{TN}{TN + TP} = \frac{3843}{3843 + 44} = 0.99 = 99\%$$

PPV = Positive Predictive Value

$$= \frac{\text{Px Sensitivity}}{\text{P} \times \text{sensitivity} + \text{(1-P) (1-sensitivity)}} \quad 100; \text{ P is the prevalence}$$

= TP/ (TP+FP) =1169/1213 =96.4%

NPV = Negative Predictive Value.

$$= \frac{\text{(1-p)} \times \text{specificity}}{\text{(I-P) Specificity + P (1-sensitivity)}} \quad 100 \text{ ; P is the prevalence}$$

$$= \frac{TN}{TN + FN} = \frac{3843}{4563} = 84.2\%.$$

The sensitivity and specificity values gives a direct assessment of usefulness of the test in practice and are not affected by the proportion of subjects with the abnormality, i.e., the prevalence. However to know how good the test is at predicting abnormality, one has to find the probability of index test for giving correct diagnosis, whether positive or negative. These two proportions are expressed as "Positive Predictive Value" (PPV) and the "Negative Predictive Value (NPV)" the specificity and sensitivity remain unchanged despite the change in prevalence of abnormality. The predictive values, in contrast, are clinically useful but depend strongly on the prevalence. This fact should be borne in mind while interpreting their results. the predictive value of a test thus depends upon the prevalence of the abnormality being tested, which may or may not be known. The more uncommon is the true abnormality, the more certain we can be that a negative test indicates no abnormality and less sure that a positive result really indicates an abnormal patient.

Whenever a single diagnostic test is used for diagnosing any disease, its accuracy is bound to be poor if the prevalence of the disease in the population being examined is low, this is true even for a test, which is known to be highly sensitive and specific. Therefore, in order to increase the accuracy, the prevalence among examined would have to be increased. This can be done by pre-selection of the subjects.

The simplest diagnostic test is one where the results of an investigation, such as an x-ray examination or biopsy, are used to classify patients into two groups according to the presence or absence of a symptom or sign. For example, the table shows the relation between the results of a test, a liver scan, and the correct diagnosis based on either necropsy, biopsy, or surgical inspection. How good is the liver scan at diagnosis of abnormal pathology?

Relation between results of liver scan and correct diagnosis			
	Pathology		
Liver scan	Abnormal (+)	Normal (-)	Total
Abnormal(+)	231	32	263
Normal(-)	27	54	81
Total	258	86	344

One approach is to calculate the proportions of patients with normal and abnormal liver scans who are correctly "diagnosed" by the scan. The terms positive and negative are used to refer to the presence or absence of the condition of interest, here abnormal pathology. Thus there are 258 true positives and 86 true negatives. The proportions of these two groups that were correctly diagnosed by the scan were 231/258=0.90 and 54/86=0.63 respectively. These two proportions have confusingly similar names.

Sensitivity is the proportion of true positives that are correctly identified by the test.

Specificity is the proportion of true negatives that are correctly identified by the test.

We can thus say that, based on the sample studied, we would expect 90% of patients with abnormal pathology to have abnormal (positive) liver scans, while 63% of those with normal pathology would have normal (negative) liver scans.

The sensitivity and specificity are proportions, so confidence intervals can be calculated for them using standard methods for proportions.

Sensitivity and specificity are one approach to quantifying the diagnostic ability of the test. In clinical practice, however, the test result is all that is known, so we want to know how good the test is at predicting abnormality. In other words, what proportion of patients with abnormal test results are truly abnormal? This question is addressed in a subsequent note.

The whole point of a diagnostic test is to use it to make a diagnosis, so we need to know the probability that the test will give the correct diagnosis. The sensitivity and specificity do not give us this information. Instead we must approach the data from the direction of the test results, using predictive values.

Positive predictive value is the proportion of patients with positive test results who are correctly diagnosed.

Negative predictive value is the proportion of patients with negative test results who are correctly diagnosed.

Using the same data as in the previous note, we know that 231 of 263 patients with abnormal liver scans had abnormal pathology, giving the proportion of correct diagnoses as 231/263 = 0.88. Similarly, among the 81 patients with normal liver scans the proportion of correct diagnoses was 54/81 = 0.59. These proportions are of only limited validity, however. The predictive values of a test in clinical practice depend critically on the prevalence of the abnormality in the patients being tested; this may well differ from the prevalence in a published study assessing the usefulness of the test.

In the liver scan study the prevalence of abnormality was 0.75. If the same test was used in a different clinical setting where the prevalence of abnormality was 0.25 we would have a positive predictive value of 0.45 and a negative predictive value of 0.95. The rarer the abnormality the more sure we can be that a negative test indicates no abnormality, and the less sure that a positive result really indicates an abnormality. Predictive values observed in one study do not apply universally.

The positive and negative predictive values (PPV and NPV) can be calculated for any prevalence as follows:

$$\text{PPV} = \frac{\text{Sensitivity x prevalence}}{\text{Sensitivity x prevalence + (1 - specificity) x (1 - prevalence)}}$$

$$\text{NPV} = \frac{\text{Specificity x (1 - prevalence)}}{\text{(1 - sensitivity) x prevalence + specificity x (1– prevalence)}}$$

If the prevalence of the disease is very low, the positive predictive value will not be closc to 1 even if both the sensitivity and specificity are high. Thus in screening the general population it is inevitable that many people with positive test results will be false positives.

The prevalence can be interpreted as the probability before the test is carried out that the subject has the disease, known as the prior probability of disease. The positive and negative predictive values are the revised estimates of the same probability for those subjects who are positive and negative on the test, and are known as posterior probabilities. The difference between the prior and posterior probabilities is one way of assessing the usefulness of the test.

For any test result we can compare the probability of getting that result if the patient truly had the condition of interest with the corresponding probability if he or she were healthy. The ratio of these probabilities is called the likelihood ratio, calculated as sensitivity/ (1 - specificity).

The likelihood ratio indicates the value of the test for increasing certainty about a positive diagnosis. For the liver scan data the prevalence of abnormal pathology was 0.75, so the pre-test odds of disease were 0.75/(1 -0.75) = 3.0. The sensitivity was 0.895 and the specificity was 0.628. The post-test odds of disease given a positive test is 0.878/(1 -0.878) = 7.22, and the likelihood ratio is 0.895/(1 - 0.628) = 2.41. The post test odds of having the disease is the pre-test odds multiplied by the likelihood ratio.

A high likelihood ratio may show that the test is useful, but it does not necessarily follow that a positive test is a good indicator of the presence of disease.

We have previously considered diagnosis based on tests that give a yes or no answer. Many diagnostic tests, however, are quantitative, notably in clinical chemistry. The same statistical approach can be used only if we can select a cut off point to distinguish "normal" from "abnormal", which is not a trivial problem. Firstly, we can investigate to what extent the test results differ among people who do or do not have the diagnosis of interest. The receiver operating characteristic (ROC) plot is one way to do this. These plots were developed in the 1950s for evaluating radar signal detection. Only recently have they become commonly used in medicine.

We assume that high values are more likely among those dubbed "abnormal". The usefulness of the test for predicting graft versus host disease will clearly relate to the degree of non-overlap between the two distributions.

CHAPTER 8 VITAL STATISTICS

8.1 INTRODUCTION

Vital statistics are derived from information obtained at the time when the occurrences of vital events and their characteristics are inscribed in a civil register. Vital acts and events are the births, deaths, fetal deaths, marriages, and all such events that have something to do with an individual's entrance and departure from life together with the changes in civil status that may occur to a person during his lifetime. Recording of these events in the civil register is known as vital or civil registration and the resulting documents are called vital records.

8.2 STRUCTURE OF VITAL STATISTICS SYSTEM

The production of vital statistics comprised a system of operations in which the registration of vital events is an important component. The system begins with the registration followed by the processing and controlling of vital records and ends with the compilation and analysis of vital statistics. Under Commonwealth Act (CA) 591, the Bureau of Census [now National Statistics Office - (NSO)] is mandated to generate general purpose statistics and to carry out and administer Act No. 3753. Under the same law, the head of the NSO is also the Civil Registrar General (CRG) who directs and supervises the local civil registration activities in the country. The CRG in this regard is empowered to prepare and issue implementing rules and regulations on civil registration and to prepare and order printed the necessary forms for proper compliance. The set-up of vital statistics system involves different entities and cuts across different departments and personalities. For the registration of vital events, the Local Civil Registry Offices (LCROs), which are the registration units in the country and headed by the City/Municipal Civil Registrars (C/MCRs), are under the Local Government Units (LGUs). The hospitals, clinics, rural health units and similar institutions including barangay secretaries, practising physicians, midwives, nurses, traditional midwives, solemnizing officers from various religious sects and denomination are required to assist in the reporting of vital events for registration at the LCROs. The concerned parents, next of kin, contracting parties, a witness or the person who has full knowledge of the occurrence of the event are also required to report the event, in default of the first mentioned set of informants. The processing and controlling of vital documents are done at the LCROs and at the NSO Provincial and Central Offices. The compilation and analysis of vital statistics is taken cared of by the NSO Central Office under the Vital Statistics Division (VSD) of the Civil Registration Department. Handling of documents through automated processing of data entry, data cleaning, file updating, and generation of preliminary tables at the LCRO level are done through the use of Civil Registry Information System (CRIS). This system enhances the capability of LCROs to attend to the growing demand for birth, marriage and death certification and information on these vital events on for local and policy makers. However, only LCROs with computers are able to avail of the CRIS. At NSO, the automation is made possible through the use of Decentralized Vital Statistics System (DVSS). For this report, two versions of DVSS were used. For the processing of January to December 2003 registrations, the DOS based DVSS was utilized while the January to March 2004 documents, the enhanced windows based DVSS called DVSS 2000 or DVSS2K, was used. Such enhancements were made possible through the civil registration system information technology project or CRS - ITP.

8.3 REGISTRATION METHOD

As mandated in Act 3753, all vital events that marked the entry and departure of a person in his lifetime and the changes in his/her civil status shall be registered. The registration method is defined as the continuous, permanent and compulsory recording of the occurrences and characteristics of vital events, primarily for their value as legal documents and secondary for their usefulness as a source of statistics.

Place Where to Register the Event

As a general rule, the place of registration is the LCRO of the city of municipality where the vital events occur. Out of town reporting of vital event occurs when the documents presented to the civil registrar of LCRO, which is not the place of occurrence, not for registration but to be forwarded to the civil registrar of LCRO where the event occurred and where it should be registered.

Forms to Use

The civil register consists of certificates and the registry book. It also includes the actual copies of the registrable court decisions and the legal instruments concerning the civil status of persons. The certificates are loose-leaf forms in a set of four copies except for the Certificate of Foundling which is in a set of three.

Person Who Will Report the Event

The informant is the one who reports the event for registration and who gives information to be recorded in the civil register. In case of live birth, the law requires the hospital or clinic administrator or his representative if the birth occurred in the hospital or clinic. If the birth occurred elsewhere, the attendant who may either be a physician, nurse, license midwife or traditional birth attendant makes the report. In default of the hospital authority, or the attendant, the responsibility of reporting the births devolves upon either or both parents or upon a person who has full knowledge of the facts of birth and filiation of the child. For death occurrences, the report shall be made by the hospital or clinic administrator if the person dies in the hospital or clinic, or by attending physician or by the nearest relative or by any interested party who has knowledge of the occurrence of death. In all cases, the report shall be submitted to the Local Health Officer (LHO) who shall direct and order the C/MCR to enter the death in the civil register. In case of marriages, the solemnizing officer is required by law to report the event. In default of the solemnizing officer, the duty is lodged upon contracting parties.

Period When to Report the Event

Live births shall be reported for registration to C/MCR not later than thirty days from the date of birth.

Death or fetal death shall be reported to LHO within forty eight hours from the time of death and the LHO shall direct or cause the registration to the C/MCR not later than thirty days from date of death.

Marriages that require the issuance of marriages license shall be reported to C/MCR for registration not later than fifteen days from the date of marriage. However, marriages that do not require a license such as marriage at the point of death; marriages in remote places; marriages between members of ethnic cultural community and marriages between men and women who have lived together for at least five years, shall be reported not later than thirty days after the date of marriage.

Any report made to the LCROs beyond the regulatary period are considered late and can be entered only in the civil register after the informant complies with the requirements for delayed registration.

Operative Act of Registration

The C/MCR sees to it that appropriate form it used; form is properly and completely filled-up; and proper attachments are submitted. In case, the entries are found incomplete, the C/MCR has to require the person concerned to fill up the document completely or to correct the entries.

When the document is accepted for registration, the date of receipt is recorded in the space provided and the documents received for the day are entered immediately in the appropriate civil registry book, assigning therein the corresponding registry number. After registration entry/entries found erroneous can only be corrected through RA 9048, except sex, nationality, age and status which require court approval.

Distribution of Registered Documents

Upon registration, the C/MCR distributes the copies accordingly: the first copy to the informant; the second copy to the CRG; the third copy shall be retained by the LCRO; and the fourth copy to the attendant or solemnizing officer, as the case may be. The CRG copy is the source of vital statistics for the report

8.4 DEFINITION OF TERMS AND CONCEPTS

Significant terminologist and descriptions in the foregoing highlights and tables are defined below. Included are some items found in the certificates and summary measure used in describing the facts of events.

Live Birth is a complete expulsion or extraction from its mother of a product of conception, irrespective of the duration of the pregnancy, which after such separation, breathes or shows any other evidence of life, such as beating of the heart, pulsation of the umbilical cord, or definite movement of voluntary muscles, whether or not the umbilical cord has been cut or the placenta is attached; each product of such a birth is considered live born.

Marriage is a contract of permanent union between a man and a woman entered into in accordance with law for the establishment of conjugal and family life.

Death refers to the permanent disappearance of all evidence of life at any time after live birth has taken place (postnatal cessation of vital function without capability of resuscitation).

Fetal Death refers to death prior to the complete expulsion or extraction of a product of conception from its mother, irrespective of the duration of pregnancy; the death is indicated by the fact that after such separation, the fetus does not breathe or show any other evidence of life, such as beating of the heart, pulsation of the umbilical cord, and definite movement of voluntary muscles.

Early Neonatal Death refers to death among live births during the first 7 days of life.

Infant Mortality refers to deaths of infants under one year of age.

Peri natal Mortality refers to the deaths of fetuses, weighing at least 500 grams or had 22 completed weeks of gestation, and of infants 7 days of age.

Maternal Mortality refers to the death of a woman while pregnant or within 42 days of termination of pregnancy, irrespective of the duration and the site of the pregnancy, from any cause related to or aggravated by the pregnancy or its management, but not from accidental or incidental causes.

Neonatal Mortality refers to deaths among live births during the first 28 completed days of life.

Crude Birth Rate (CBR) refers to the number of live births per 1,000 mid-year population.

Crude Marriage Rate (CMR) is a gross measure of the level of the relative frequency of marriages in an area for a given year. It expresses additions, by the formal means of legal marriage, being made to the married segment of the total population. This refers to the number of marriages per 1,000 mid-year population.

Crude Death Rate (CDR) refers to the number of deaths per 1,000 mid-year population.

Infant Mortality Rate (IMR) refers to the number of infant deaths per 1,000 live births in a given year.

Maternal Mortality Rate (MMR) refers to the number of maternal deaths in a given year per 100,000 live births in that year.

Total Fertility Rate (TFR) refers to the average number of children a woman would have by the time she reached age of 50, if she were to experience the Average Specific Fertility Rates of a given year.

Age Specific Fertility Rate (ASFR) refers to the number of live births born to a woman of a given age or age group by the mid-year female population of the same age or age group during the same year. This refers to average number of births per 1,000 females of specific age group.

Crude Rate of Natural Increase (CRNI) refers to the difference between crude birth rate and crude death rate.

Natural Increase refers to the excess of births over deaths.

Birth Order refers to the numerical order of a child in relation to all previous pregnancies of the mother.

Daily Average refers to the arithmetic mean of birth, death or marriage occurrences per day.

Daily Index is the increase/decrease from the overall daily average of event occurrences.

Period of Gestation refers to the number of completed weeks which have elapsed between the first day of the last normal menstrual period and the date of delivery irrespective of whether the product of conception was live-born or born without evidence of life.

Sex Ratio refers to the number of males per one hundred females.

Usual Residence refers to the place where the person habitually or permanently resides.

Place of Occurrence refers to the place where the vital event took place.

Content and Coverage of Publication

Vital registration is a continuous process. Hence, there is a need to establish certain cut-off period. For example if the data presented are vital events that occurred in 2003 and were registered in January 2003 to March 2004. Events occurring in 2003 but were registered beyond March 2004 were no longer included in the generation of 2003 Vital Statistics. For interpretation of data, caution is necessary since information presented is not adjusted for under registration. Observed marked fluctuations in vital events for specific areas may not necessarily reflect differentials, but rather an indication of variations in registration/registered submission of events.

8.5 SOURCES OF DATA

Vital Statistics data come from Certificates of Live Birth, Certificates of Fetal Death, Certificates of Death, Certificates of Marriage and Certificates of Dissolution. The forms for these certificates are provided by State Department of Health. The following table describes who completes the forms and where they are filed:

Filing of State Vital Statistics		
Certificate	**Completed by**	**Initially filed with**
Live Birth	Hospital or Birth Attendant	State Dept. of Health
Fetal Death	Hospital or Birth Attendant	Local Health Jurisdiction
Death	Funeral Director, Physician, Coroner or Medical Examiner	Local Health Jurisdiction
Marriage	Person Performing the Marriage	County Auditor
Dissolution	Clerk of Court, Petitioner's Attorney	County Clerk
Abortions	Abortion Providers	State Dept. of Health

The registration and reporting of vital statistics requires births, fetal deaths, deaths, marriages, and dissolutions of marriage to be reported within a timely fashion. Birth and death certificates are designed to gather information in a manner consistent with federal reporting requirements of the National Center for Health Statistics.

The Registrar General of India for Health Statistics actually registers only those vital events occurring in country. However, a formal interstate exchange agreement governs the mutual exchange of information on births and deaths between states and other countries so that events occurring to Indian residents elsewhere are also reported to this office. Such an interstate exchange agreement does not exist, however, for marriages and divorces. Therefore, the Center for Health Statistics does not have the records for all of the state's residents since some may have gone elsewhere to be married or divorced. Interstate agreement between most states ensures comparative arrangement between vital records offices.

Data may either be tabulated by residence (where the person lived) or by occurrence (where the event occurred). City data are generally less reliable than county data. The city of residence is assigned by whether or not the person reportedly lived within city limits using responses to an item on the certificate: "Inside city limits– yes/no." If the response to this item is "yes", "unknown", or blank, the place of residence is assigned to the reported city. If the response is "no", the place of residence is assigned a "balance of county" code. Reporting on this item has been found to be somewhat unreliable when compared to locating addresses within city boundaries using geocoding software. For city of occurrence there is no "inside city limits" item to use for coding. If a city is given on the certificate, the event is coded as occurring within city limits of that city. However, if the place of occurrence lists a rural road, state park, or other remote location, the place of occurrence is coded to "balance of county".

Numbers vs. Crude or Age-Adjusted Rates

When should numbers or rates be used? The number of events can be used to determine the size of a problem in any area (e.g., how many people die of cancer) or to estimate population changes due to birth and death. But, using just numbers, we cannot readily compare two areas or two time periods. Such comparisons should take the size of the population into account to avoid erroneous conclusions.

To eliminate the effect of different sized populations, we compare rates. A rate is the number of vital events (such as deaths) in a specified time period divided by the number of people at risk of these events in that period (typically, a state or county population, or the number of births in the case of infant death). This figure is generally multiplied by a constant such as 1,000 or 100,000 to get a number that is easy to read and compare and is reported as "per 1,000" or "per 100,000".

Rates calculated in this manner are called **crude rates**. They adjust for differences in population size but not differences in population characteristics. These population characteristics also need to be considered in interpreting comparisons. For example, since death rates increase with increasing age, a county with an older population may have higher death rates just because its population is older.

To compare rates and see if the county is high just because of its older population, we need to use **age-adjusted death rates**. These rates are computed by taking a county's death rates for each age group and applying them to a standard population. When comparing age-adjusted rates, it is important to compare rates that use the same standard population.

The age-adjusted death rate tells us what the county's death rate would be if it had the same age distribution as the standard population. The major use of age-adjusted death rates is to allow comparisons between different areas and/or over various periods of time. Users should be aware that an age-adjusted death rate has no absolute meaning; it is an artificial number based on a hypothetical population and is only useful for comparing with other rates calculated in the same manner.

Although reports often focus on which population has the highest rate, one should remember that rates can mask differences in numbers that may be needed for policy decisions. For example, the infant mortality rate is considerably higher for many people of color than for whites. However, due to the state's racial composition, most infants who die in this state are white. To reduce racial disparity, one would focus on reducing infant mortality among people of color. Such a reduction, however, would not necessarily have much effect on the state's overall infant mortality rate. In determining the burden of a health problem in a community, numbers are usually the most appropriate measure.

Small Numbers

How should small numbers be handled? If the state collects all births and deaths in a year, then aren't the birth and death rates exactly as calculated?

It's certainly true that vital statistics are not based on samples of the population, as many research data are. We do know the actual number of births, deaths, and population (assuming complete reporting of events), so we can calculate an exact birth or death rate for any one year. However, the data may still be affected by random fluctuations in the number of events between successive measurements (e.g., for different years).

The effect of such random fluctuations on birth or death rates is proportionately larger when the number of events is small. For example, one more infant death has a larger numerical impact on an area with 3 deaths than it does on an area with 300 deaths. Because of these random fluctuations, the rates based on small numbers may not be as reliable as those based on larger numbers in the sense that they may have limited predictive value.

Cause of Death

The causes of death presented in this chapter are classified in accordance with the International Classification of Diseases, Tenth Revision published by the World Health Organization. The State of Washington began using this revision on January 1, 1999. The ninth revision was used for 1980-1998. The change to ICD-10 will create a discontinuity in trends that must be accounted for when comparing 1999 mortality to prior years. To put it another way, **1999 cause-of-death data are not comparable to prior years**, unless adjustments are made for the coding and classification changes. Without adjustment, it is impossible to know whether an observed increase or decrease in deaths due to a particular cause is "real" or merely the result of the changes in classification and coding.

Tabulated causes of death in this chapter are based on the underlying cause of death. The underlying cause of death is defined as "(a) the disease or injury which initiated the train of events leading directly to death or (b) the circumstances of the accident or violence which produced the fatal injury." International (World Health Organization) rules are used to determine the underlying cause of death using data supplied by the certifier in the "cause of death" and "other significant conditions" sections of the death certificate.

Due to the detailed nature of the ICD classification system, it is common to group ICD codes into more general categories for analysis and comparison purposes. The National Center for Health Statistics (NCHS) provides one of the most commonly used classification systems in which causes of deaths for adults are grouped into 113 separate groups and deaths for infants into 130 groups.

Some Definitions

Birth Weight - Weight of fetus or infant at time of delivery (normally recorded in pounds and ounces).

Fetal Death - Death prior to the complete expulsion or extraction from its mother of a product of human conception, irrespective of the duration of pregnancy. The death is indicated by the fact that after such expulsion or extraction the fetus does not breathe or show any other evidence of life such as beating of the heart, pulsation of the umbilical cord, or definite movement of voluntary muscles. Reporting official deaths to the state is required only when the gestational period is twenty weeks or more.

Infant Death - Death of a child under one year of age.

Live Birth - The complete expulsion or extraction from its mother of a product of human conception, irrespective of the duration of pregnancy, which, after such expulsion or extraction, breathes, or shows any other evidence of life such as beating of the heart, pulsation of the umbilical cord, or definite movement of voluntary muscles, whether or not the umbilical cord has been cut or the placenta is attached.

Abortion - The termination (spontaneous or induced) of a pregnancy before the fetus has attained viability. Consistent with common usage and understanding, when the term abortion is used in this report, it refers to induced abortion.

Gestational Period - Number of weeks elapsed between the first day of the last menstrual period and date of delivery or date of pregnancy termination. The term gestational period is interchangeable with weeks of gestation, gestational age, and duration of pregnancy. This report uses the physician's estimate of gestational age.

Induced Abortion - The purposeful interruption of pregnancy, irrespective of the duration of pregnancy, with the intention other than to produce a live born infant or to remove a dead fetus, the result of which is not a live birth. Procedures for false pregnancy, ectopic pregnancy, and miss abortion (dead ovum retained in uterus in intended pregnancy) are not included in the definition. The term is used in this report interchangeably with induced termination of pregnancy, induced termination and abortion.

Live Birth Order - Total number of live births to a given mother, including current birth.

Maternal Death - Death attributed to complications of pregnancy, childbirth, or the puerperium (ICD-10 O00-O99) for women of childbearing age; includes abortion-related death.

Neonatal Death - Death of an infant within the first 27 days of life.

Nulliparous - Having never given birth to a liveborn infant.

Occurrence Data - Data allocated by place where the event occurred, regardless of the person's place of residence.

Parity - Total number of previous live births; does not include the current birth.

Perinatal Death - Fetal deaths of 20 or more weeks' gestation plus infant deaths of less than seven days. This is one of four definitions used by the National Center for Health Statistics. Caution should be used in comparing perinatal death rates with rates from other sources unless it is certain that the same definition has been used.

Plurality - The number of siblings born as the result of a single pregnancy (e.g., twins, triplets).

Postneonatal Death - Death of an infant of 28-364 days of age.

Pregnancy - The sum of abortions (induced terminations), live births, and fetal deaths (spontaneous terminations) reported to the state. This figure underestimates the actual number of pregnancies because fetal deaths are required to be reported to the state only for gestational ages of 20 weeks or more. Thus, early fetal deaths (commonly called 'miscarriages') are not included in the total.

Premature Birth - A live birth weighing 2,500 grams (5-1/2 pounds) or less. If birth weight is not stated, length of gestation (under 37 weeks) is used.

Residence Data - Data allocated by place of residence of the child's mother (births, fetal deaths), or by place of residence of the decedent (deaths), regardless of where the event occurred.

Underlying Cause of Death - The disease or injury which initiated the train of morbid events leading directly or indirectly to death or the circumstances of the accident or violence which produced the fatal injury.

Rates and Ratios

Rounding of Rates - Rates are rounded to the nearest tenth. When the rate or percent is less than one-tenth, the entry is 0. Rates are not calculated when the number of events is less than 5.

Rates and ratios are calculated by dividing the number of events of concern by the population at risk (or a related population) and multiplying by a standard constant (i.e., 1,000 or 10,000 or 100,000).

What is Incidence?

Incidence is a measure of disease that allows us to determine a person's probability of being diagnosed with a disease during a given period of time. Therefore, incidence is the number of newly diagnosed cases of a disease. An incidence rate is the number of new cases of a disease divided by the number of persons at risk for the disease. If, over the course of one year, five women are diagnosed with breast cancer, out of a total female study population of 200 (who do not have breast cancer at the beginning of the study period), then we would say the incidence of breast cancer in this population was 0.025 (or 2,500 per 100,000 women-years of study).

What is Prevalence?

Prevalence is a measure of disease that allows us to determine a person's likelihood of having a disease. Therefore, the number of prevalent cases is the total number of cases of disease existing in a population. A prevalence rate is the total number of cases of a disease existing in a population divided by the total population. So, if a measurement of cancer is taken in a population of 40,000 people and 1,200 were recently diagnosed with cancer and 3,500 are living with cancer, then the prevalence of cancer is 0.118 (or 11,750 per 100,000 persons).

What is Morbidity?

Morbidity is another term for illness. A person can have several co-morbidities simultaneously. So, morbidities can range from Alzheimer's disease to cancer to traumatic brain injury. Morbidities are NOT deaths. Prevalence is a measure often used to determine the level of morbidity in a population.

What is Mortality?

Mortality is another term for death. A mortality rate is the number of deaths due to a disease divided by the total population. If there are 25 lung cancer deaths in one year in a population of 30,000, then the mortality rate for that population is 83 per 100,000.

8.6 DEMOGRAPHY

Map of countries by population

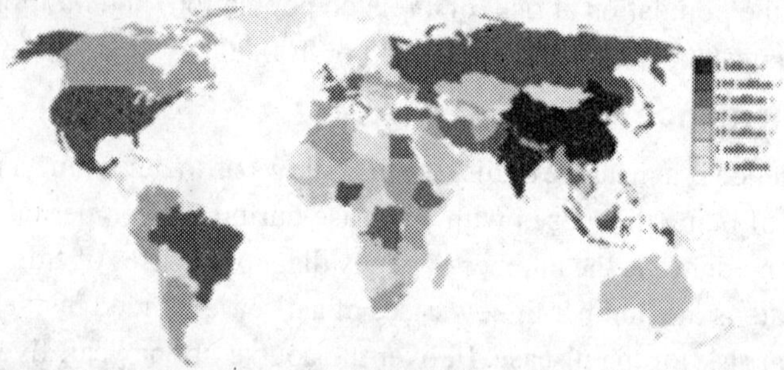

Map of countries by population

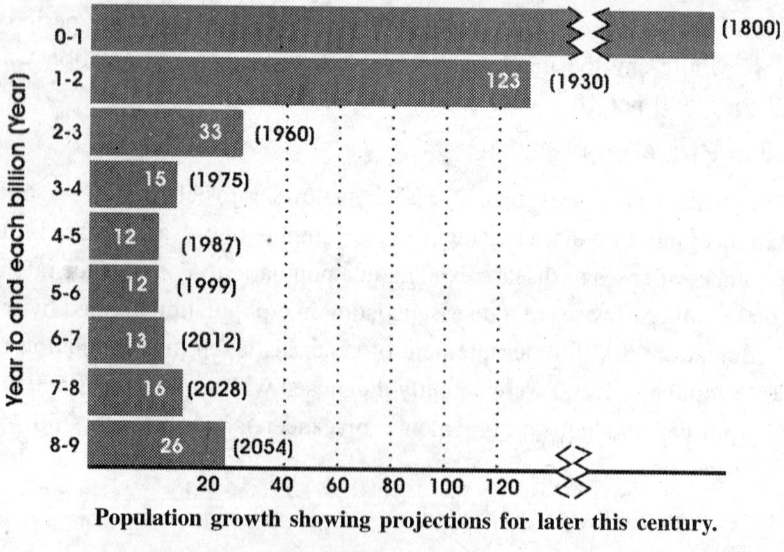

Population growth showing projections for later this century.

Demography is the statistical study of all populations. It can be a very general science that can be applied to any kind of dynamic population, that is, one that changes over time or space . It encompasses the study of the size, structure and distribution of populations, and spatial and/or temporal changes in them in response to birth, death, migration and aging.

Human demography is the most well known discipline of demography, and typically what people refer to when using the term demography. Demographic analysis can be applied to whole societies or to groups defined by criteria such as education, nationality, religion and ethnicity. In academia, demography is often regarded as a branch of either anthropology, economics, or sociology. **Formal demography** limits its object of study to the measurement of populations processes, while the more broad field of social demography population studies also analyze the relationships between economic, social, cultural and biological processes influencing a population.

The term demographics is often used erroneously for demography, but refers rather to selected population characteristics as used in government, marketing or opinion research, or the demographic profiles used in such research.

Data and Methods

There are two methods of data collection: Direct and indirect. Direct data come from vital statistics registries that track all births and deaths as well as certain changes in legal status such as marriage, divorce, and migration (registration of place of residence). In developed countries with good registration systems (such as the United States and much of Europe), registry statistics are the best method for estimating the number of births and deaths.

The census is the other common direct method of collecting demographic data. A census is usually conducted by a national government and attempts to enumerate every person in a country. However, in contrast to vital statistics data, which are typically collected continuously and summarized on an annual basis, censuses typically occur only every 10 years or so, and thus are not usually the best source of data on births and deaths. Analyses are conducted after a census to estimate how much over or undercounting took place. Censuses do more than just count people. They typically collect information about families or households, as well as about such individual characteristics as age, sex, marital status, literacy/education, employment status and occupation, and geographical location. They may also collect data on migration (or place of birth or of previous residence), language, religion, nationality (or ethnicity or race), and citizenship. In countries in which the vital registration system may be incomplete, the censuses are also used as a direct source of information about fertility and mortality; for example the censuses of the People's Republic of China gather information on births and deaths that occurred in the 18 months immediately preceding the census.

Indirect methods of data collections are required in countries where full data are not available, such as is the case in much of the developing world. One of these techniques is the sister method, where survey researchers ask women how many of their sisters have died or had children and at what age. With these surveys, researchers can then indirectly estimate birth or death rates for the entire population. Other indirect methods include asking people about siblings, parents and children.

Important Concepts

Important concepts in demography include which we have discussed above:

- The **crude birth rate**, the annual number of live births per 1000 people.
- The **general fertility rate**, the annual number of live births per 1000 women of childbearing age (often taken to be from 15 to 49 years old, but sometimes from 15 to 44).
- **Age-specific fertility** rates, the annual number of live births per 1000 women in particular age groups (usually age 15-19, 20-24 etc).
- The **crude death rate**, the annual number of deaths per 1000 people.
- The **infant mortality rate**, the annual number of deaths of children less than 1 year old per 1000 live births.

- The **expectation of life** (or life expectancy), the number of years which an individual at a given age could expect to live at present mortality levels.
- The **total fertility rate**, the number of live births per woman completing her reproductive life, if her childbearing at each age reflected current age-specific fertility rates.
- The **gross reproduction rate**, the number of daughters who would be born to a woman completing her reproductive life at current age-specific fertility rates.
- The **net reproduction ratio** is the expected number of daughters, per newborn prospective mother, who may or may not survive to and through the ages of childbearing.

Note that the crude death rate as defined above and applied to a whole population can give a misleading impression. For example, the number of deaths per 1000 people can be higher for developed nations than in less-developed countries, despite standards of health being better in developed countries. This is because developed countries have relatively more older people, who are more likely to die in a given year, so that the overall mortality rate can be higher even if the mortality rate at any given age is lower.

The fertility rates can also give a misleading impression that a population is growing faster than it in fact is, because measurement of fertility rates only involves the reproductive rate of women, and does not adjust for the sex ratio. For example, if a population has a total fertility rate of 4.0 but the sex ratio is 66/34 (twice as many men as women), this population is actually growing at a slower natural increase rate than would a population having a fertility rate of 3.0 and a sex ratio of 50/50. This distortion is greatest in India and Myanmar, and is present in China as well.

Science of Population

Population change through three processes: fertility, mortality and migration. Fertility involves the number of children that women have and is to be contrasted with fecundity (a woman's childbearing potential). Mortality is the study of the causes, consequences, and measurement of processes affecting death to members of the population. Demographers most commonly study mortality using the Life Table, a statistical device which provides information about the mortality conditions (most notably the life expectancy) in the population. Migration refers to the movement of persons from an origin place to a destination place across some pre-defined, political boundary. Migration researchers do not designate movements 'migrations' unless they are somewhat permanent. Thus demographers do not consider tourists and travellers to be migrating. While demographers who study migration typically do so through census data on place of residence, indirect sources of data including tax forms and labor force surveys are also important.

Demography is today widely taught in many universities across the world, attracting students with initial training in social sciences, statistics or health studies. Being at the crossroads of several disciplines such as geography, economics, sociology or epidemiology, demography offers tools to approach a large range of population issues by combining a more technical quantitative approach that represents the core of the discipline with many other methods borrowed from social or other sciences. Demographic research is conducted in universities, in research institutes as well as in statistical departments and in several international agencies. Population institutions are part of the Cicred (International Committee for Coordination of Demographic Research) network while most individual scientists engaged in demographic research are members of the IUSSP (International Union for the Scientific Study of Population).

Demographics of India

Population growth, from 443 million in 1960 to 1,004 million in 2000.

The **Demographics of India** are overall remarkably diverse. India's population of approximately 1.13 billion people (estimate for March 10, 2008) comprises approximately one-sixth of the world's population. India is expected to overtake China by 2030 and will then be the most populated country in the world. India has more than two thousand ethnic groups, and every major religion is represented, as are four major families of languages (Indo-European, Dravidian, Austro-Asiatic and Tibeto-Burman languages) as well as a language isolate (the Nihali language spoken in parts of Maharashtra). Further complexity is lent by the great variation that occurs across this population on social parameters such as income and education. Only the continent of Africa exceeds the linguistic, cultural and genetic diversity of the nation of India.

Salient Features

Although India occupies only 2.4% of the world's land area, it supports over 17.5% of the world's population. 31.8% of Indians are younger than 15 years of age. As per the 2001 census, 72.22% of the people live in more than 550,000 villages, and the remainder in more than 2000 towns and cities.

Although 80.5% of the people are Hindus, India, with 13.4% of its population Muslim, is also home to the third-largest Muslim population in the world after Indonesia and Pakistan. India also contains the majority of the world's Zoroastrians, Sikhs and Jains. Other religious groups include Christians (2.3%), Buddhists (0.8%), Jews and Bahá'ís.

Census

The most recent census of India was performed in 2001 for enumeration as of March 1 of that year. It was the 14th census in an unbroken series, and the 6th after independence in 1947 (with the exception that census could not be held for Assam in the 1981 and Jammu & Kashmir in 1991). Eight censuses were performed under the British Raj, the first one was carried out throughout the 1860s and completed in 1872. After this, there has been one census every decade starting in 1881.

The 2001 census was conducted in two phases, the first being Housenumbering and Houselisting operations, carried out in May 2000, and the second being population enumeration, carried out from February 9 to 28, 2001. The reference time for the census is 1 March, 2001. The homeless population was enumerated on 28 February. A revisional round was undertaken 1 to 5 March 2001 to account for mutations between the time of visit in February and 1 March.

The total population calculated for 1 March 2001 was 1,027,015,247, making the 2001 census the first to count more than a billion Indians. The population had risen by 21.34% compared to the 1991 total. The female population had increased by 0.3 percentage points to 48.4%. Maharashtra has the largest urban agglomeration while Delhi is the most urbanised market at over 93% urbanization.

Key Data

Total Population: 1,129.9 million (July 1, 2007 est. CIA) 1,028.7 million (2001 Census final figures, March 1 enumeration and estimated 124,000 in areas of Manipur that could not be covered in the enumeration).

Rural Population: 72.2%, male: 381,668,992, female: 360,948,755 (2001 Census).

Population History

Year	Total Population
1950	357,000,000
1960	443,000,000
1970	553,000,000
1980	684,000,000
1990	838,141,000
2000	1,004,591,054
2005	1,095,054,669
2007	1,129,866,154

Population Projections (in millions)

Year	Under 15	15-64	65+	Total
2000	361	604	45	1010
2005	368	673	51	1093
2010	370	747	58	1175
2015	372	819	65	1256
2020	373	882	76	1331

Source: Based on P.N. Mari Bhat, "Indian Demographic Scenario 2025", Institute of Economic Growth, New Delhi, Discussion Paper No. 27/2001.

Urban Population

Age structure:

0–14 years : 30.8%, male: 188,208,196, female: 171,356,024

15–64 years : 64.3%, male: 386,432,921, female: 364,215,759

65+ years : 4.9%, male: 27,258,259, female: 30,031,289 (2007 est.)

The average age of Indians is 24.8 years.

Population growth rate: 1.38% (2007 est.)

Birth rate: 22.69 births/1,000 population (2007 est.)

Death rate: 6.58 deaths/1,000 population (2006 est.)

Literacy rate: 79.9%

Percent of the population under the poverty line: 22% (2006 est.)

Unemployment Rate: 7.8%

Net migration rate: -0.05 migrant(s)/1,000 population (2007 est.)

Sex Ratio

At birth : 1.12 male(s)/female

Under 15 years : 1.098 male(s)/female

15–64 years : 1.061 male(s)/female

65 years and over : 0.908 male(s)/female

Total population : 1.064 male(s)/female (2006 est.)

Infant mortality rate: Total: 34.61 deaths/1,000 live births (2007 est.) female: 29.23 deaths/1,000 live births male: 39.42 deaths/1,000 live births

Life Expectancy at Birth

Total population : 68.59 years

Male : 66.28 years

Female : 71.17 years (2007 est.)

Total fertility rate: 2.81 children born/woman (2007 est.) The TFR (Total number of children born per women) according to Religion in 2001 was: Hindus - 2.27, Muslims - 3.06, Sikhs - 1.86, Christians - 2.06, Buddhists

- 2.29, Jains - 1.50, Animists and Others - 2.99, Tribals - 3.16, Scheduled Castes - 2.89.

Nationality

Noun : Indian(s)

Adjective : Indian

Religions: Hindu 80.5%, Muslim 13.4%, Christian 2.3%, Sikh 1.8%, Buddhists 0.8%, Jains 0.4%, Others 0.7%, Unspecified 0.1% (2001 Census).

Scheduled Castes and Tribes: Scheduled Castes: 16.2% (2001 Census). Scheduled Tribes: 8.2% (2001 Census).

Languages: There are 216 languages with more than 10,000 native speakers in India. The largest of these is Hindi with some 337 million (the second largest being Bengali with some 207 million). 22 languages are recognized as official languages. In India, there are 1,652 languages and dialects in total.

Religious Breakdown

Censuses were conducted in parts of India in the ancient times with examples such as Kautilya's *Arthashastra* which describes the collection of population statistics for taxation in 4th century B.C. The British census in 1865-1872 was the first conducted in modern times in India.

The 2001 census figures released by the India Census Commission give a breakdown by various parameters including religion.

1. All figures in %.
2. Gender Ratio*: No. of females/1000 males
3. *Others* including Bahá'ís, Jews and Parsis.
4. Tribal Animists (and non religious) are grouped under Others after 1926 (1931 census onwards)

It should also be noted that about 40% of the Hindus speak Hindi while the rest speak Bengali, Telugu, Marathi, Tamil, Gujarati,Kannada and other languages. Almost 70% of the Muslims speak Urdu while the rest speak

Census information for 2001

Composition	Hindus	Muslims	Christians	Sikhs	Buddhist	Jains	Others
% total of population 2005	80.4%	13.4%	2.3%	1.9%	1.1%	0.4%	0.5%
10-Yr Growth % (est '91–'01)	20.3%	29.5%	22.6%	18.2%	24.5%	26.0%	103.1%
Sex ratio* (avg. 944)	935	940	1009	895	955	940	100
Literacy rate (avg. 79.9)	75.5	60.0	90.3	70.4	73.0	95.0	50.0
Work Participation Rate	40.4	31.3	39.7	37.7	40.6	32.9	48.4
Rural sex ratio	944	953	1001	895	958	937	995
Urban sex ratio	922	907	1026	886	944	941	966
Child sex ratio (0–6 yrs)	925	950	964	786	942	870	976

Source: The First Report on Religion: Census of India 2001.

α = The data excludes Mao-Maram, Paomata and Purul subdivisions of Senapati District of Manipur.

β = The data is "unadjusted" (without excluding Assam and Jammu and Kashmir); 1981 census was not conducted in Assam and 1991 census was not conducted in Jammu and Kashmir.

Kashmiri, Bengali, Malayalam, Tamil, Gujarati and other languages. About one-third of the Christians speak Malayalam, one-sixth speak Tamil while the rest speak a variety of languages.

CHAPTER 9 APPLICATION OF STATISTICS IN OPERATIONAL RESEARCH

9.1 AN OVERVIEW

The terms operations research and management science are often used synonymously. When a distinction is drawn, management science generally implies a closer relationship to the problems of business management. Operations research also closely relates to Industrial engineering. Industrial engineering takes more of an engineering point of view, and industrial engineers typically consider OR techniques to be a major part of their toolset.

Some of the primary tools used by operations researchers are statistics, optimization, stochastics, queueing theory, game theory, graph theory, decision analysis, and simulation. Because of the computational nature of these fields, OR also has ties to computer science, and operations researchers regularly use custom-written or off-the-shelf software.

Operations research is distinguished by its ability to look at and improve an entire system, rather than concentrating only on specific elements (though this is often done as well). An operations researcher faced with a new problem is expected to determine which techniques are most appropriate given the nature of the system, the goals for improvement, and constraints on time and computing power. For this and other reasons, the human element of OR is vital. Like any other tools, OR techniques cannot solve problems by themselves.

9.2 SCOPE OF OPERATIONS RESEARCH

A few examples of applications in which operations research is currently used include:

- Designing the layout of a hospital for efficient flow of facilities to the more number of patients.
- Constructing a telecommunications network at low cost while still guaranteeing QoS (quality of service) or QoE (Quality of

experience) if particular connections become very busy or get damaged.

- Designing the layout of a computer chip to reduce manufacturing time (therefore reducing cost).
- Managing the flow of raw materials and products in a supply chain based on uncertain demand for the finished products
- Efficient messaging and customer response tactics.
- Roboticizing or automating human-driven operations processes
- Globalizing operations processes in order to take advantage of cheaper materials, labor, land or other productivity inputs.
- Blending of raw materials in oil refineries.

Operations research is also used extensively in government where evidence-based policy is used.

History

Some say that Charles Babbage (1791-1871) is the "father of operations research" because his research into the cost of transportation and sorting of mail led to England's universal "Penny Post" in 1840. The modern field of operations research arose during World War II. Scientists in the United Kingdom including Patrick Blackett, Cecil Gordon, C. H. Waddington, Owen Wansbrough-Jones and Frank Yates, and in the United States with George Dantzig looked for ways to make better decisions in such areas as logistics and training schedules. After the war it began to be applied to similar problems in industry.

Blackett's team made a number of crucial analyses which aided the war effort. Britain introduced the convoy system to reduce shipping losses, but while the principle of using warships to accompany merchant ships was generally accepted, it was unclear whether it was better for convoys to be small or large. Convoys travel at the speed of the slowest member, so small convoys can travel faster. It was also argued that small convoys would be harder for German U-boats to detect. On the other hand, large convoys could deploy more warships against an attacker. Blackett's staff showed that the losses suffered by convoys depended largely on the number of escort vessels present, rather than on the overall size of the convoy. Their conclusion, therefore, was that a few large convoys are more defensible than many small ones.

In another piece of work, Blackett's team analysed a report of a survey carried out by RAF Bomber Command. For the survey, Bomber Command inspected all bombers returning from bombing raids over Germany over a particular period. All damage inflicted by German air defenses was noted and the recommendation was given that armour be added in the most heavily damaged areas. Their suggestion to remove some of the crew so that an aircraft loss would result in fewer personnel loss was rejected by RAF command. Blackett's team instead made the surprising and counter-intuitive recommendation that the armour be placed in the areas which were completely untouched by damage, according to the survey. They reasoned that the survey was biased, since it only included aircraft that successfully came back from Germany. The untouched areas were probably vital areas, which, if hit, would result in the loss of the aircraft.

When the Germans organised their air defences into the Kammhuber Line, it was realised that if the RAF bombers were to fly in a bomber stream they could overwhelm the night fighters who flew in individual cells directed to their targets by ground controllers. It was then a matter of calculating the statistical loss from collisions against the statistical loss from night fighters to calculate how close the bombers should fly to minimise RAF losses.

It is known as "operational research" in the United Kingdom ("operational analysis" within the UK military and UK Ministry of Defence, where OR stands for "Operational Requirement") and as "operations research" in most other English-speaking countries, though OR is a common abbreviation everywhere. With expanded techniques and growing awareness, OR is no longer limited to only operations, and the proliferation of computer data collection has relieved analysts of much of the more mundane research. But the OR analyst must still know how a system operates, and learn to perform even more sophisticated research than ever before. In every sense the name OR still applies, more than a half century later.

9.3 STATISTICS IN OPERATIONAL RESEARCH

Statistics is a mathematical science pertaining to the collection, analysis, interpretation or explanation, and presentation of data. It is applicable to a wide variety of academic disciplines, from the natural and social sciences to the humanities, and to government and business.

Statistical methods can be used to summarize or describe a collection of data; this is called **descriptive statistics**. In addition, patterns in the data may be modeued in a way that accounts for randomness and uncertainty in the observations, and then used to draw inferences about the process or population being studied; this is called **inferential statistics**. Both descriptive and inferential statistics comprise **applied statistics**. There is also a discipline called **mathematical statistics**, which is concerned with the theoretical basis of the subject.

The word ***statistics*** is also the plural of ***statistic*** (singular), which refers to the result of applying a statistical algorithm to a set of data, as in economic statistics, crime statistics, etc.

Statistics arose, no later than the 18th century, from the need of states to collect data on their people and economies, in order to administer them. Its meaning broadened in the early 19th century to include the collection and analysis of data in general. Today statistics is widely employed in government, business, and the natural and social sciences.

Because of its origins in government and its data-centric world view, statistics is considered to be not a subfield of mathematics but rather a distinct field that uses mathematics. Its mathematical foundations were laid in the 17th and 18th centuries with the development of probability theory. The method of least squares, a central technique of the discipline, was invented in the early 19th century by several authors. Since then new techniques of probability and statistics have been in continual development. Modern computers have expedited large-scale statistical computation, and have also made possible new methods that would be impractical to perform manually.

Overview

In applying statistics to a scientific, industrial, or societal problem, one begins with a process or population to be studied. This might be a population of people in a country, of crystal grains in a rock, or of goods manufactured by a particular factory during a given period. It may instead be a process observed at various times; data collected about this kind of "population" constitute what is called a time series.

For practical reasons, rather than compiling data about an entire population, one usually studies a chosen subset of the population, called a sample. Data are collected about the sample in an observational or experimental setting. The data are then subjected to statistical analysis, which serves two related purposes: description and inference.

- Descriptive statistics can be used to summarize the data, either numerically or graphically, to describe the sample. Basic examples of numerical descriptors include the mean and standard deviation. Graphical summarizations include various kinds of charts and graphs.
- Inferential statistics is used to model patterns in the data, accounting for randomness and drawing inferences about the larger population. These inferences may take the form of answers to yes/no questions (hypothesis testing), estimates of numerical characteristics (estimation), descriptions of association (correlation), or modeling of relationships (regression). Other modelling techniques include ANOVA, time series, and data mining.

The concept of correlation is particularly noteworthy. Statistical analysis of a data set may reveal that two variables (that is, two properties of the population under consideration) tend to vary together, as if they are connected. For example, a study of annual income and age of death among people might find that poor people tend to have shorter lives than affluent people. The two variables are said to be correlated. However, one cannot immediately infer the existence of a causal relationship between the two variables (see Correlation does not imply causation). The correlated phenomena could be caused by a third, previously unconsidered phenomenon, called a lurking variable.

If the sample is representative of the population, then inferences and conclusions made from the sample can be extended to the population as a whole. A major problem lies in determining the extent to which the chosen sample is representative. Statistics offers methods to estimate and correct for randomness in the sample and in the data collection procedure, as well as methods for designing robust experiments in the first place.

The fundamental mathematical concept employed in understanding such randomness is probability. Mathematical statistics (also called statistical theory) is the branch of applied mathematics that uses probability theory and analysis to examine the theoretical basis of statistics.

The use of any statistical method is valid only when the system or population under consideration satisfies the basic mathematical assumptions of the method. Misuse of statistics can produce subtle but serious errors in description and interpretation — subtle in that even experienced professionals sometimes make such errors, and serious in that they may affect social policy, medical practice and the reliability of structures such as bridges and nuclear power plants. Even when statistics is correctly applied, the results can be difficult to interpret for a non-expert. For example, the statistical significance of a trend in the data — which measures the extent to which the trend could be caused by random variation in the sample — may not agree with one's intuitive sense of its significance. The set of basic statistical skills (and skepticism) needed by people to deal with information in their everyday lives is referred to as statistical literacy.

9.4 STATISTICAL METHODS

Experimental and Observational Studies

A common goal for a statistical research project is to investigate causality, and in particular to draw a conclusion on the effect of changes in the values of predictors or independent variables on response or dependent variables. There are two major types of causal statistical studies, experimental studies and observational studies. In both types of studies, the effect of differences of an independent variable (or variables) on the behaviour of the dependent variable are observed. The difference between the two types is in how the study is actually conducted. Each can be very effective.

An experimental study involves taking measurements of the system under study, manipulating the system, and then taking additional measurements using the same procedure to determine if the manipulation may have modified the values of the measurements. In contrast, an observational study does not involve experimental manipulation. Instead data are gathered and correlations between predictors and the response are investigated.

An example of an experimental study is the famous Hawthorne studies which attempted to test changes to the working environment at the Hawthorne plant of the Western Electric Company. The researchers were interested in whether increased illumination would increase the productivity of the assembly line workers. The researchers first measured productivity in the plant then modified the illumination in an area of the plant to see if changes in illumination would affect productivity. As it turns out, productivity improved under all the experimental conditions (see Hawthorne effect). However, the study is today heavily criticized for errors in experimental procedures, specifically the lack of a control group and blindedness.

An example of an observational study is a study which explores the correlation between smoking and lung cancer. This type of study typically uses a survey to collect observations about the area of interest and then perform statistical analysis. In this case, the researchers would collect observations of both smokers and non-smokers, perhaps through a case-control study, and then look at the number of cases of lung cancer in each group.

The basic steps for an experiment are to:

1. Plan the research including determining information sources, research subject selection, and ethical considerations for the proposed research and method,
2. Design the experiment concentrating on the system model and the interaction of independent and dependent variables,
3. Summarize a collection of observations to feature their commonality by suppressing details (descriptive statistics),
4. Reach consensus about what the observations tell us about the world we observe (statistical inference),
5. Document and present the results of the study.

Levels of Measurement

There are four types of measurements or measurement scales used in statistics. The four types or levels of measurement (nominal, ordinal, interval and ratio) have different degrees of usefulness in statistical research. Ratio measurements, where both a zero value and distances between different measurements are defined, provide the greatest flexibility in statistical methods that can be used for analyzing the data. Interval measurements have meaningful distances between measurements but no meaningful zero value (such as IQ measurements or temperature measurements in Fahrenheit). Ordinal measurements have imprecise differences between consecutive values but a meaningful order to those values. Nominal measurements have no meaningful rank order among values.

Variables conforming only to nominal or ordinal measurements are together sometimes called categorical variables, since they cannot reasonably be numerically measured, whereas ratio and interval measurements are grouped together as quantitative or continuous variables due to their numerical nature.

Statistical Techniques

Some well-known statistical tests and procedures for research observations are:

- Student's t-test
- Chi-square test
- Analysis of variance (ANOVA)
- Mann-Whitney U
- Regression analysis
- Factor analysis
- Correlation
- Pearson product-moment correlation coefficient
- Spearman's rank correlation coefficient
- Time series analysis
- All these tehniques have been disussed in earlier chapters.

Statistical Computing

The rapid and sustained increases in computing power starting from the second half of the 20th century have had a substantial impact on the practice of statistical science. Early statistical models were almost always from the class of linear models, but powerful computers, coupled with suitable numerical algorithms, caused a resurgence of interest in nonlinear models (especially neural networks and decision trees) and the creation of new types, such as generalised linear models and multilevel models.

Increased computing power has also led to the growing popularity of computationally-intensive methods based on resampling, such as permutation tests and the bootstrap, while techniques such as Gibbs sampling have made Bayesian methods more feasible. The computer revolution has implications for the future of statistics, with a new emphasis on "experimental" and "empirical" statistics. A large number of both general and special purpose statistical packages are now available to practitioners.

There is a general perception that statistical knowledge is all-too-frequently intentionally misused, by finding ways to interpret the data that are favourable to the presenter. A famous saying attributed to Benjamin Disraeli is, "There are three kinds of lies: lies, damned lies and statistics." And Harvard President Lawrence Lowell wrote in 1909 "That statistics like veal pies, are good if you know the person that made them, and are sure of the ingredients."

If various studies appear to contradict one another, then the public may come to distrust such studies. For example, one study may suggest that a given diet or activity raises blood pressure, while another may suggest that it lowers blood pressure. The discrepancy can arise from subtle variations in experimental design, such as differences in the patient groups or research protocols, that are not easily understood by the non-expert. (Media reports sometimes omit this vital contextual information entirely).

By choosing (or rejecting, or modifying) a certain sample, results can be manipulated; throwing out outliers is one means of doing so. Such manipulations need not be malicious or devious; they can arise from unintentional biases of the researcher. The graphs used to summarize data can also be misleading.

Deeper criticisms come from the fact that the hypothesis testing approach, widely used and in many cases required by law or regulation, forces one hypothesis (the null hypothesis) to be "favored", and can also seem to exaggerate the importance of minor differences in large studies. A difference that is highly statistically significant can still be of no practical significance.

One response has been a greater emphasis on the *p*-value over simply reporting whether a hypothesis was rejected at the given level of significance. The *p*-value, however, does not indicate the size of the effect. Another increasingly common approach is to report confidence intervals. Although these are produced from the same calculations as hypothesis tests or *p*-values, they describe both the size of the effect and the uncertainty surrounding it. The details of the use and applications of operational research has not been discussed here. However, a broad overview on this subject is presented for medical students for their knowledge.

CHAPTER 10

STATISTICS AND NATIONAL HEALTH

10.1 NATIONAL HEALTH POLICY AND STATISTICS – AT A GLANCE

A National Health Policy was last formulated in 1983, and since then there have been marked changes in the determinant factors relating to the health sector. Some of the policy initiatives outlined in the NHP-1983 have yielded results, while, in several other areas, the outcome has not been as expected.

The NHP-1983 gave a general exposition of the policies which required recommendation in the circumstances then prevailing in the health sector. The noteworthy initiatives under that policy were:

(i) A phased, time-bound programme for setting up a well-dispersed network of comprehensive primary health care services, linked with extension and health education, designed in the context of the ground reality that elementary health problems can be resolved by the people themselves.

(ii) Intermediation through 'Health volunteers' having appropriate knowledge, simple skills and requisite technologies.

(iii) Establishment of a well-worked out referral system to ensure that patient load at the higher levels of the hierarchy is not needlessly burdened by those who can be treated at the decentralized level.

(iv) An integrated network of evenly spread speciality and super-speciality services; encouragement of such facilities through private investments for patients who can pay, so that the draw on the Government's facilities is limited to those entitled to free use.

Government initiatives in the public health sector have recorded some noteworthy successes over time. Smallpox and guinea worm disease have been eradicated from the country. Polio is on the verge of being eradicated; leprosy, kala azar and filariasis can be expected to be eliminated in the foreseeable future. There has been a substantial drop in the Total Fertility Rate and Infant Mortality Rate. The success of the initiatives taken in the public health field are reflected in the progressive improvement of many demographic/ epidemiological / infrastructural indicators over time – (Box-I).

Box-I : Achievements Through The Years - 1951-2000

Indicator	1951	1981	2000
Demographic Changes			
Life Expectancy	36.7	54	64.6(RGI)
Crude Birth Rate	40.8	33.9(SRS)	26.1(99 SRS)
Crude Death Rate	25	12.5(SRS)	8.7(99 SRS)
IMR	146	110	70 (99 SRS)
Epidemiological Shifts			
Malaria (cases in million)	75	2.7	2.2
Leprosy cases per 10,000 population	38.1	57.3	3.74
Smallpox (no. of cases)	>44,887	Eradicated	
Guineaworm (no. of cases)		>39,792	Eradicated
Polio		29709	265
Infrastructure			
SC/PHC/CHC	725	57,363	1,63,181 (99-RHS)
Dispensaries and Hospitals (all)	9209	23,555	43,322 (95–96-CBHI)
Beds (Pvt & Public)	117,198	569,495	8,70,161 (95-96-CBHI)
Doctors (Allopathy)	61,800	2,68,700	5,03,900 (98-99-MCI)
Nursing Personnel	18,054	1,43,887	7,37,000 (99-INC)

While noting that the public health initiatives over the years have contributed significantly to the improvement of these health indicators, it is to be acknowledged that public health indicators / disease-burden statistics are the outcome of several complementary initiatives under the wider umbrella of the developmental sector, covering Rural Development, Agriculture, Food Production, Sanitation, Drinking Water Supply, Education, etc. Despite the impressive public health gains as revealed in the statistics in Box-I, there is no gainsaying the fact that the morbidity and mortality levels in the country are still unacceptably high. These unsatisfactory health indices are, in turn, an indication of the limited success of the public health system in meeting the preventive and curative requirements of the general population.

Out of the communicable diseases which have persisted over time, the incidence of malaria staged a resurgence in the 1980s before stabilising at a fairly high prevalence level during the 1990s. Over the years, an increasing level of insecticide-resistance has developed in the malarial vectors in many parts of the country, while the incidence of the more deadly P-Falciparum Malaria has risen to about 50 percent in the country as a whole. In respect of TB, the public health scenario has not shown any significant decline in the pool of infection amongst the community, and there has been a distressing trend in the increase of drug resistance to the type of infection prevailing in the country. A new and extremely virulent communicable disease – HIV/AIDS– has emerged on the health scene since the declaration of the NHP-1983. As there is no existing therapeutic cure or vaccine for this infection, the disease constitutes a serious threat, not merely to public health but to economic development in the country. The common water-borne infections – Gastroenteritis, cholera, and some forms of Hepatitis – continue to contribute to a high level of morbidity in the population, even though the mortality rate may have been somewhat moderated.

The period after the announcement of NHP-83 has also seen an increase in mortality through 'life-style' diseases–diabetes, cancer and cardiovascular diseases. The increase in life expectancy has increased the requirement for geriatric care. Similarly, the increasing burden of trauma cases is also a significant public health problem.

Another area of grave concern in the public health domain is the persistent incidence of macro and micro nutrient deficiencies, especially among women and children. In the vulnerable sub-category of women and the girl child, this has the multiplier effect through the birth of low birth weight babies and serious ramifications of the consequential mental and physical retarded growth.

In retrospect, it is observed that the financial resources and public health administrative capacity which it was possible to marshal, was far short of that necessary to achieve such an ambitious and holistic goal. Against this backdrop, it is felt that it would be appropriate to pitch NHP-2002 at a level consistent with our realistic expectations about financial resources, and about the likely increase in public health administrative capacity. The recommendations of NHP-2002, therefore, attempt to maximize the broad-based availability of health services to the citizenry of the country on the basis of realistic considerations of capacity.

10.2 NATIONAL HEALTH POLICY IN INDIA (2002)–AN OVERVIEW

The public health investment in the country over the years has been comparatively low, and as a percentage of GDP has declined from 1.3 percent in 1990 to 0.9 percent in 1999. The aggregate expenditure in the health sector is 5.2 percent of the GDP. Out of this, about 17 percent of the aggregate expenditure is public health spending, the balance being out-of-pocket expenditure. The NHP-2002 has been formulated taking into consideration these ground realities in regard to the availability of resources.

Box- II : Differentials in Health Status Among States

Sector	Population BPL (%)	IMR/ per 1000 live births (1999 -SRS)	<5 Mortality per 1000 (NFHS II)	Weight for Age- % of Children under 3 years (<-2SD)	MMR/ Lakh (Annual Report 2000)	Leprosy cases per 10000 population	Malaria +ve cases in year 2000 (in thousands)
India	26.1	70	94.9	47	408	3.7	2200
Rural	27.09	75	103.7	49.6	-	-	-
Urban	23.62	44	63.1	38.4	-	-	-

contd.

contd.

Better Performing States							
Kerala	12.72	14	18.8	27	87	0.9	5.1
Maharashtra	25.02	48	58.1	50	135	3.1	138
TN	21.12	52	63.3	37	79	4.1	56
Low Performing States							
Orissa	47.15	97	104.4	54	498	7.05	483
Bihar	42.60	63	105.1	54	707	11.83	132
Rajasthan	15.28	81	114.9	51	607	0.8	53
UP	31.15	84	122.5	52	707	4.3	99
MP	37.43	90	137.6	55	498	3.83	528

Also, the statistics bring out the wide differences between the attainments of health goals in the better– performing States as compared to the low-performing States. It is clear that national averages of health indices hide wide disparities in public health facilities and health standards in different parts of the country. Given a situation in which national averages in respect of most indices are themselves at unacceptably low levels, the wide inter-State disparity implies that, for vulnerable sections of society in several States, access to public health services is nominal and health standards are grossly inadequate. Despite a thrust in the NHP-1983 for making good the unmet needs of public health services by establishing more public health institutions at a decentralized level, a large gap in facilities still persists.

Access to, and benefits from, the public health system have been very uneven between the better-endowed and the more vulnerable sections of society. This is particularly true for women, children and the socially disadvantaged sections of society. The statistics given in Box-III highlight the handicap suffered in the health sector on account of socio-economic inequity.

Box-III : Differentials in Health Status Among Socio-Economic Groups

Indicator	Infant Mortality /1000	Under 5 Mortality/1000	% Children Underweight
India	70	94.9	47
Social Inequity			
Scheduled Castes	83	119.3	53.5

contd.

contd.

Scheduled Tribes	84.2	126.6	55.9
Other Disadvantaged	76	103.1	47.3
Others	61.8	82.6	41.1

It is a principal objective of NHP-2002 to evolve a policy structure which reduces these inequities and allows the disadvantaged sections of society a fairer access to public health services.

DELIVERY OF NATIONAL PUBLIC HEALTH PROGRAMMES

It is self-evident that in a country as large as India, which has a wide variety of socio-economic settings, national health programmes have to be designed with enough flexibility to permit the State public health administrations to craft their own programme package according to their needs. Also, the implementation of the national health programme can only be carried out through the State governments' decentralized public health machinery. Since, for various reasons, the responsibility of the Central Government in funding additional public health services will continue over a period of time, the role of the Central Government in designing broad-based public health initiatives will inevitably continue. Moreover, it has been observed that the technical and managerial expertise for designing large-span public health programmes exists with the Central Government in a considerable degree; this expertise can be gainfully utilized in designing national health programmes for implementation in varying socio-economic settings in the States. With this background, the NHP-2002 attempts to define the role of the Central Government and the State governments in the public health sector of the country.

Over the last decade or so, the Government has relied upon a 'vertical' implementational structure for the major disease control programmes. Through this, the system has been able to make a substantial dent in reducing the burden of specific diseases. However, such an organizational structure, which requires independent manpower for each disease programme, is extremely expensive and difficult to sustain. Over a long time-range, 'vertical' structures may only be affordable for those diseases which offer a reasonable possibility of elimination or eradication in a foreseeable time-span.

It is a widespread perception that, over the last decade and a half, the rural health staff has become a vertical structure exclusively for the implementation of family welfare activities. As a result, for those public health programmes where there is no separate vertical structure, there is no identifiable service delivery system at all. The policy will address this distortion in the public health system.

STATE OF PUBLIC HEALTH INFRASTRUCTURE

It would detract from the quality of the exercise if, while framing a new policy, it were not acknowledged that the existing public health infrastructure is far from satisfactory. For the outdoor medical facilities in existence, funding is generally insufficient; the presence of medical and para-medical personnel is often much less than that required by prescribed norms; the availability of consumables is frequently negligible; the equipment in many public hospitals is often obsolescent and unusable; and, the buildings are in a dilapidated state. In the indoor treatment facilities, again, the equipment is often obsolescent; the availability of essential drugs is minimal; the capacity of the facilities is grossly inadequate, which leads to overcrowding, and consequentially to a steep deterioration in the quality of the services. As a result of such inadequate public health facilities, it has been estimated that less than 20 percent of the population, which seek OPD services, and less than 45 percent of that which seek indoor treatment, avail of such services in public hospitals. This is despite the fact that most of these patients do not have the means to make out-of-pocket payments for private health services except at the cost of other essential expenditure for items such as basic nutrition.

EXTENDING PUBLIC HEALTH SERVICES

While there is a general shortage of medical personnel in the country, this shortfall is disproportionately impacted on the less developed and rural areas. No incentive system attempted so far, has induced private medical personnel to go to such areas; and, even in the public health sector, the effort to deploy medical personnel in such under-served areas, has usually been a losing battle. In such a situation, the possibility needs to be examined of entrusting some limited public health functions to nurses, paramedics and other personnel from the extended health sector after imparting adequate training to them.

India has a vast reservoir of practitioners in the Indian Systems of Medicine and Homoeopathy, who have undergone formal training in their own disciplines. The possibility of using such practitioners in the implementation of State/Central Government public health programmes, in order to increase the reach of basic health care in the country, is addressed in the NHP-2002.

ROLE OF LOCAL SELF-GOVERNMENT INSTITUTIONS

Some states have adopted a policy of devolving programmes and funds in the health sector through different levels of the Panchayati Raj Institutions. Generally, the experience has been an encouraging one. The adoption of such an organisational structure has enabled need-based allocation of resources and closer supervision through the elected representatives. The Policy examines the need for a wider adoption of this mode of delivery of health services, in rural as well as urban areas, in other parts of the country.

NORMS FOR HEALTH CARE PERSONNEL

It is observed that the deployment of doctors and nurses, in both public and private institutions, is ad-hoc and significantly short of the requirement for minimal standards of patient care. This policy will make a specific recommendation in regard to this deficiency.

EDUCATION OF HEALTH CARE PROFESSIONALS

Medical and Dental Colleges are not evenly spread across various parts of the country. Apart from the uneven geographical distribution of medical institutions, the quality of education is highly uneven and in several instances even sub-standard. It is a common perception that the syllabus is excessively theoretical, making it difficult for the fresh graduate to effectively meet even the primary health care needs of the population. There is a general reluctance on the part of graduate doctors to serve in areas distant from their native place. NHP-2002 suggest policy initiatives to rectify the resultant disparities.

Certain medical disciplines, such as molecular biology and gene-manipulation, have become relevant in the period after the formulation of the previous National Health Policy. The components of medical research in recent years have changed radically. In the foreseeable future such research will rely increasingly on the new disciplines. It is observed that the current undergraduate medical syllabus does not cover such emerging subjects. The Policy will make appropriate recommendations in respect of such deficiencies.

Also, certain speciality disciplines – Anesthesiology, Radiology and Forensic Medicine – are currently very scarce, resulting in critical deficiencies in the package of available public health services. This Policy will recommend some measures to alleviate such critical shortages.

NEED FOR SPECIALISTS IN 'PUBLIC HEALTH' AND 'FAMILY MEDICINE'

In any developing country with inadequate availability of health services, the requirement of expertise in the areas of 'public health' and 'family medicine' is markedly more than the expertise required for other clinical specialities. In India, the situation is that public health expertise is non-existent in the private health sector, and far short of requirement in the public health sector. Also, the current curriculum in the graduate/post-graduate courses is outdated and unrelated to contemporary community needs. In respect of 'family medicine', it needs to be noted that the more talented medical graduates generally seek specialization in clinical disciplines, while the remaining go into general practice. While the availability of postgraduate educational facilities is 50 percent of the total number of qualifying graduates each year, and can be considered adequate, the distribution of the disciplines in the postgraduate training facilities is overwhelmingly in favour of clinical specializations. NHP-2002 examines the possible means for ensuring adequate availability of personnel with specialization in the 'public health' and 'family medicine' disciplines, to discharge the public health responsibilities in the country.

Nursing Personnel

The ratio of nursing personnel in the country vis-à-vis doctors/beds is very low according to professionally accepted norms. There is also an acute shortage of nurses trained in super-speciality disciplines for deployment in tertiary care facilities. NHP-2002 addresses these problems.

Urban Health

In most urban areas, public health services are very meagre. To the extent that such services exist, there is no uniform organizational structure. The urban population in the country is presently as high as 30 percent and is likely to go up to around 33 percent by 2010. The bulk of the increase is likely to take place through migration, resulting in slums without any infrastructure support. Even the meagre public health services which are available do not percolate to such unplanned habitations, forcing people to avail of private health care through out-of-pocket expenditure.

The rising vehicle density in large urban agglomerations has also led to an increased number of serious accidents requiring treatment in well-equipped trauma centres. NHP-2002 is address itself to the need for providing this unserved urban population a minimum standard of broad-based health care facilities.

Mental Health

Mental health disorders are actually much more prevalent than is apparent on the surface. While such disorders do not contribute significantly to mortality, they have a serious bearing on the quality of life of the affected persons and their families. Sometimes, based on religious faith, mental disorders are treated as spiritual affliction. This has led to the establishment of unlicensed mental institutions as an adjunct to religious institutions where reliance is placed on faith cure. Serious conditions of mental disorder require hospitalization and treatment under trained supervision. Mental health institutions are woefully deficient in physical infrastructure and trained manpower. NHP-2002 address itself to these deficiencies in the public health sector.

Information, Education and Communication

A substantial component of primary health care consists of initiatives for disseminating to the citizenry, public health-related information. IEC initiatives are adopted not only for disseminating curative guidelines (for the TB, Malaria, Leprosy, Cataract Blindness Programmes), but also as part of the effort to bring about a behavioural change to prevent HIV/AIDS and other life-style diseases. Public health programmes, particularly, need high visibility at the decentralized level in order to have an impact. This task is difficult as 35 percent of our country's population is illiterate. The present IEC strategy is too fragmented, relies too heavily on the mass media and does not address the needs of this segment of the population. It is often felt that the effectiveness of IEC programmes is difficult to judge; and consequently it is often asserted that accountability, in regard to the productive use of such funds, is doubtful. The Policy, while projecting an IEC strategy, will fully address the inherent problems encountered in any IEC programme designed for improving awareness and bringing about a behavioural change in the general population.

It is widely accepted that school and college students are the most impressionable targets for imparting information relating to the basic principles of preventive health care. The policy will attempt to target this group to improve the general level of awareness in regard to 'health-promoting' behaviour.

Health Research

Over the years, health research activity in the country has been very limited. In the Government sector, such research has been confined to the research institutions under the Indian Council of Medical Research, and other institutions funded by the States/Central Government. Research in the private sector has assumed some significance only in the last decade. In our country, where the aggregate annual health expenditure is of the order of Rs. 80,000 crores, the expenditure in 1998-99 on research, both public and private sectors, was only of the order of Rs. 1150 crores. It would be reasonable to infer that with such low research expenditure, it is virtually impossible to make any dramatic breakthrough within the country, by way of new molecules and vaccines; also, without a minimal back-up of applied and operational research, it would be difficult to assess whether the health expenditure in the country is being incurred through optimal applications and appropriate public health strategies. Medical research in the country needs to be focused on therapeutic drugs/vaccines for tropical diseases, which are normally neglected by international pharmaceutical companies on account of their limited profitability potential. The thrust will need to be in the newly-emerging frontier areas of research based on genetics, genome-based drug and vaccine development, molecular biology, etc. NHP-2002 address these inadequacies and spell out a minimal quantum of expenditure for the coming decade, looking to the national needs and the capacity of the research institutions to absorb the funds.

Health Statistics

The absence of a systematic and scientific health statistics database is a major deficiency in the current scenario. The health statistics collected are not the product of a rigorous methodology. Statistics available from different parts of the country, in respect of major diseases, are often not obtained in a manner which make aggregation possible or meaningful.

Further, the absence of proper and systematic documentation of the various financial resources used in the health sector is another lacuna in the existing health information scenario. This makes it difficult to understand trends and levels of health spending by private and public providers of health care in the country, and, consequently, to address related policy issues and to formulate future investment policies.

NHP-2002 address itself to the programme for putting in place a modern and scientific health statistics database as well as a system of national health accounts.

The Impact of Globalization on the Health Sector

There are some apprehensions about the possible adverse impact of economic globalisation on the health sector. Pharmaceutical drugs and other health services have always been available in the country at extremely inexpensive prices. India has established a reputation around the globe for the innovative development of original process patents for the manufacture of a wide-range of drugs and vaccines within the ambit of the existing patent laws. With the adoption of Trade Related Intellectual Property Rights (TRIPS), and the subsequent alignment of domestic patent laws consistent with the commitments under TRIPS, there will be a significant shift in the scope of the parameters regulating the manufacture of new drugs/vaccines. Global experience has shown that the introduction of a TRIPS-consistent patent regime for drugs in a developing country results in an across-the-board increase in the cost of drugs and medical services. NHP-2002 address itself to the future imperatives of health security in the country, in the post-TRIPS era.

Population Growth and Health Standards

Efforts made over the years for improving health standards have been partially neutralized by the rapid growth of the population. It is well recognized that population stabilization measures and general health initiatives, when effectively synchronized, synergistically maximize the socio-economic well-being of the people. Government has separately announced the 'National Population Policy 2000'. The principal common features covered under the National Population Policy-2000 and NHP-2002, relate to the prevention and control of communicable diseases; giving priority to the containment of HIV/AIDS infection; the universal immunization of children against all major preventable diseases; addressing the unmet needs for basic and reproductive health services, and supplementation of infrastructure. The synchronized implementation of these two policies – National Population Policy – 2000 and National Health Policy-2002– the very cornerstone of any national structural plan to improve the health standards in the country.

Objectives

The main objective of this policy is to achieve an acceptable standard of good health amongst the general population of the country. It is expected that this initiative will strengthen the capacity of the public health administration at the State level to render effective service delivery. The contribution of the private sector in providing health services would be much enhanced, particularly for the population group which can afford to pay for services. NHP-2002 will endeavour to achieve the time-bound goals mentioned in Box-IV.

Box-IV: Goals to be Achieved by 2000-2015

Eradicate Polio and Yaws	2005
Eliminate Leprosy	2005
Eliminate Kala Azar	2010
Eliminate Lymphatic Filariasis	2015
Achieve Zero Level Growth of HIV/AIDS	2007
Reduce Mortality by 50% on Account of TB, Malaria and Other Vector and Water Borne Diseases	2010
Reduce Prevalence of Blindness to 0.5%	2010
Reduce IMR to 30/1000 and MMR to 100/Lakh	2010
Increase Utilization of Public Health Facilities from Current Level of <20 to >75%	2010
Establish an Integrated System of Surveillance, National Health Accounts and Health Statistics	2005
Increase Health Expenditure by Government as a % of GDP from the Existing 0.9 % to 2.0%	2010

Contd.

contd.

Increase Share of Central Grants to Constitute at least 25% of Total Health Spending	2010
Increase State Sector Health Spending from 5.5% to 7% of the Budget	2005
Further Increase to 8%	2010

NHP-2002–Policy Prescriptions

Global experience has shown that the quality of public health services, as reflected in the attainment of improved public health indices, is closely linked to the quantum and quality of investment through public funding in the primary health sector. Box-V gives statistics which clearly show that standards of health are more a function of the accurate targeting of expenditure on the decentralised primary sector (as observed in China and Sri Lanka), than a function of the aggregate health expenditure.

Box-V: Public Health Spending in Select Countries

Indicator	%Population with income of <$1 day	Infant Mortality Rate/1000	%Health Expenditure to GDP	%Public Expenditure on health to Total health
India	44.2	70	5.2	17.3
China	18.5	31	2.7	24.9
Sri Lanka	6.6	16	3	45.4
UK	-	6	5.8	96.9
USA	-	7	13.7	44.1

Therefore the Policy, while committing additional aggregate financial resources, places great reliance on the strengthening of the primary health structure for the attaining of improved public health outcomes on an equitable basis. Further, it also recognizes the practical need for levying reasonable user-charges for certain secondary and tertiary public health care services, for those who can afford to pay.

10.3 SUMMATION

The crafting of a National Health Policy is a rare occasion in public affairs when it would be legitimate, indeed valuable, to allow our dreams to mingle with our understanding of ground realities. Based purely on the clinical facts defining the current status of the health sector, we would have arrived at a certain policy formulation; but, buoyed by our dreams, we have ventured slightly beyond that in the shape of NHP-2002, which, in fact, defines a vision for the future.

The health needs of the country are enormous and the financial resources and managerial capacity available to meet them, even on the most optimistic projections, fall somewhat short. Broadly speaking, NHP – 2002 focuses on the need for enhanced funding and an organizational restructuring of the national public health initiatives in order to facilitate more equitable access to the health facilities. Also, the Policy is focused on those diseases which are principally contributing to the disease burden – TB, Malaria and Blindness from the category of historical diseases; and HIV/AIDS from the category of 'newly emerging diseases'. This is not to say that other items contributing to the disease burden of the country will be ignored; but only that the resources, as also the principal focus of the public health administration, will recognize certain relative priorities.

The Policy highlights the expected roles of different participating groups in the health sector. Further, it recognizes the fact that, despite all that may be guaranteed by the Central Government for assisting public health programmes, public health services would actually need to be delivered by the State administration, NGOs and other institutions of civil society. The attainment of improved health levels would be significantly dependent on population stabilization, as also on complementary efforts from other areas of the social sectors – like improved drinking water supply, basic sanitation, minimum nutrition, etc.–to ensure that the exposure of the populace to health risks is minimized.

Any expectation of a significant improvement in the quality of health services, and the consequential improved health status of the citizenry, would depend not only on increased financial and material inputs, but also on a more empathetic and committed attitude in the service providers, whether in the private or public sectors. In some measure, this optimistic policy document is based on the understanding that the citizenry is increasingly demanding more by way of quality in health services, and the health delivery system, particularly in the public sector, is being pressed to respond. In this backdrop, it needs to be recognized that any policy in the social sector is critically dependent on the service providers treating their responsibility not as a commercial activity, but as a service, albeit a paid one. In the area of public health, an improved standard of governance is a prerequisite for the success of any health policy.

GLOSSARY OF STATISTICAL TERMS

Statistics

Statistics is the use of data to help the decision maker to reach better decisions.

Data

It is any group of measurements that interests us. These measurements provide information for the decision maker. (i) The data that reflects non-numerical features or qualities of the experimental units, is known as qualitative data. (ii) The data that possesses numerical properties is known as quantitative data.

Population

Any well defined set of objects about which a statistical enquiry is being made is called a population or universe.

The total number of objects (individuals) in a population is known as the size of the population. This may be finite or infinite.

Individual

Each object belonging to a population is called as an individual of the population.

Sample

A finite set of objects drawn from the population with a particular aim, is called a sample.

The total number of individuals in a sample is called the sample size.

Characteristic

The information required from an individual, from a population or from a sample, during the statistical enquiry (survey) is known as the characteristic of the individual. It is either numerical or non-numerical. For e.g. the size of liver is a numerical characteristic which refers to a quantity, whereas the mother tongue of a person is a non-numerical characteristic which refers to a quality. Thus we have quantitative and qualitative types of characteristics.

Variate

A quantitative characteristic of an individual which can be expressed numerically is called a variate or a variable. It may take different values at different times, places or situations.

Attribute

A qualitative characteristic of an individual which can be expressed numerically is called an attribute. For e.g. the mother-tongue of a person, the color of eyes or the color of hair of a person etc.

Discrete Variate

A variable that is not capable of assuming all the values in a given range is a discrete variate.

Continuous Variate

A variate that is capable of assuming all the numerical values in a given range, is called a continuous variate. Consider two examples carefully, viz. the number of students of a class and their heights. Both variates differ slightly, in the sense that, the number of students present in a class is a number say between 0 and 50; always a whole number. It can never be 1.5, 4.33 etc. This type of variate can take only isolated values and is called a discrete variate. On the other hand heights ranging from 140 cm to 190 cm can take values like 140.7, 135.8, 185.1 etc. Such a variate is a continuous variate.

Absolute Risk

Probability of an event over a period of time; expressed as a cumulative incidence like 10-year risk of 10% (meaning 10% of individuals in the group of interest will develop the condition in the next 10year period). It shows the actual likelihood of contracting the disease and provides more realistic and comprehensible risk than relative risk/odds ratio.

Addition Rule

The probability of any of one of several mutually exclusive events occurring is equal to the sum of their individual probabilities. A typical example is the probability of a baby to be homozygous or heterozygous for a Mendelian recessive disorder when both parents are carriers. This equals to 1/4 + 1/2 =

3/4. A baby can be either homozygous or heterozygous but not both of them at the same time; thus, these are mutually exclusive events (see also multiplication rule).

Adjusted Odds Ratio

In a multiple logistic regression model where the response variable is the presence or absence of a disease, an odds ratio for a binomial exposure variable is an adjusted odds ratio for the levels of all other risk factors included in a multivariable model. It is also possible to calculate the adjusted odds ratio for a continuous exposure variable. An adjusted odds ratio results from the comparison of two strata similar at all variables except exposure (or the marker of interest). It can be calculated when stratified data are available as contingency tables by Mantel-Haenszel test.

Affected Family-Based Controls (AFBAC) Method

One of several family-based association study designs (Thomson, 1995). This one uses affected siblings as controls and examines the sharing between two affected family members. The parental marker alleles not transmitted to an affected child or never transmitted to an affected sib pair form the so-called affected family-based controls (AFBAC) population.

Age-Standardized Rate

An age-standardized rate is a weighted average of the age-specific rates, where the weights are the proportions of a standard population in the corresponding age groups. The potential confounding effect of age is removed when comparing age-standardized rates computed using the same standard population.

Alternative Hypothesis

In practice, this is the hypothesis that is being tested in an experiment. It is the conclusion that is reached when a null hypothesis is rejected. It is the opposite of null hypothesis, which states that there is a difference between the groups or something to that effect.

Analysis of Molecular Variance (AMOVA)

A statistical (analysis of variance) method for analysis of molecular genetic data. It is used for partitioning diversity within and among populations using nucleotide sequence or other molecular data. AMOVA produces estimates of variance components and F-statistic analogs (designated as phi-statistics). The significance of the variance components and phi-statistics is tested using a permutational approach, eliminating the normality assumption that is inappropriate for molecular data (Excoffier, 1992). AMOVA can be performed on Arlequin. For examples, see Roewer, 1996; Stead, 2003; Watkins, 2003).

ANOVA (Analysis of Variance)

A test for significant differences between multiple means by comparing variances. It concerns a normally distributed response (outcome) variable and a single categorical explanatory (predictor) variable, which represents treatments or groups. ANOVA is a special case of multiple regression where indicator variables (or orthogonal polynomials) are used to describe the discrete levels of factor variables. The term analysis of variance refers not to the model but to the method of determining which effects are statistically significant. Major assumptions of ANOVA are the homogeneity of variances (it is assumed that the variances in the different groups of the design are similar) and normal distribution of the data within each treatment group. Under the null hypothesis (that there are no mean differences between groups or treatments in the population), the variance estimated from the within-group (treatment) random variability (residual sum of squares = RSS) should be about the same as the variance estimated from between-groups (treatments) variability (explained sum of squares = ESS). If the null hypothesis is true, mean ESS / mean RSS (variance ratio) should be equal to 1. This is known as the F test or variance ratio test (see also one-way and two-way ANOVA). The ANOVA approach is based on the partitioning of sums of squares and degrees of freedom associated with the response variable. ANOVA interpretations of main effects and interactions are not so obvious in other regression models. An accumulated ANOVA table reports the results from fitting a succession of regression models to data from a factorial experiment. Each main effect is added on to the constant term followed by the interaction(s). At each level an F test result is also reported showing the extra effect of adding each variable so it can be worked out which model would fit best. In a two-way ANOVA with equal replications, the order of terms added to the model does not matter, whereas, this is not the case if there are unequal replications. When the assumptions of ANOVA are not met, its non-parametric equivalent Kruskal-Wallis test may be used.

Arithmetic Mean

$M = (x_1 + x_2 + ... x_n) / n$ (n = sample size).

Association

A statistically significant correlation between an environmental exposure or a biochemical/genetic marker and a disease or condition. An association may be an artifact (random error-chance, bias, confounding) or a real one. In population genetics, an association may be due to population stratification, linkage disequilibrium, or direct causation. A significant association should be presented together with a measure of the strength of association (odds ratio, relative risk or relative hazard and its 95% confidence interval) and when appropriate a measure of potential impact (attributable risk, prevented fraction, attributable fraction/etiologic fraction).

Assumptions

Certain conditions of the data that are required to be met for validity of a statistical test. ANOVA generally assumes normal distribution of the data within each treatment group, homogeneity of the variances in the treatment groups, and independence of the observations. In regression analysis, main assumptions are the normal distribution of the response variable, constant variance across fitted values, independence of error terms, and the consistency of underlying hazard rate over time (proportionality assumption) in Cox Proportional Hazard Models.

Asymptotic

Refers to a curve that continually approaches either the x or y axis but does not actually reach it until x or y equals infinity. The axis so approached is the asymptote. An example is the normal distribution curve.

In point estimation, the property that the bias approaches zero as the sample size (N) increases. Therefore, estimators with this property improve as N increases.

Attributable Risk (AR)

Also called excess risk or risk difference. A measure of potential impact of an association. It quantifies the additional risk of disease following exposure over and above that experienced by individuals who are not exposed. It shows how much of the disease is eliminated if no one had the risk factor (unrealistic). The information contained in AR combines the relative risk and the risk factor prevalence. The larger the AR, the greater the effect of the risk factor on the exposed group.

Attributable Fraction (Etiologic Fraction)

It shows what proportion of disease in the exposed individuals is due to the exposure.

Balanced Design

An experimental design in which the same number of observations is taken for each combination of the experimental factors.

Bartlett's Test

A test for homogeneity of variance.

Bayesian Inference

An inference method radically different from the classical frequentist approach which takes into account the prior probability for an event. Established as a new method by Reverend Thomas Bayes. See a slide presentation on Introduction to Bayesian Statistics; +Plus: Bayesian Statistics Explained; Bayesian Revolution in Genetics; BMJ Collection on Bayesian Statistics; Books; Partition Software for Online Bayesian Analysis; Bayesian Calculator; A Bayesian Perspective on Interpreting Statistical Significance (InStat) and Bayesian Calculator.

Bayes' Method in Genetic Counseling

This method uses available additional information to modify risks calculated purely by Mendelian probabilities. It combines prior and conditional probabilities to give joint and posterior probabilities of unknown events. See Bayesian Methods in Genetic Risk Calculation, Bayesian Analysis and Risk Assessment in Genetic Counseling and Testing and A Unified Approach to Bayesian Risk Calculations.

Bernoulli distribution models the behaviour of data taking just two distinct values (0 and 1).

Bias

An estimator for a parameter is unbiased if its expected value is the true value of the parameter. Otherwise, the estimator is biased. It is the quantity E = (q -hat) - q. If the estimate of q is the same as actual but unknown q, the estimate is unbiased (as in estimating the mean of normal, binomial and poisson distributions). If bias tends to decrease as n gets larger, this is called asymptotic unbiasedness. See reviews on epidemiologic meaning of bias: Bias in Clinical Trials, Bias and Confounding in Molecular Epidemiolog.

Binary (Dichotomous) Variable

A discrete random variable that can only take two possible values (success or failure).

Binomial Distribution

The binomial distribution gives the probability of obtaining exactly successes in independent trials, where there are two possible outcomes one of which is conventionally called success (Binomial Distribution).

Blocks

Homogeneous grouping of experimental units (subjects) in experimental design. Groups of experimental units that are relatively homogeneous in that the responses on two units within the same block are likely to be more similar than the responses on two units in different blocks. Dividing the experimental units into blocks is a way of improving the accuracy between treatments. Blocking will minimize variation between subjects that is not attributable to the factors under study. Blocking is similar to matching in two-sample tests or stratification to control for confounding.

Blocking

When the available experimental units are not homogeneous, grouping them into blocks of homogeneous units (stratification) will reduce the experimental error variance. This is called blocking where differences between experimental units other than those caused by treatment factors are taken into account. This is like comparing age-matched groups (blocks) of a control group with the corresponding blocks in the patients group in an investigation of the side effects of a drug as age itself may cause differences in the experiment. Block effects soak up the extra, uninteresting and already known variability in a model. Blocking is preferable to randomization when the factors that might affect the outcome are known.

Bootstrap

An application of resampling statistics. It is a data-based simulation method used to estimate variance and bias of an estimator and provide confidence intervals for parameters where it would be difficult to do so in the usual way.

Canonical

Something that has been reduced to its simplest form.

Carryover Effect

Any effect of a drug that lasts beyond the period of treatment. This is a worry in drug trials with crossover design and the reason for the washout period between treatments.

Case-Control Study

A design preferred over cohort studies for relatively rare diseases in which cases with a disease or exposure are compared with controls randomly selected from the same study base. This design yields odds ratio as opposed to relative risk from cohort studies.

Causal Relationship

It does not matter how small it is, a P-value does not signify causality. To establish a causal relationship, the following non-statistical evidence is required: consistency (reproducibility), biological plausibility, dose-response, temporality (when applicable) and strength of the relationship (as measured by odds ratio/relative risk/hazard ratio). See Hills's criteria of causality; Seven Common Errors in Statistics; and Causality by DR Cox, JR Stat Soc A 1992;155:291 (JSTOR-UK link). The original reference for Hill's criteria is Hill AB: The environment and disease: association or causation. Proc R Soc Medicine 1965;58:295-300.

Categorical (Nominal) Variable

A variable that can be assigned to categories. A non-numerical (qualitative) variable measured on a (discrete) nominal scale such as gender, drug treatments, disease subtypes; or on an ordinal scale such as low, median or high dosage. A variable may alternatively be quantitative (continuous or discrete).

Censored Observation

Observations that survived to a certain point in time before dropping out from the study for a reason other than having the outcome of interest (lost to follow up or not enough time to have the event). Thus, censoring is simply an incomplete observation that has ended before time-to-event. These observations are still useful in survival analysis.

Central Limit Theorem

The means of a relatively large (>30) number of random samples from any population (not necessarily a normal distribution) will be approximately normally distributed with the population mean being their mean and variance being the (population variance /n). This approximation will improve as the sample size (the number of samples) increases. See Mathematical Basis; Quick Time Demonstration; JAVA Demonstration; Simulation.

Chi-Squared Distribution

A distribution derived from the normal distribution. Chi-squared (χ^2) is distributed with v degrees of freedom with mean = v and variance = 2v.

Chi-Squared Test

The most commonly used test for frequency data and goodness-of-fit. In theory, it is nonparametric but because it has no parametric equivalent, it is not classified as such. It is not an exact test and with the current level of computing facilities, there is not much excuse not to use Fisher's exact test for 2x2 contingency table analysis instead of Chi-squared test. Also for larger contingency tables, the G-test (log-likelihood ratio test) may be a better choice. The Chi-square value is obtained by summing up the values (residual2/fit) for each cell in a contingency. In this formula, residual is the difference between the observed value and its expected counterpart and fit is the expected value.

Cochran's Q Test

A nonparametric test examining change in a dichotomous variable across more than two observations. If there are two observations, McNemar's test should be used.

Coefficient of Variation

It is a measure of spread for a set of data. It is a measure of variation in relation to the mean. Calculated as standard deviation divided by the mean (x100).

Cohort Effect

The tendency for persons born in certain years to carry a relatively higher or lower risk of a given disease. This may have to be taken into account in case-control studies.

Conditional (Fixed-Effects) Logistic Regression

The conditional logistic regression (CLR) model is used in studies where cases and controls can be matched (as pairs) with regard to variables believed to be associated with the outcome of interest. The model creates a likelihood that conditions on the matching variable. It is the preferred method for the analysis of nested case-control studies when matching is done at the individual level (there may be more than one control per case). In economic analysis, it is called fixed-effects logit for panel data.

Confounding Variable

A variable that is associated with both the outcome and the exposure variable. A classic example is the relationship between heavy drinking and lung cancer. Here, the data should be controlled for smoking as it is related to both drinking and lung cancer. A positive confounder is related to exposure and response variables in the same direction (as in smoking); a negative confounder shows an opposite relationship to these two variables (age in a study of association between oral contraceptive use and myocardial infarction is a negative confounder). The data should be stratified before analyzing it if there is a confounding effect. Mantel-Haenszel test is designed to analyze stratified data to control for a confounding variable. Alternatively, a multivariable regression model can be used to adjust for the effects of confounders.

Conservative Test

A test where the chance of type I error (false positive) is reduced and type II error risk is increased. Thus, these tests tend to give larger Pvalues compared to non-conservative (liberal) tests for the same comparison.

Contrast

A contrast is combinations of treatment means, which is also called the main effect in ANOVA. It measures the change in the mean response when there is a change between the levels of one factor. For example, in an analysis of three different concentrations of a growth factor on cell growth in cell culture with means m1, m2, m3, against a control value (mo) without any growth factor, a contrast would be:

$$q = mo - 1/3\ (m1+ m2+ m3)$$

The important point is that the coefficients sum to zero (1/1 - 1/3 - 1/3 - 1/3). If the value of the contrast (q) is zero or not significantly different from zero, there is no main effect, i.e., the combined growth factor mean is not different (positive or negative) from the no growth factor mean.

Correlation Coefficient

Pearson's correlation coefficient (r), Spearman's rank correlation (rho) and multiple regression correlation coefficient (R2).

Correspondence Analysis

In population genetics, a complementary analysis to genetic distances and dendrograms. It displays a global view of the relationships among populations (Greenacre MJ, 1984; Greenacre and Blasius, 1994; Blasius and Greenacre, 1998). With its visual output, it supplements more formal inferential analyzes. This type of analysis tends to give results similar to those of dendrograms as expected from theory (Cavalli-Sforza & Piazza, 1975), but is more informative and accurate than dendrograms especially when there is considerable genetic exchange between close geographic neighbours (Cavalli-Sforza etal. 1994). Cavalli-Sforza et.al. concluded in their enormous effort to work out the genetic relationships among human populations that two-dimensional scatter plots obtained by correspondence analysis frequently resemble geographic maps of the populations with some distortions

(Cavalli-Sforza etal. 1994). Using the same allele frequencies that are used in phylogenetic tree construction, correspondence analysis can be performed on ViSta (v7.0), VST, Statistica, SAS but most conveniently on MultiVariate Statistical Package (MVSP).

Cox Proportional Hazards Model

A regression method described by D.R. Cox (J Royal Stat Soc, Series B 1972;34:187-220; JSTOR-UK) for modeling survival times (for significance of the difference between survival times, log-rank test is used). It is also called proportional hazards model because it estimates the ratio of the risks (hazard ratio or relative hazard). As in any regression model, there are multiple predictor variables (such as prognostic markers whose individual contribution to the outcome is being assessed in the presence of the others) and the outcome variable (e.g., whether the patients survived five years, or died during follow-up, etc). The model assumes that the underlying hazard rate (rather than survival time) is a function of the independent variables and consistent over time (proportionality assumption, i.e. the survival functions of the groups are approximately parallel). There is no assumption for the shape and nature of the underlying survival function. Cox's regression model has been the most widely used method in survival data analysis regardless of whether the survival time is discrete or continuous and whether there is censoring (Lee & Go, 1997). Cox regression uses the maximum likelihood method rather than the least squares method.

Covariate

Generally used to mean explanatory variable, less generally an additional explanatory variable is of no interest but included in the model. More specifically, it denotes a 'continuous' explanatory variable which is unaffected by treatments and has a linear relationship to the response. The intention is to produce more precise estimates of the effect of the explanatory variable of main interest. In the analysis, a model is first fitted using the covariate (and the blocking factor, if any). Then the main explanatory variable is added and its additional effect is assessed statistically. Whether the use of a covariate is wise can be judged by checking its effect on the residual (error) mean square (variance). If the addition of covariate reduces it remarkably, it will improve the analysis.

Covariance (Covariation)

It is a measure of the association between a pair of variables: the expected value of the product of the deviation of two random variables from their respective means. It is also called a measure of 'linear dependence' between the two random variables. If the two variables are independent (no linear correlation), then their covariance is zero but for non-zero values covariance is unstandardized (unlike correlation coefficient); there is no limit to possible values. Because of this, it is difficult to compare covariances. A negative value means that for small values of X, there are large values of Y (inverse association). It is calculated as the mean sum-of-products using each xi and yi values, their means mx and my, and (n-1). (The covariance standardized to lie between -1 and +1 is Pearson's correlation coefficient.)

Covariance Models

Models containing some quantitative and some qualitative explanatory variables, where the chief explanatory variables of interest are qualitative and the quantitative variables are introduced primarily to reduce the variance of the error terms. [Models in which all explanatory variables are qualitative are called analysis of variance–ANOVA–models.] Analysis of covariance–ANCOVA–combines features of ANOVA and regression. It augments the ANOVA model containing the factor effects with one or more additional quantitative variables that are related to the response variable. The intention is to make the analysis more precise by reducing the variance of the error terms. Each continuous quantitative variable added to the ANOVA model is called a concomitant variable (and sometimes also covariates). If qualitative variables are added to an ANOVA model to reduce error variance, the model remains to be ANOVA. By adding extra variables, the results are said to be controlled or adjusted for the additional variables (like age or sex).

Apart from the above use of the term, analysis of covariance is more generally used for almost any analysis assessing the relationship between a response variable and a number of explanatory variables. In a multiple regression model, additional variables, which are known not to have any effect on the response variable, such as age and sex, are sometimes added to the model to adjust the response for these variables (age and sex in this case).

Such variables are called confounders (or covariates). When the response is normally distributed, this is the preferred method over a simple t-test when the two groups compared differ, say, in their age and sex distribution (or any other confounding variable). The result is then controlled (or adjusted) for age and sex. When such adjustments are made, the regression coefficient for the significant effect variable will be (most probably) different from the one obtained from a univariable model involving only that variable (say the effect of a disease on pulse rate as compared to healthy controls).

Cramer's Coefficient of Association (C)

Also known as contingency coefficient. While Chi-squared is used to determine significance of an association (and varies by sample size for the same association), Cramer's C is a measure of association varying from 0 (no association) to 1 (perfect association) that is independent of the sample size. However, it seldom reaches its upper limit. It allows direct comparison of the degree of association between different contingency tables. It is calculated directly from the Chi-squared value and the total sample size as (C2/C2+N) ½.

Cramer's V

A measure of the strength association for any size of contingency tables. It can be seen as a correction of the Chi-squared value for sample size. For a 2x2 table, Cramer's V is equal to the Phi coefficient. Cramer's V is most useful for large contingency tables.

Crossover Design

A clinical trial design during which each subject crosses over from receiving one treatment to another one.

Cross-Sectional Data

Data collected at one point in time (as opposed to longitudinal/cohort data for example).

Degrees of Freedom (df)

The number of independent units of information in a sample used in the estimation of a parameter or calculation of a statistic. In the simplest example of a 2x2 table, if the marginal totals are fixed, only one of the four cell frequencies is free to vary and the others will be dependent on this value not to alter the marginal totals. Thus, the df is only 1. Similarly, it can easily be worked out that in a contingency table with r rows and c columns, the df = (r-1)(c-1). In parametric tests, the idea is slightly different that the n bits of data have n degrees of freedom before we do any statistical calculations. As soon as we estimate a parameter such as the mean, we use up one of the df, which was initially present. This is why in most formulas, the df is (n-1). In the case of a two-sample t-test with n1 and n2 observations, to do the test we calculate both means. Thus, the df = (n1 + n2 - 2). In linear regression, when the linear equation y = a + bx is calculated, two parameters are estimated (the intercept and the slope). The df used up is then 2: df = (n1 + n2 - 2). Non-parametric tests do not estimate parameters from the sample data, therefore, df do not occur in them.

In simple linear regression, the df is partitioned similar to the total sum of squares (TSS). The df for TSS is N-k. Although there are n deviations, one df is lost due to the constraint they are subject to: they must sum to zero. TSS equals to RSS + ESS. In one-way ANOVA, the df for RSS is N-2 because two parameters are estimated in obtaining the fitted line. ESS has only one df associated with it. This is because the n deviations between the fitted values and the overall mean are calculated using the same estimated regression line, which is associated with two df (see above). One of them is lost because of the constraint that the deviations must sum to zero. Thus, there is only one df associated with ESS. Just like TSS = RSS + ESS, their df have the same relationship: N-1 = (N-2) + 1.

Deletion (or Deleted) Residual

A modified version of the standardized residual, which uses an estimate of s2 from a regression in which point i has been deleted. It is used in calculation of the modified Cook's distance instead of standardized residuals. Deletion residuals are also known as likelihood residuals.

Descriptive Statistics

Summary of available data. Examples are male-to-female ratio in a group; numbers of patients in each subgroup; the mean weight of male and female students in a class, etc. Only when the distribution is symmetric, mean and standard deviation can be used. Otherwise (as in survival data), mean and percentiles/range should be used to describe the data.

Discrete Variable

A variable of countable number of integer outcomes. Examples include -ordinal multinomial–several prognostic outcomes (such as poor, median and good) as a function of treatment modalities, stage of the disease, age etc., or –multinomial– people's choices of hospitals (hospital A, B or C) as a function of their income level, age, education etc. A discrete variable may be binomial: diseased or non-diseased in a cohort or case-control study. The nature of the outcome variable as discrete or continuous is crucial in the choice of a regression model.

Dummy Variables

A binary variable that is used to represent a given level of a categorical variable. In genetic data analysis, for example, it is created for each allele at a multiallelic locus. The most common choices as dummy variables are 0 and 1. For each level of the variable, 1 denotes having the feature and 0 denotes all other levels. Also called indicator variables. If an indicator variable is used, the regression coefficient gives the change per unit compared to the reference value. Creating dummy variables on Stata: Stata & UCLA Statistics: STATA Dummy Variables.

Dunn's Test

This test is used when a difference between the groups is found in a non-parametric ANOVA test. Dunn's test is a post hoc test that makes pairwise (multiple) comparisons to identify the different group.

Dunnett's Test

When ANOVA shows a significant difference between groups, if one of the groups is a control (reference) group, Dunnett's Test is used as a post hoc test. This multiple comparison test can be used to determine the significant differences between a single control group mean and the remaining treatment group means in an analysis of variance setting. It is one of the least conservative post hoc tests.

Ecological Study

Analyses based on data grouped to the municipal, provincial or national level.

Ecological Fallacy

The aggregation bias, which is the unfortunate consequence of making inferences for individuals from aggregate data. It results from thinking that relationships observed for groups necessarily hold for individuals. The problem is that it is not valid to apply group statistics to an individual member of the same group.

Edwards' Test

A statistical test for seasonality that looks for a one-cycle sinusoidal deviation from the null distribution.

Effect Modification

The situation in which a measure of effect changes over values of another variable (the association estimates are different in different subpopulations of the sample). The relative risk or odds ratio associated with exposure will be different depending on the value of the effect modifier. For example if in a disease association study, the odds ratios are different in different age groups or in different sexes, age or sex are effect modifiers. Effect modification is highly related to statistical interaction in regression models. If where an exposure decreases risk for one value of the effect modifier and increases risk for another value of effect modifier, this is called crossover.

Eigenvalues (Latent Values)

In multivariate statistics, eigenvalues give the variance of a linear function of the variables. Eigenvalues measure the amount of the variation explained by each principal component (PC) and will be largest for the first PC and smaller for the subsequent PCs. An eigenvalue greater than 1 indicates that PCs account for more variance than accounted by one of the original variables in standardized data. This is commonly used as a cut-off point for which PCs are retained.

EM Algorithm

A method for calculating maximum likelihood estimates with incomplete data. E (expectation)-step computes the expected values for missing data and M (maximization)-step computes the maximum likelihood estimates assuming complete data. It was first used in genetics (Ceppellini R *et.al.*, 1955) to estimate allele frequency for phenotype data when genotypes are not fully observable (this requires the assumption of HWE and calculation of expected genotypes from phenotype frequencies).

Empirical P-Value

A P-value obtained by a simulation program such as Monte Carlo statistics. This is less likely to be affected by multiple comparisons.

Empirical Rule

In variables normally distributed, 68% of the data values are within 1SD of the mean; 95% are within 2SD of the mean; and 99.7% (nearly all) are within 3SD of the mean.

Epidemiologic Flaws and Fallacies

Beware of confounders, selection bias, response bias, variable observer, Hawthorne effect (changes caused by the observer in the observed values), diagnostic accuracy bias, regression to the mean, significance Turkey, nerd of nonsignificance, cohort effect, ecological fallacy, Berkson bias (selection bias in hospital-based studies) and others.

Epi-Info

An epidemiologic data management and analysis package freely available from the CDC website. Originally a DOS program, the latest version (3.3.2) is designed for Microsoft Windows 95-XP (release date: Feb. 9, 2005). There are also tutorials available online: CDC, Nebraska University, Dalhousie University and Henry Ford Health Systems.

Error Terms

Residuals in regression models. Shown as Wi or ei. Their expected value is zero, thus, they vary around zero with a variance equal to s2: N(0, s2). They are assumed to be normally distributed, have equal variance for all fitted values, and independent. Normality is a reasonable assumption in many cases. The assumption of equal variance implies that every observation on the dependent variable contains the same amount of information. The impact of heterogeneous variances is a loss of precision of estimates compared to the precision that would have been realized if the hetrogeneous variances had been taken into account. Transformation of the dependent variable may help to homogenize the unequal variances. Correlated errors are most frequent in time sequence data and they also cause the loss in precision in the estimates.

Explained (Regression) Sum of Squares (ESS)

The measure between treatments sum of squares (variability) in ANOVA. If the means of treatment groups are different, the ESS would be greater than RSS to yield a high variance ratio. The bigger the ESS, the better explained the data by the model.

Exploratory Data Analysis

An initial look at the data with minimal use of formal mathematics or statistical methods, but more with an informal graphical approach. Scatter plots, correlation matrices and contingency tables (for binary data) can be used to get an initial idea for relationships between explanatory variables (for collinearity) or between an explanatory variable(s) and a response variable(s) (correlation). In ANOVA, normality can be checked by box-plots. It gives some indication of which variables should be in the model and which one of them should be put into the model first, and whether linear relationship is adequate.

Exponential Distribution

The (continuous) distribution of time intervals between independent consecutive random events like those in a Poisson process.

Exponential Family

A family of probability distributions in the form

$$f(x) = \exp\{a(q)b(x) + c(q) + d(x)\}$$

where q is a parameter and a, b, c, d are known functions. This family includes the normal distribution, binomial distribution, Poisson distribution and gamma distribution as special cases.

Exposure

In an epidemiologic study, exposure may represent an environmental exposure, an intervention or the presence of a marker (biomarker/genetic marker).

Factor

A categorical explanatory variable with small number of levels such that each item classified belongs to exactly one level for that category. If the factor is 'sex', the levels are 'male' and 'female'; if the factor is 'drug received', the levels are 'drug A', 'drug B', 'drug C', etc. A set of factor levels, uniquely defining a single treatment, is called a cell. A cell may have just one observation (no replication) or multiple observations (replications).

Factorial Experiments

In some data, the explanatory (predictor) variables are all categorical (i.e., factors) and the response variable is quantitative. When there are two or more categorical predictor variables, the data are called factorial. The different possible values of the factors are often assigned numerical values known as levels.

Factorial Analysis of Variance

An analysis in which the treatments differ in terms of two or more factors (with several levels) as opposed to treatments being different levels of a single factor as in one-way ANOVA.

F Distribution

A continuous probability distribution of the ratio of two independent random variables, each having a Chi-squared distribution, divided by their respective degrees of freedom. The most common use is to assign P values to mean square ratios (variance ratios) in ANOVA. In regression analysis, the F-test can be used to test the joint significance of all variables of a model (Tables of critical values of t, F and Chi-square).

Fisher's Exact Test

An exact significance test to analyze 2x2 tables for any sample size. It is a misconception that it is suitable only for small sample sizes. This arises from the demanding computational procedure for large samples, which is no longer an issue. It is the only test for a 2x2 table when an expected number in any cell is smaller than 5.

Friedman Test

This non-parametric test is an extension of Wilcoxon matched pairs signed ranks test which is concerned with more than two time periods of data collection or conditions, and groups of three or more matched subjects.

F Test

The F test for linear regression tests whether the slope is significantly different from 0, which is equivalent to testing whether the fit using non-zero slope is significantly better than the null model with 0 slope.

Gaussian Distribution

Another name for the normal distribution.

G Statistics

An application of the log-likelihood ratio statistics for the hypothesis of independence in an r x c contingency table. It can also be used to test goodness-of-fit. The G-test should be preferred over Chi-squared test when for any cell in the table, ½ O-E½ > E. The Chi-squared distribution is usually poor for the test statistics G2 when N/rc is smaller than five (preferable to the Chi-squared test in Hardy-Weinberg Equilibrium (HWE) test as long as this condition is met). HyperStat and StatXact perform G statistics.

General Linear Model

A group of linear regression models in which the response variable is continuous and normally distributed, the response variable values are predicted from a linear combination of predictor variables, and the linear combination of values for the predictor variables is not transformed (i.e., there is no link function as in generalized linear models). Linear multiple regression is a typical example of general linear models whereas simple linear regression is a special case of generalized linear models with the identity link function.

Generalized Linear Model (GLM)

A model for linear and non-linear effects of continuous and categorical predictor variables on a discrete or continuous but not necessarily normally distributed dependent (outcome) variable. (Note that in the general linear model, the dependent (outcome) variable should be normally distributed). Normal, binary (or linear logistic; when the outcome variable is a proportion), binomial or Poisson (when the outcome variable is a count), exponential and gamma (when the outcome variable is continuous and non-negative) models are different versions of generalized linear models. Particular types of models arise by specifying an appropriate link function, variance and distribution. For example, normal linear regression corresponds to an identity link function, constant variance and a normal distribution. Logistic regression arises from a logit link function and a binomial distribution (the variance of the response (npq) is related to its mean (np): variance = mean (1 - (mean/n)). Loglinear models are used for binomial or Poisson counts. Standard techniques for analyzing censored survival data, such as the Cox regression, can also be handled within the GLM framework.

Genetic Distance

A measurement of genetic relatedness of populations. The estimate is based on the number of allelic substitutions per locus that have occurred during the separate evolution of two populations.

Geometric Mean

G = (x1.x2...xn)1/n where n is the sample size. This can also be expressed as antilog ((1/n) S log x), which means the antilog of the mean of the logs of each value.

Half-Normal Plot

A diagnostic test for model inadequacy or revealing the presence of outliers. It compares the ordered residuals from the data to the expected values of ordered observations from a normal distribution. While the full-normal plots use the signed residuals, half-normal plots use the absolute values of the residuals. Outliers appear at the top right of the plot as distinct points, and departures from a straight line mean that the model is not satisfactory. It is appropriate to use a half-normal plot only when the distribution is symmetrical about zero because any information on symmetry will be lost.

Haplotype Relative Risk Method

This method uses non-inherited parental haplotypes of affected persons as the control group and thus eliminates the risks and bias associated with using unrelated individuals as controls in case-control association studies, as well as the higher cost (see Falk & Rubinstein, 1987; Knapp, 1993; Terwilliger & Ott, 1992).

Harmonic Mean

Of a set of numbers (y1 to yn), the harmonic mean is the reciprocal of the arithmetic mean of the reciprocal of the numbers [H = N / (1/(y1 + y2 + ... yn))]. The harmonic mean is either smaller than or equal to the arithmetic mean. It is a measure of position.

Hazard Function (Instantaneous Failure Rate, Conditional Failure, Intensity, or Force of Mortality Function)

The function that describes the probability of failure during a very small time increment (assuming that no failures have occurred prior to that time). Hazard is the slope of the survival curve – a measure of how rapidly subjects are having the event (dying, developing an outcome etc).

Hazard Rate

It is a time-to-failure function used in survival analysis. It is defined as the probability per time unit that a case that has survived to the beginning of the respective interval will fail in that interval. Specifically, it is computed as the number of failures per time units in the respective interval, divided by the average number of surviving cases at the mid-point of the interval.

Hazard Ratio (Relative Hazard)

Hazard ratio compares two groups differing in treatments or prognostic variables etc. If the hazard ratio is 2.0, then the rate of failure in one group is twice the rate in the other group. The computation of the hazard ratio assumes that the ratio is consistent over time, and that any differences are due to random sampling. Before performing any tests of hypotheses to compare survival curves, the proportionality of hazards assumption should be checked (and should hold for the validity of Cox's proportional hazard models).

Hetereoscedastic Data

Data that have non-constant (heterogeneous) variance across the predicted values of y. In this case, residual graph will show varying variability across the fitted values. This is a regression diagnostic problem and should be fixed by transforming the data.

Heuristics

A term in computer science that refers to guesses made by a program to obtain approximately accurate results. Frequently used in phylogenetics and computational biology.

Hierarchical Model

In linear modeling, models which always include all the lower-order interactions and main effects corresponding to any interaction they include.

Historical Fallacy

The mistake of assuming that an association observed in cross-sectional data will be similar to that observed in longitudinal data or vice versa.

Homoscedasticity (Homogeneity of Variance)

Normal-theory-based tests for the equality of population means such as the t-test and analysis of variance, assume that the data come from populations that have the same variance, even if the test rejects the null hypothesis of equality of population means. If this assumption of homogeneity of variance is not met, the statistical test results may not be valid. Heteroscedasticity refers to lack of homogeneity of variances.

Hotelling's T2 Test

This is a generalization of Student's t-test for multivariate data. Designed to provide a global significance test for the difference between two groups with simultaneously measured multiple dependent/outcome variables and multiple explanatory/independent variables. It can also be used for one group with simultaneously measured multiple dependent outcome variables (another test similar to Hotelling's T2 test is Mahalanobis's D2 test).

Hypergeometric Distribution

A probability distribution of a discrete variable generally associated with sampling from a finite population without replacement. An example may be that given a lot with 25 good units and five faulty. The probability that a sample of five will yield not more than one faulty item follows a hypergeometric distribution.

Index Plot

An index plot plots each residual, leverage, or Cook's distance against the corresponding observation (row) number (i or index) in the dataset. In many cases, the row number corresponds to the order in which the data were collected. If this is the case, this would be similar to plotting the residuals (or another diagnostic quantity) against time. The index plot is a helpful diagnostic test for normal linear and particularly generalized linear models. Both outliers and influential points can be detected by the index plot. It is particularly useful when the data is in time order so that pattern in the residuals, etc. over time can be detected. If a residual index plot is showing a trend in time, then they are not independent (violation of a major assumption of linear regression).

Inferential Statistics

Making inferences about the population from which a sample has been drawn and analyzed.

Influential Points

Observations that actually dominate a regression analysis (due to high leverage, high residuals or their combination). The method of ordinary least squares gives equal weight to every observation. However, every observation does not have equal impact on the least squares results. The slope, for example, is influenced most by the observations having values of the independent variable farthest from the mean. An observation is influential if deleting it from the dataset would lead to a substantial change in the fit of the generalized linear model. High-leverage points have the potential to dominate a regression analysis but not necessarily exert an influence (i.e., a point may have high leverage but low influence as measured by Cook statistics). Cook statistics is used to determine the influence of a data point on the model.

Interaction

If the effect of one factor depends on the level of another factor, the two factors involved are said to interact, and a contrast involving all these levels is called their interaction. Factors A and B interact if the effect of factor A is not independent of the level of factor B. For example, when there are two main effects on a response variable, if their combined effect is higher than the sum of their main effects due to a bonus (say, the effects of a kind of exercise and a kind of diet on blood lipid levels), they have an interaction (meaning a simple additive model is not sufficient to account for the observed data and a multiplicative term must be added). Briefly, interaction is a deviation from additivity. Also, there would be an interaction between the factors sex and treatment if the effect of treatment was not the same for males and females in a drug trial. Interaction is closely linked with effect modification in epidemiology

Intercept

In linear regression, the intercept is the mean value of the response variable when the explanatory variable takes the value of zero (the value of y when x=0).

Interpolation

Making deductions from a model for values that lie between data points. Deductions for values beyond the data points is called extrapolation and the results are not valid.

Interquartile Range (dQ)

dQ is a measure of spread and is the counterpart of the standard deviation for skewed distributions. dQ is the distance between the upper and lower quartiles (QU-QL).

Interval Variable (Equivalent to Continuous Variable)

A quantitative variable measured on a scale with constant intervals (like days, milliliters, kilograms, miles so that equal-sized differences on different parts of the scale are equivalent) where the zero point and unit of measurement are arbitrary. When temperature is measured on two scales, Fahrenheit and Centigrade, the zero points in these two scales do not correspond, and a 10% increase in Fahrenheit (from 500 to 550) is not a 10% increase in the corresponding Centigrade scale (10o to 12.8o = 2.8%); these two measurements cannot be mixed or compared. For estimation of correlation coefficients, data should be interval.

Kolmogorov-Smirnov Two-Sample Test:

A non-parametric test applicable to continuous frequency distributions. It is considered to be the equivalent of the C2-test for quantitative data and has greater power than the G-statistics or C2-test for goodness of fit especially when the sample size is small. It can be used to compare two independent groups. The test is based on differences between two cumulative relative frequency distributions (it compares the distributions not the parameters). Thus, the Kolmogorov-Smirnov test is also sensitive to differences in the general shapes of the distributions in the two samples such as differences in dispersion, skewness. Its interpretation is similar to that of the Wald-Wolfowitz runs test.

Kruskal-Wallis Test (One-way ANOVA by Ranks)

It is one of the non-parametric tests equivalent to one-way ANOVA that are used to compare multiple independent samples (another one is the Median test). This test assesses the hypothesis that the different samples in the comparison were drawn from the same distribution or from distributions with the same median. It can be used to analyze ordinal variables. It is an extension of the Mann-Whitney (U) test. The interpretation of the Kruskal-Wallis test is identical to that of one-way ANOVA, but is based on ranks rather than means

Kurtosis

Kurtosis is a measure of whether the data are peaked or flat in its distribution relative to a normal distribution (whose kurtosis is zero). Positive kurtosis indicates a 'peaked' distribution and negative kurtosis indicates a 'flat' distribution (data sets with high kurtosis have a distinct peak near the mean and decline rapidly; data sets with low kurtosis tend to have a flat top near the mean rather than a sharp peak).

Large Sample Effect

In large samples, even small or trivial differences can become statistically significant. This should be distinguished from biological/clinical importance.

Least Squares Method

A method of fitting a straight line or curve based one minimization of the sum of squared differences (residuals) between the predicted and the observed points. Given the data points (xi, yi), it is possible to fit a straight line using a formula, which gives the y=a+bx. The gradient of the straight line b is given by [S(xi - mx)(yi-my)] / [(S(x-mx))2], where mx and my are the means for xi and yi. The intercept a is obtained by my - bmx.

Leverage Points

In regression analysis, these are the observations that have an extreme value on one or more explanatory variable. The leverage values indicate whether or not X values for a given observation are outlying (far from the main body of the data). A high leverage value indicates that the particular observation is distant from the centre of the X observations. High-leverage points have the potential to dominate a regression analysis but not necessarily influential. If the residual of the same data point and Cook's distance are also high, then it is an influential point.

Likelihood

The probability of a set of observations given the value of some parameter or set of parameters. For example, the likelihood of a random sample of n observations (x1 to xn) with probability distribution f(x; q) is given by: L = P f(xi; q 0). This function, which applies equally to continuous density and discrete mass functions, is the basis of maximum likelihood estimation.

Likelihood Ratio Test

A general purpose test of hypothesis Ho against an alternative H_1 based on the ratio of two likelihood functions one derived from each of Ho and H_1. The statistics l is given by l = -2 ln (LH0 / LH1) has approximately a C_2 distribution with df equal to the difference in the number of parameters in the two hypotheses. One application of this test is the G-test, which is used in categorical data analysis as a goodness-of-fit or independence test (the tests statistics has a Chi-squared distribution).

Linear Expression

A polynomial expression with the degree of polynomial being 1. It will be something like, f(x)=2x1+3, but not x2+2x+4.

Linear Logistic Model

A linear logistic model assumes that for each possible set of values for the independent (X) variables, there is a probability p that an event (success) occurs. Then the model is that Y is a linear combination of the values of the X variables: Y = bo + b1*X1 + b2*X2 + b3*X3 + … bk*Xk, where Y is the logit transformation of the probability p. Logistic in statistical usage stems from logit and has nothing to do with the military use of the word which means the provision of material.

Linear Regression Models

In the context of linear statistical modeling, 'linear' means linear in the parameters (coefficients), not the explanatory variables. The explanatory variables can be transformed (say, x2), but the model will still be linear if the coefficients remain linear. When the overall function (Y) remains a sum of terms that are each an X variable multiplied by a coefficient, the function Y is said to be linear in the coefficients. A non-linear model is different in that it has a non-constant slope.

Log 0 is Undefined

If we need to use a log transformation but some data values are 0, the usual way to get round this problem is to add a small positive quantity (such as 1/2) to all the values before taking logs.

Log Transformation

This transformation pulls smaller data values apart and brings the larger data values together and closer to the smaller data values (shrinkage effect). Thus, it is mostly used to shrink highly positively skewed data.

Logistic (Binary) Regression

A statistical analysis most frequently models the relationship between a dichotomous (binary) outcome variable (such as diseased or healthy; dead or alive; relapsed or not relapsed), and a set of explanatory variables of any kind (such as age, HLA type, blood pressure, kind of treatment, disease stage etc). It can also be used when the outcome variable is polytomous (several categories of the prognosis; including ordinal response 'ordinal logistic regression' or 'proportional odds ratio model'), and when there are several outcome variables (multinomial logistic regression–a special class of loglinear models). Analysis of data from case-control studies via logistic regression can proceed in the same way as cohort studies.

Logit Transformation

The logit (or logistic) transformation Y of a probability p of an event is the logarithm of the ratio between the probability that the event occurs (p) and that the event does not occur (1-p): $Y = \ln (p/(1-p))$. Thus it is a transformation of a binary (dichotomous) response variable. The logit transformation of p is also known as the log odds of p, since it is the logarithm of the odds. There are other link functions for binary response variables.

Loglinear Model

Multinomial data (from contingency tables) can be fitted by using a generalized linear model with a Poisson response distribution and a log link function. The resulting models for counts in the cells of a contingency table are known as loglinear models in which the logarithm of the expected value of a count variable is modeled as a linear function of parameters. Loglinear models try to model all important associations among all variables. In this respect, they are related to ANOVA models for quantitative data. Loglinear modeling allows more than two discrete variables to be analyzed and interactions between any combination of them to be identified. Associations between variables in log–linear models are analogous to interactions in ANOVA models.

The aim is to find a small model, which achieves a reasonable fit (small residual). Data sets with a binary response (outcome) variable and a set of explanatory variables that are all categorical can be modeled either by logistic regression or by loglinear modeling.

Longitudinal Data

Data collected over a period of time as in cohort studies. These data are usually analyzed by using survival analysis techniques.

Mann-Whitney (U) Test

A non-parametric test for comparing the distribution of a continuous variable between two independent groups. It is analogous to the independent two-sample t-test, so that it can be used when the data are ordinal or not normally distributed. The Wilcoxon signed ranks T-test for independent samples is another non-parametric alternative to the t-test in this context (for paired samples, Wilcoxon matched pairs signed rank test should be used).

Mantel-Haenszel C2 Test

Test for a null hypothesis of no overall relationship in a series of 2x2 tables for stratified data derived either from a cohort or a case-control study. It allows analysis of confounding and gives an adjusted odds ratio or relative risk. It can be used on categorical or categorized continuous data. The test is only valid when the variance of observed data is 5. It is inappropriate when the association changes dramatically across strata. It is, however, applicable for sparse data sets for which asymptotic theory does not hold for G2. The test statistics, M2, has approximately a Chi-squared distribution with df = 1. Increasingly more frequently called Cochran-Mantel-Haenszel (CMH) test.

Maximum Likelihood

This method is a general method of finding estimated values of parameters. It yields values for the unknown parameters, which maximize the probability of obtaining the observed values. The estimation process involves considering the observed data values as constants and the parameter to be estimated as a variable, and then using differentiation to find the value of the parameter that maximizes the likelihood function. First a likelihood function is set up which expresses the probability of the observed data as a function of the unknown parameters. The maximum likelihood estimators of these parameters are chosen to be those values, which maximize this function. The resulting estimators are those, which agree most closely with the observed data. This method works best for large samples, where it tends to produce estimators with the smallest possible variance. The maximum likelihood estimators are often biased in small samples. Another method for point estimation is the method of moments.

McNemar's Test

A special form of the Chi-squared test used in the analysis of paired (not independent) proportions. This non-parametric test compares two correlated dichotomous responses and finds its most frequent use in situations where the same sample is used to find out the agreement (concordance) of two diagnostic tests or difference (discordance) between two treatments. If the pairs of data points are the measurements on two matched people (such as affected and unaffected siblings) in a case-control study, or two measurements on the same person, the appropriate test for equality of proportions is the McNemar's test. It can be used to assess the outcome of two treatments applied to the same individuals or the significance of the agreement between two detection methods of a physical sign. If there are more than two periods of data collection (such as pretest, posttest and follow-up), Cochran's Q test should be used.

Mean (or Average)

A measure of location for a batch of data values; the sum of all data values divided by the number of elements in the distribution. Its accompanying measure of spread is usually the standard deviation. Unlike the median and the mode, it is not appropriate to use the mean to characterize a skewed distribution.

Mean Squares

A sum of squares divided by its associated df is a mean square. In ANOVA, the regression (explained) mean square is ESS/k-1, and the residual (error) mean square is RSS/N-k. Note that the mean squares are not additive, i.e., they do not add up to TSS/N-1. Importantly, the residual (error) mean square is an unbiased estimator of the variance (s2) in ANOVA. The regression (explained) mean square equals to the variance only when the slope (b) is zero. Their ratio (mean square ratio = regression MS / residual MS) is therefore provides a test for the null hypothesis that b = 0. Large F values support the alternative hypothesis that the slope is not zero. This is the basis of the F test in ANOVA.

Measurement Type

The data may be measured in the following scales: nominal, ordinal, interval or ratio scales (known as Stevens' typology). The scale of the measurements may be (other than nominal scale measurements) either continuous or discrete, and either bounded or unbounded.

Measures of Association

These measures include the Phi coefficient of association, Cramer's contingency coefficient (C) and V, Kendall's tau-b and (Stuart's) tau-c, Somers' D (a modification of Kendall's tau-b), Yule's Q, gamma, Spearman's rank correlation coefficient (rho), Pearson's correlation coefficient, lambda (symmetric and asymmetric), uncertainty coefficients (symmetric and asymmetric), Guttman's coefficient of predictability (lambda)/Goodman-Kruskal's lambda, Goodman-Kruskal's gamma and Goodman-Kruskal's tau (concentration coefficient).

Measures of Central Tendency

These are parameters that characterize an entire distribution. These include mode, median and mean.

Median

Another measure of location just like the mean. The value that divides the frequency distribution in half when all data values are listed in order. It is insensitive to small numbers of extreme scores in a distribution. Therefore, it is the preferred measure of central tendency for a skewed distribution (in which the mean would be biased) and is usually paired with the interquartile range (dQ) as the accompanying measure of spread.

Median Test

This is a crude version of the Kruskal-Wallis ANOVA in that it assesses the difference in samples in terms of a contingency table. The number of cases in each sample that fall above or below the common median is counted and the Chi-square value for the resulting 2xk samples contingency table is calculated. Under the null hypothesis (all samples come from populations with identical medians), approximately 50% of all cases in each sample are expected to fall above (or below) the common median. The median test is particularly useful when the scale contains artificial limits, and many cases fall at either extreme of the scale. In this case, the median test is the most appropriate method for comparing samples.

Meta-Analysis

A systematic approach yielding an overall answer by analyzing a set of studies that address a related question. This approach is best suited to questions, which remain unanswered after a series of studies. Meta-analysis provides a weighted average of the measure of effect (such as odds ratio). The rationale is to increase the power by analyzing the sets of data. The selection of studies to include in a meta-analysis study is the main problem with this approach. Funnel Plot is an informal method to assess the effect of publication bias in this context.

Mode

The observed value that occurs with the greatest frequency. The mode is not influenced by small numbers of extreme values.

Model Building

The traditional approach to statistical model building is to find the most parsimonious model that still explains the data. The more variables included in a model (overfitting), the more likely it becomes mathematically unstable, the greater the estimated standard errors become, and the more dependent the model becomes on the observed data. Choosing the most adequate and minimal number of explanatory variables helps to find out the main sources of influence on the response variable, and increases the predictive ability of the model. Ideally, there should be more than 10 observations for each variable in the model. The usual procedures used in variable selection in regression analysis are: univariate analysis of each variable (using C2 test), stepwise method (backward or forward elimination of variables; using the deviance difference), and best subsets selection. Once the essential main effects are chosen, interactions should be considered next. As in all model building situations in biostatistics, biological considerations should play a role in variable selection.

Multicolinearity

In multiple regression, two or more X variables are colinear if they show strong linear relationships. This makes estimation of regression coefficients impossible. It can also produce unexpectedly large estimated standard errors for the coefficients of the X variables involved. This is why an exploratory analysis of the data should be first done to see if any collinearity among explanatory variables exists. Multicolinearity is suggested by non-significant results in individual tests on the regression coefficients for important explanatory (predictor) variables. Multicolinearity may make the determination of the main predictor variable having an effect on the outcome difficult.

Multiple Regression

To quantify the relationship between several independent (explanatory) variables and a dependent (outcome) variable. The coefficients (a, b1 to bi) are estimated by the least squares method, which is equivalent to maximum likelihood estimation. A multiple regression model is built upon three major assumptions:

1. The response variable is normally distributed,
2. The residual variance does not vary for small and large fitted values (constant variance),
3. The observations (explanatory variables) are independent.

Multiple regression is the prototype for general linear models because the response variable should be normally distributed and there is no link function, whereas, simple linear regression is a special case for generalized linear models. The extension of multiple regression to multivariate data analysis is called canonical correlation.

Multiplication Rule

The probability of two or more statistically independent events all occurring is equal to the product of their individual probabilities. If the probability of having trisomy 21 is a, and trisomy 6 is b, assuming independence of these two events, for a baby the probability of having both trisomies is (a x b). One of the most critical errors of judgment in the use of independence assumption relates to a court case in the UK (Watkins, 2000).

Multivariable Analysis

As opposed to univariable analysis, statistical analysis performed in the presence of more than one explanatory variable to determine the relative contributions of each to a single event is (or should be) called multivariable analysis (in practice, however, it is called univariate and multivariate analysis more frequently). It is a method to simultaneously assess contributions of multiple variables or adjust for the effects of confounders. Multiple linear regression, multiple logistic regression, proportional hazards analysis are examples of multivariable analysis, which has no similarity whatsoever to multivariate analysis.

Multivariate Analysis

Methods to deal with more than one related 'outcome/dependent variable' (like two outcome measures from the same individual) simultaneously with adjustment for multiple confounding variables (covariates). When there is more than one dependent variable, it is inappropriate to do a series of univariate tests. Hotelling's T2 test is used when there are two groups (like cases and controls) with multiple dependent measures (may be more than two), and multivariate analysis of variance (MANOVA) is used for more than two groups. Wilks' lambda is the most common parameter used to quantitate the significance of the result of a multivariate procedure (others are Roy's largest criterion, Hotelling-Lawley trace, and Pillai-Bartlett trace). Unfortunately, the word 'multivariate' is most frequently used instead of 'multivariable' analysis (which means multiple independent/explanatory variables but one outcome/dependent variable). Canonical correlation, cluster analysis, factor analysis (FA) and principal component analysis (PCA) are types of multivariate analysis. PCA aims at reducing a large set of variables to a small set that still contains most of the information in the large set. While PCA summarizes or approximates the data using fewer dimensions (to visualize it, for example), FA provides an explanatory model for the correlations among the data

Multivariate Analysis of Variance (MANOVA)

An extension of Hotelling's T2 test to more than two groups with related 'multiple' outcome measures. Groups are compared on all variables simultaneously as a global test (rather than one-by-one as ANOVA does).

Negative Predictive Value

Probability of a true negative as in a person identified healthy by a test is really free from the disease.

Nested Model

Models that are related where one model is an extension of the other.

Nominal Variable

A qualitative variable defined by mutually exclusive unordered categories such as blood groups, races, sex etc.

Nonlinear Regression

Regression analysis in which the fitted (predicted) value of the response variable is a nonlinear function of one or more X variables.

Nonparametric Methods (Distribution Free Methods)

Statistical methods to analyze data from populations, which do not assume a particular population distribution. Mann-Whitney U test, Kruskal-Wallis test and Wilcoxon's (T) test are examples. Such tests do not assume a distribution of the data specified by certain parameters (such as mean or variance). For example, one of the assumptions of the Student's t-test and ANOVA is normal distribution of the data. If this is not valid, a non-parametric equivalent must be used. If a wrong choice of test has been made, it does not matter very much if the sample size is large (a non-parametric test can be used where a parametric test might have been used but a parametric test can only be used when the assumptions are met). For a small sample size, non-parametric tests tend to give a larger P value. In general, parametric tests are more robust, more complicated to compute and have greater power efficiency. Parametric tests compare parameters such as the mean in t-test and variance in F-test as opposed to non-parametric tests that compare distributions. Non-parametric methods are most appropriate when the sample sizes are small. In large (e.g., $n > 100$) data sets, it makes little sense to use nonparametric statistics.

Normal Distribution

(Gaussian distribution) is a model for values on a continuous scale. A normal distribution can be completely described by two parameters: mean (m) and variance (s2). It is shown as C ~ N(m, s2). The distribution is symmetrical with mean, mode and median all equal at m. In the special case of m = 1 and s2 = 1, it is called the standard normal distribution.

Normal Probability Plot of the Residuals

A diagnostic test for the assumption of normal distribution of residuals in linear regression models. Each residual is plotted against its expected value under normality. A plot that is nearly linear suggests normal distribution of the residuals. A plot that obviously departs from linearity suggests that the error distribution is not normal.

Null Model

A model in which all parameters except the intercept are 0. It is also called the intercept–only model. The null model in linear regression is that the slope is 0, so that the predicted value of Y is the mean of Y for all values of X. The F test for the linear regression tests whether the slope is significantly different from 0, which is equivalent to testing whether the fit using non-zero slope is significantly better than the null model with 0 slope.

Number Needed to Treat

The reciprocal of the reduction in absolute risk between treated and control groups in a clinical trial. It is interpreted as the number of patients who need to be treated to prevent one adverse event.

Odds

The odds of a success is defined as the ratio of the probability of a success to the probability of a failure (p/(1-p)). If a team has a probability of 0.6 of winning the championship, the odds for winning is 0.6/(1-0.6) = 3:2. Similarly, the odd in a case-control study is the frequency of the presence of the marker divided by the frequency of absence of the marker (in cases or controls separately). The link function logit (or logistic) is the loge of the odds.

Odds Multiplier

In logistic regression, b = loge (odds ratio), thus exp b = odds ratio. For a continuous (explanatory) variable, exp b is called the odds multiplier and corresponds to the odds ratio for a unit increase in the explanatory variable. The odds multiplier of the coefficient is the odds ratio for its level relative to the reference level. If x increases from a to b by c, the odds multiplier becomes exp (cb). The resulting value shows the proportional change in the odds associated with x = b relative to x = a. It follows that for binary variables where x can only get values of 0 and 1, exp b = odds ratio.

Odds Ratio (OR)

Also known as relative odds and approximate relative risk. It is the ratio of the odds of the risk factor in a diseased group and in a non-diseased (control) group (the ratio of the frequency of presence/absence of the marker in cases to the frequency of presence/absence of the marker in controls). The interpretation of the OR is that the risk factor increases the odds of the disease 'OR' times. OR is used in retrospective case-control studies (relative risk (RR) is the ratio of proportions in two groups which can be estimated in a prospective–cohort–study). These two and relative hazard (or hazard ratio) are measures of the strength/magnitude of an association. As opposed to the P value, these do not change with the sample size. OR and RR are considered interchangeable when certain assumptions are met, especially for large samples and rare diseases. Odds ratio is calculated as ad/bc where a,b,c,d are the entries in a 2x2 contingency table (hence the alternative definition as the cross-product ratio). In logistic regression, the coefficient b corresponds to the loge of the odds ratio. There are statistical methods to test the homogeneity of odds ratios.

One-Way ANOVA

A comparison of several groups of observations, all of which are independent and subjected to different levels of a single treatment (such as cells exposed to different dosage of a growth factor). It may be that different groups were exposed to the same treatment (different cell types exposed to a new agent). The main interest focuses on the differences among the means of groups.

Ordinal Variable

An ordered (ranked) qualitative/categorical variable. The degree of HLA matching (one, two, three or four antigen matching in two loci) in transplant pairs, or HLA sharing in parents (one-to-four shared antigens) are ordinal variables although the increments do not have to be equal in magnitude (see interval and ratio variables). An ordinal variable may be a categorized quantitative variable. When two groups are compared for an ordinal variable, it is inappropriate to use ordinary Chi-squared test but the trend test or its equivalents must be used.

Outcome (Response, Dependent) Variable

The observed variable, which is shown on y axis. A statistical model shows this as a function of predictor variable(s).

Outlier

An extreme observations that is well separated from the remainder of the data. In regression analysis, not all outlying values will have an influence on the fitted function. Those outlying with regard to their X values (high leverage), and those with Y values that are not consistent with the regression relation for the other values (high residual) are expected to be influential. The test the influence of such values, the Cook statistics is used.

Overdispersion

Dispersion is a measure of the extent to which data are spread about an average. Overdispersion is the situation that occurs most frequently in Poisson and binomial regression when variance is much higher than the mean (normally, it should be similar). It is evident with a high (>2) residual mean deviance (which should normally be around one) and the presence of too many outliers. The reasons for overdispersion may be outliers, misspecification of the model, variation between the response probabilities and correlation between the binary responses. It distorts standard error and confidence interval estimations. In the analysis, overdispersion may be taken into account by estimating a dispersion parameter.

Overfitting

In a multivariable model, having more variables than can be justified from sample size. The statistical rule of thumb is to have at least ten subjects for each variable investigated.

Overmatching

When cases and controls are matched by an unnecessary non-confounding variable, this is called overmatching and causes underestimation of an association. For example, matching for a variable strongly correlated with the exposure but not with the outcome will cause loss of efficiency. Another kind of overmatching is matching for a variable which is in the causal chain or closely linked to a factor in the causal chain. This will also obscure evidence for a true association. Finally, if a too strict matching scheme is used, it will be very hard to find controls for the study.

Parameter

A numerical characteristic of a population specifying a distribution model (such as normal or Poisson distribution). This may be the mean, variance, degrees of freedom, the probability of a success in a binomial distribution, etc.

Pearson's Correlation Coefficient (r)

A measure of the strength of the 'linear' relationship between two quantitative variables. A major assumption is the normal distribution of variables. If this is not met (for example, due to outliers), the non-parametric equivalent Spearman's rank correlation should be used. The r represents C2 obtained from the 2x2 table, corrected for the total sample size. It can then be calculated as ±(C2/N)1/2. This formula is equivalent to covariance divided by the product of the standard deviations of the two variables. The correlation coefficient, r, can take any value between -1 and +1; 0 meaning no "linear" relationship (there may still be a strong non-linear relationship). It is the absolute value of r showing the strength of relationship. An associated P value can be computed for the statistical significance (a small P value does not necessarily mean a strong relationship). The square of the r, is r2 (coefficient of determination). It is also shown as R2, and used in regression analysis.

Poisson Distribution

The probability distribution of the number of (rare) occurrences of some random event in an interval of time or space. Poisson distribution is used to represent distribution of counts like number of defects in a piece of material, customer arrivals, insurance claims, incoming telephone calls, or alpha particles emitted. A transformation that often changes Poisson data approximately normal is the square root.

Polynomial

A sum of multiples of integer powers of a variable. The highest power in the expression (n) is the degree of the polynomial. When n=1, for example, f(x)=2x1+3, this is a linear expression. If n=2, it is quadratic (for example, x2 + 2x + 4); if n=3, it is cubic, if n=4, it is quartic and if n=5, it is quintic.

Population

The population is the universe of all the objects from which a sample could be drawn for an experiment.

Population Attributable Risk

The proportion of a disease in a specified population attributable to a specific factor (such as a genetic risk factor).

Population Stratification (Substructure)

An example of 'confounding by ethnicity' in which the co-existence of different disease rates and allele frequencies within population sub-sections lead to an association between the two at a whole population level. Differing allele frequencies in ethnically different strata in a single population may lead to a spurious association or mask an association by artificially modifying allele frequencies in cases and controls when there is no real association (for this to happen, the subpopulations should differ not only in allele frequencies but also in baseline risk to the disease being studied).

Positive Predictive Value

Probability of a true positive as in a person identified as diseased by a test is really diseased.

Predictor (Explanatory, Independent) Variable

The variable already in hand in the beginning of an experiment or observation and whose effect on an outcome variable is being modeled.

Predictive Value

The probability that a person with a positive test if affected by the disease (positive predictive value) or the probability that a person with a negative test does not have the disease (negative predictive value). Estimation requires sensitivity, specificity and disease prevalence.

Prevented Fraction

The amount of a health problem that actually has been prevented by a prevention strategy in real world.

Probability

The ratio of the number of likely outcomes to the number of possible outcomes.

Probability Density Function

When a curve is used to model the variation in a population and the total area between the curve and the x-axis is 1, then the function that defines the curve is a probability density function.

Probability Distribution Function

A function which gives for each number x, the probability that the value of a continuous random variable X is less than or equal to x. For discrete random variables, the probability distribution function is given as the probability associated with each possible discrete value of the variable.

Proportional Odds Ratio

When the response variable in an ordered/ordinal logistic regression model has more than two ordered response categories, odds ratio obtained for each category is called a proportional odds ratio

P-value (SP = Significance Probability)

The P value gives the probability that the null hypothesis is correct; therefore, if it is a small value (like <0.05), null hypothesis is rejected. More technically, it is the probability of the observed data or more extreme outcome would have occurred by chance, i.e., departure from the null hypothesis when the null hypothesis is true. In a genetic association study, the P value represents the probability of error in accepting the alternative hypothesis (or rejecting the null hypothesis) for the presence of an association. For example, the P level of 0.05 (i.e., 1/20) indicates that assuming there was no relation between those variables whatsoever (the null hypothesis is correct), and we were repeating experiments like ours one after another, we could expect that approximately in every 20 replications of the experiment, there would be one in which the relation between the variables in question would be equal to or more extreme than what has been found. In the interpretation of a P value, it is important to know the accompanying measure of association and the biological/clinical significance of the significant difference. However small, a P value does not indicate the size of an effect (odds ratio/relative risk/hazard ratio do). A P value >0.05 does not necessarily mean lack of association. It does so only if there is enough power to detect an association. Most statistical nonsignificance is due to lack of power to detect an association (poor experimental design). Both 'p' and 'P' are used to indicate significance probability but the international standard is P.

Qualitative

Qualitative (categorical) variables define different categories or classes of an attribute. Examples are gender, blood groups or disease states. A qualitative (categorical) variable may be nominal or ordinal. When there are only two categories, it is termed binary (like sex, dead or alive).

Quantitative

Quantitative variables are variables for which a numeric value representing an amount is measured. They may be discrete (for example, taking values of integers) or continuous (such as weight, height, blood pressure). If a quantitative variable is categorized, it becomes an ordinal variable.

Random Sampling

A method of selecting a sample from a target population or study base using simple or systematic random methods. In random sampling, each subject in the target population has equal chance of being selected to the sample. Sampling is a crucially important point in selection of controls for a case-control study. By randomization, systematic effects are turned into error (term), and there is an expected balancing out effect: known and unknown factors that might influence the outcome are assigned equally to the comparison groups. One disadvantage of randomization is generation of a potentially large error term. This can be avoided by using a block design.

Randomized (Complete) Block Design

An experimental design in which the treatments in each block are assigned to the experimental units in random order. Blocks are all of the same size and each treatment appears in the same number of times within each block (usually once). A different level of the factor is assigned to each member of the block randomly. The data can be analyzed using the paired t-test (when there are two units per block) or by randomized block ANOVA (in blocks of any size). The results are substantially more precise than a completely randomized design of comparable size. In studies with a block design, more assumptions are required for the model: no interactions between treatments and blocks, and constant variance from block to block.

Ratio Variable

A quantitative variable that has a zero point as its origin (like 0 cm = 0 inch) so that ratios between values are meaningfully defined. Unlike the interval variables, which do not have a true zero point, the ratio of any two values in the scales is independent of the unit of measurement. For example, 2/12 cm has the same ratio as the corresponding values in inch (but the same cannot be said for 2/12 Celsius and 2/12 Fahrenheit which are interval variables).

Regression Diagnostics

Tests to identify the main problem areas in regression analysis: normality, common variance and independence of the error terms; outliers, influential data points, collinearity, independent variables being subject to error, and inadequate specification of the functional form of the model. The purpose of the diagnostic techniques is to identify weaknesses in the regression model or the data. Remedial measures, correction of errors in the data, elimination of true outliers, collection of better data, or improvement of the model, will allow greater confidence in the final product. See also error terms, residuals (including likelihood distance test), leverages and Cook statistics.

Regression Modeling

Formulating a mathematical model of the relationship between a response (outcome, dependent) variable, Y, and a set of explanatory (predictor, independent, regressor) variables, x. Depending on the characteristics of the variables, the choice of model can be simple linear regression, multiple regression, logistic (binary) regression, Poisson regression, etc. In any regression problem, the key quantity is the mean value of the outcome variable, given the value of the independent variable(s). This quantity is called the conditional mean and expressed as "E (Y½x)" where Y is the response (outcome), x is the explanatory (predictor) variable. The question is whether the variable(s) in question tells us more about the outcome variable than a model that does not include that variable. In other words, whether the coefficient of the variable(s) is zero and the outcome is equal to a constant (which is the mean for Y) or not. The aim of model building is to arrive at a meaningful (say, biologically relevant) and parsimonious model that explains the data. The model may be linear if the parameters are linear, or nonparametric if the parameters are not linear. No matter how strong is the statistical relationship between x and Y, no cause-and-effect pattern is necessarily implied by the regression models.

Relative Risk (RR)

Also known as risk ratio. The RR shows how many times more or less the individuals with the risk factor are likely to get the disease relative to those who do not have the risk factor. RR gives the strength of association in prospective cohort studies. It cannot be estimated in retrospective case-control studies, and its use to describe the cross-product ratio (as frequently done in HLA association studies) is inappropriate.

Resampling Statistics

Data-based simulation procedures that sample (with replacement) repeatedly from observed data to generate empirical estimates of results that would be expected by chance. Examples include bootstrapping and permutation tests.

Residuals

Residuals reflect the overall badness-of-fit of the model. They are the differences between the observed values of the outcome variable and the corresponding fitted values predicted by the regression line (the vertical distance between the observed values and the fitted line). In a regression analysis, a large residual for a data point indicates that the data point concerned is not close to its fitted value. If there are too many large (standardized) residuals either the model fitted is not adequate or there is overdispersion of the data. Ideally, the residuals should have constant variance along the line. This can be checked by a normal probability plot of the residuals. In the plot of residuals against the explanatory variable (or the fitted values), there should not be any pattern if the assumption of constant variation is met, i.e., residuals do not tend to get larger as the variable values get larger or smaller.

Residual Plot

A graph that plots residuals against fitted values. It is used to check equal variance assumption of the error terms in linear regression. Residual analysis for logistic regression is more difficult than for general linear regression models because the responses Yi can take only the values 0 and 1. Consequently, the residuals will not be normally distributed. Plots of residuals against fitted values or explanatory variables will be uninformative. Residual plots are generally unhelpful for generalized linear models (where index plots and half-normal plots are preferred).

Residual (Error) Sum of Squares (RSS)

The measure of within treatment groups sum of squares (variability) in ANOVA. It is the deviation around the fitted regression line. The sum of squared differences between each observed Y value (Yi) and the fitted Y value (Yi -hat) equals to the residual (error) sum of squares.

Regression (Explained) Sum of Squares (ESS)

The measure of between treatment groups sum of squares (variability) in ANOVA. It is the deviation of fitted regression value around mean. The sum of squared differences between each fitted Y value (Yi-hat) and the overall mean of the Y values equals to the explained (regression) sum of squares. The sum of ESS and RSS gives the total sum of squares (TSS) which equals to the sum of squared differences between each observed Y value (Yi) and the overall mean (total deviation).

Risk Ratio (Relative Risk)

The risk ratio is the percentage difference in classification between two groups obtained as the ratio of two risks or proportions. For example, the proportion of people recovering after stroke with one treatment equals 0.10, while the proportion after a different treatment equals 0.16. The risk ratio equals 0.625 (0.10/0.16); 37.5% ((1-0.625)*100 or (0.16-0.10)/0.16) fewer patients treated by the first method recover. The risk ratio takes on values between zero ('0') and infinity. One ('1') is the neutral value and means that there is no difference between the groups compared.

Robustness

A statistical test or procedure is robust when violation of assumptions has little effect on the results. Student's t-test, for example, is robust against departures from normality.

Sample Size Determination

Mathematical process of deciding how many subjects should be studied (at the planning phase of a study). Among the factors to consider are the incidence or prevalence of the condition, the magnitude of difference expected between cases and controls, the power that is desired and the allowable magnitude of type I error (pre-determined significance probability).

SAS (Statistical Analysis System)

A comprehensive computer software system for data processing and analysis. It can be used for almost any type of statistical analysis. Produced by SAS.

Scales of Measurement

The type of data is always one of the following four scales of measurement: nominal, ordinal, interval, or ratio. Each of these can be discrete or continuous.

Sensitivity

Sensitivity is the proportion of true positives that are correctly identified by a diagnostic test. Those that produce few false negatives have higher sensitivity.

Sign Test

A test based on the probabilities of different outcomes for any number of pluses and minuses, i.e., observations below or above a prespecified value. The sign test can be used to investigate the significance of the difference between a population median and a specified value for it, or between the observed sex/transmission ratio and the 50:50 expected value. It can also be used for paired data. This time, the differences between the pairs will be either negative or positive, and the smaller of the two total negatives or positives plus the total number of pairs will form the test statistics. For example, when the total number is 20, if the number for the less frequent sign is 5 or smaller, $P < 0.05$ (two-tailed) A sign test in disguise is McNemar's test, which is used for paired data for dichotomous response.

Simple Linear Regression Model

The linear regression model for a normally distributed outcome (response) variable and a single predictor (explanatory) variable. The straight line models the mean value of the response variable for each value of the explanatory variable. The major assumption is constant variation of residuals along the fitted line which points out that the model is equally good across all x values. The null hypothesis stating that the explanatory variable has no effect on the response (in other words, the slope of the fitted line is zero) can be tested statistically. The two main aims of regression analysis are to predict the response and to understand the relationships between variables. As in all linear models, the error term (shown as Wi or ei) is additive (as opposed to multiplicative, i.e., yi = a + bxi + ei) and independent, and they are assumed to have a normal distribution. As an exception, the simple linear regression is a special case for generalized linear models.

Skewness

The degree of (lack of) asymmetry about a central value of a distribution. A distribution with many small values and few large values is positively (right) skewed (long tail in the distribution curve or stemplot is to the right); the opposite (left tail) is negatively (left) skewed. The measures of location median, midinterquartile range (midQ) and midrange decrease in this order for a left-skewed distribution.

Spearman's Rank Correlation

A non-parametric correlation coefficient (rho) that is calculated by computing the Pearson's correlation coefficient (r) for the association between the ranks given to the values of the variables involved. It is used for ordinal data and interval/ratio data. It is also possible to compare two correlation coefficients.

Specificity

Specificity is the proportion of true negatives that are correctly identified by the test. Those that produce few false positives have higher specificity.

Standard Deviation

Like variance, the standard deviation (SD) is a measure of spread (scatter) of a set of data. Unlike variance, which is expressed in squared units of measurement, the SD is expressed in the same units as the measurements of the original data. It is calculated from the deviations between each data value and the sample mean. It is the square root of the variance. For different purposes, n (the total number of values) or n-1 may be used in computing the variance/SD. If you have a SD calculated by dividing by n and want to convert it to a SD corresponding to a denominator of n-1, multiply the result by the square root of n/(n-1). If a distribution's SD is greater than its mean, the mean is inadequate as a representative measure of central tendency. For normally distributed data values, approximately 68% of the distribution falls within ± 1 SD of the mean, 95% of the distribution falls within ± 2 SDs of the mean, and 99.7% of the distribution falls within ± 3 SDs of the mean (empirical rule). SD should not be confused with the standard error of the mean (SEM), which is the SD of the sampling distribution of a statistics and quantifies how accurately the mean is known .

Standard Error

The standard error (SE) or as commonly called the standard error of the mean (SEM) is a measure of the extent to which the sample mean deviates from the true but unknown population mean. It is the standard deviation (SD) of the random sampling distribution of means (i.e., means of multiple samples from the same population). As such, it measures the precision of the statistic as an estimate of a population. The (estimated) SE/SEM is dependent on the sample size. It is inversely related to the square root of the sample size:

(Estimated) SE = SD / (N)1/2

The true value of the SE can only be calculated if the SD of the population is known. When the sample SD is used (as almost always), it is an estimate and should be called estimated standard error (ESE). When the sample size is relatively large (N ³ 100), the sample SD provides a reliable estimate of the SE.

Standard Residual

The standardized residual value (observed minus predicted divided by the square root of the residual mean square).

Stata

A powerful statistical package particularly useful for epidemiologic and longitudinal data management and analysis. It is mainly a command driven program produced by Stata Corporation.

Statistical Power

The probability that a test will produce a significant difference at a given significance levèl is called the power of the test. This is equal to the probability of rejecting the null hypothesis when it is untrue, i.e., making the correct decision. It is 1 minus the probability of a type II error. The true differences between the populations compared, the sample size and the significance level chosen affect the power of a statistical test. Ideally, power should be at least 0.80 to detect a reasonable departure from the null hypothesis.

Stepwise Regression Model

A method in multiple regression studies aimed to find the best model. This method seeks a model that balances a relatively small number of variables with a good fit to the data by seeking a model with high R2a (the most parsimonious model with the highest percentage accounted for). The stepwise regression can be started from a null or a full model and can go forward or backward, respectively. At any step in the procedure, the statistically most important variable will be the one that produces the greatest change in the log-likelihood relative to a model lacking the variable. This would be the variable, which would result in the largest likelihood ratio statistics, G (a high percentage accounted for gives an indication that the model fits well).

Stochastic Model

A probability model that includes chance events in the form of random measurement error or uncertainty. In a deterministic model, however, random error is inconsequential or nonexistent.

Stratum (Plural Strata)

When data are stratified according to its characteristics, each subgr .up is a stratum.

Student's t-Test

A parametric test for the significance between means (two independent sample t-test or paired samples t-test) or between a mean and a hypothesized value (one-sample t-test). One assumption is that the observations must be normally distributed, and the ratio of variances in two samples should not be more than three. If the assumptions are not met, there are non-parametric equivalents of the t-test to use (for example, Wilcoxon's Test). It is inappropriate to use the t-test for multiple comparisons as a post hoc test. The t-test for independent samples tests whether or not two means are significantly different from each other but only if they were the only two samples taken.

Subgroup Analysis

Analysis of subgroups of a sample either because of a prior hypothesis (gender or age-specific effect/association) or as a fishing expedition / data dredging. This practice increases type I error rates.

Survival Function

A time to failure function that gives the probability that an individual survives past a time point (does not experience an event like death, metastasis, conception etc). Where the event is death, the value of the survival function at time T is the probability that a subject will die at some time greater than T. The survival function always has a value between 0 and 1 and is non-increasing.

Treatment

In experiments, a treatment is what is administered to experimental units (explanatory variables). It does not have to be a medical treatment. Fertilizers in agricultural experiments; different books and multimedia methods in teaching; and chemotherapy of bone marrow transplantation in the treatment of leukemia are examples of treatments in regression analysis.

Trend Test for Counts and Proportions

A special application of the Chi-squared test (with a different formula) for ordinal data tabulated as a 2xk table. It should be used when the intention is not just to compare the differences between the two groups but to see whether there is a consistent trend towards decrease or increase in the difference between the groups. An example is the association of parental HLA sharing (one-to-four antigens in two loci) with fetal loss in a case-control study (those with recurrent miscarriages and normal fertile couples). A frequent application is the analysis of dose-response relationships. The Chi-squared test for trend has one degree of freedom. The associated P value obtained by the trend test is always smaller than the corresponding P value of an ordinary Chi-squared test. The trend test for counts and proportions is called

Cochrane-Armitage trend test. Alternative tests for the analysis of trend are Wilcoxon-Mann-Whitney test or the t-test with use of ordered scores.

t-Statistics

Defined as difference of sample means divided by standard error of difference of sample means.

Two-Way ANOVA

This method studies the effects of two factors (with several levels) separately (main effect) and, if desired, their effect in combination (interaction).

Type I Error

If the null hypothesis is true but we reject it this is an error of first kind or type I error (also called a error). This results in a false positive finding.

Type II Error

If the null hypothesis is accepted when it is in fact wrong, this is an error of the second kind or type II error (also called b error). This results in a false negative result.

Variable

Some characteristic that varies among experimental units (subjects) or from time to time. A variable may be quantitative or categorical. A quantitative variable is either discrete (assigning meaningful numerical values to observations: number of children, dosage in mg) or continuous (such as height, weight, temperature, blood pressure; also called interval variable). A categorical variable is either nominal (assigning observations to categories: gender, treatment, disease subtype, groups) or ordinal (ranked variables: low, median, high dosage). Conventionally, a random variable is shown by a capital letter, and the data values it takes by lower case letters.

Variance

The major measure of variability for a data set. To calculate the variance, all data values, their mean, and the number of data values are required. It is expressed in the squared unit of measurement. Its square root is the standard deviation. It is symbolized by s2 for a population and S2 for a sample.

Wilcoxon Matched Pairs Signed Rank T-test

A non-parametric significance test analogous to paired t-test. Most suitable for ordinal or interval/ratio variables. It is used to test for the significance of the difference between the distributions of two non-independent samples (repeated measures or matched pairs).

Yates's Correction

The approximation of the Chi-square statistic in small 2x2 tables can be improved by reducing the absolute value of differences between expected and observed frequencies by 0.5 before squaring. This correction, which makes the estimation more conservative, is usually applied when the table contains only small observed frequencies (<20). The effect of this correction is to bring the distribution based on discontinuous frequencies nearer to the continuous Chi-squared distribution. This correction is best suited to the contingency tables with fixed marginal totals. Its use in other types of contingency tables (for independence and homogeneity) results in very conservative significance probabilities. This correction is no longer needed since exact tests are available.

Z Score

The Z score or value expresses the number of standard errors by which a sample mean lies above or below the true population mean. Z scores are standardized for a distribution with mean = 0 and standard deviation = 1 The Z-statistics is defined as difference of sample proportions divided by standard error of difference of sample proportions.

APPENDIX

Area under standard normal curve (Z - score)

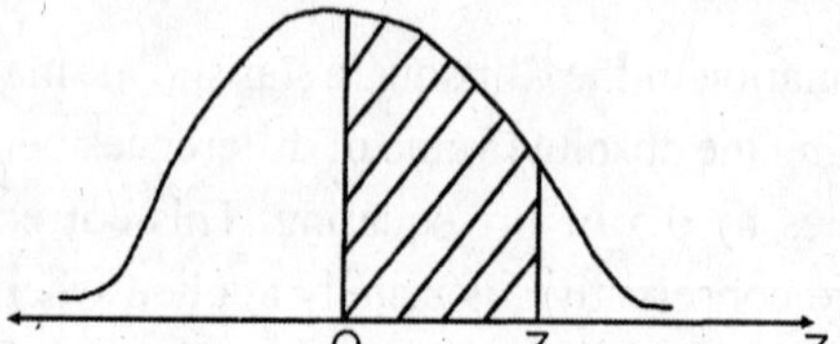

STATISTICAL TABLES

Table A

0.1	0.0398	0.0438	0.0487	0.0517	0.0557	0.0598	0.0336	0.0675	0.07114	0.0753
0.2	0.0793	0.0832	0.0871	0.0910	0.0948	0.0987	0.1026	0.1064	0.1103	0.1141
0.3	0.1179	0.1217	0.1255	0.1293	0.1331	0.1368	0.1406	0.1443	0.1480	0.1517
0.4	0.1554	0.1591	0.1628	0.1664	0.1700	0.1736	0.1772	0.1808	0.1844	0.1879
0.5	0.1915	0.1950	0.1985	0.2019	0.2054	0.2088	0.2123	0.2157	0.2190	0.2224
0.6	0.2257	0.2291	0.234	0.2357	0.2389	0.2422	0.2454	0.2486	0.2517	0.2549
0.7	0.2580	0.2611	0.2642	0.2673	0.2704	0.2734	0.2764	0.2794	0.2823	0.2852
0.8	0.2881	0.2910	0.2939	0.2967	0.2995	0.3023	0.3051	0.3078	0.3106	0.3133
0.9	0.3159	0.3186	0.3212	0.3238	0.3264	0.3289	0.3315	0.334	0.3365	0.3389
1.0	0.3413	0.3438	0.3461	0.3485	0.3508	0.3531	0.3554	0.3577	0.3599	0.3621
1.1	0.3643	0.3665	0.3686	0.3708	0.3729	0.3749	0.3770	0.3790	0.3810	0.3830
1.2	0.3849	0.3869	0.3888	0.3907	0.3925	0.3944	0.3962	0.3980	0.3997	0.4015
1.3	0.4032	0.4049	0.4066	0.4082	0.4099	0.4115	0.4131	0.4147	0.4162	0.4177
1.4	0.4192	0.4207	0.4222	0.4236	0.4251	0.4265	0.4279	0.4292	0.4306	0.4319
1.5	0.4332	0.4345	0.4357	0.4370	0.4382	0.4394	0.4406	0.4418	0.4429	0.4441
1.6	0.4452	0.4463	0.4474	0.4484	0.4495	0.4405	0.4515	0.4525	0.4535	0.4545
1.7	0.4554	0.4564	0.4573	0.4582	0.4591	0.4599	0.4608	0.4616	0.4625	0.4633
1.8	0.4641	0.4649	0.4656	0.4664	0.4671	0.4678	0.4686	0.4693	0.4699	0.4706
1.9	0.4713	0.4719	0.4726	0.4732	0.4738	0.4744	0.4750	0.4756	0.4761	0.4767
2.0	0.4772	0.4778	0.4783	0.4788	0.4793	0.4798	0.4803	0.4808	0.4812	0.4817
2.1	0.4821	0.4826	0.4830	0.4834	0.4838	0.4842	0.4846	0.4850	0.4854	0.4857
2.2	0.4861	0.4864	0.4868	0.4871	0.4875	0.4878	0.4881	0.4884	0.4887	0.4890
2.3	0.4893	0.4896	0.4898	0.4901	0.4904	0.4906	0.4909	0.4911	0.4913	0.4916
2.4	0.4918	0.4920	0.4922	0.4925	0.4927	0.4929	0.4931	0.4932	0.4934	0.4936
2.5	0.4938	0.4940	0.4941	0.4943	0.4945	0.4946	0.4948	0.4949	0.4951	0.4952
2.6	0.4953	0.4955	0.4956	0.4957	0.4959	0.4960	0.4961	0.4962	0.4963	0.4964
2.7	0.4965	0.4966	0.4967	0.4968	0.4969	0.4970	0.4971	0.4972	0.4973	0.4974
2.8	0.4974	0.4975	0.4976	0.4976	0.4977	0.4978	0.4979	0.4979	0.4980	0.4981
2.9	0.4981	0.4982	0.4982	0.4983	0.4984	0.4984	0.4985	0.4985	0.4986	0.4986
3.0	0.4987	0.4987	0.4987	0.4988	0.4988	0.4989	0.4989	0.4989	0.4990	0.4990

Values of chi-square

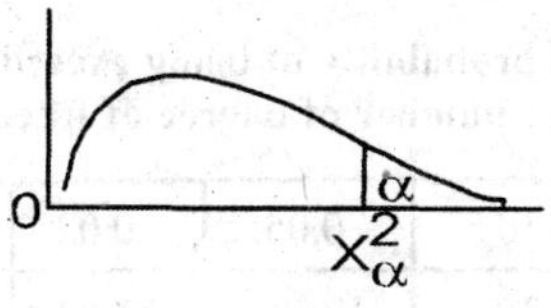

Table B

df \ α	100	0.50	0.25	0.10	0.05	0.001
1	2.71	3.84	5.02	6.63	7.88	1.8
2	4.61	5.99	7.38	9.21	10.60	13.8
3	6.25	7.81	9.35	11.30	12.80	16.3
4	7.78	9.49	11.10	13.30	14.90	18.5
5	9.24	11.10	12.80	16.10	15.70	20.5
6	10.6	12.6	14.4	16.8	18.5	22.5
7	12.0	14.1	16.0	18.5	20.3	24.3
8	13.4	15.5	17.5	20.1	22.0	26.1
9	14.7	16.9	19.0	21.7	23.6	27.9
10	16.0	18.3	20.5	23.2	25.2	29.6
11	17.3	19.7	21.9	24.7	26.8	31.3
12	18.5	21.0	23.3	26.2	28.3	32.9
13	19.8	22.4	24.7	27.7	29.8	34.5
14	21.1	23.7	26.1	29.1	31.3	36.1
15	22.3	25.0	27.5	30.6	32.8	37.7
16	23.5	26.3	28.8	32.0	34.3	39.3
17	24.8	27.8	30.2	33.4	35.7	40.8
18	26.0	28.9	31.5	34.8	37.2	42.3
19	27.2	30.1	32.0	36.2	38.6	43.8
20	28.4	31.4	34.2	37.6	40.0	45.3
21	29.6	32.7	35.5	38.9	41.4	46.8
22	30.8	33.9	36.8	40.3	42.8	48.3
23	32.0	35.2	38.1	41.6	44.2	49.7
24	33.2	36.4	39.4	43.0	45.6	51.2
25	34.4	37.7	40.6	44.3	46.9	52.6
26	35.6	38.9	41.9	45.6	48.3	54.1
27	36.6	40.1	43.2	47.0	49.6	55.5
28	37.9	41.3	44.5	48.3	51.0	56.9
29	39.1	42.6	45.7	49.6	52.3	58.3
30	40.3	43.8	47.0	50.9	53.7	59.7
35	46.4	49.8	53.2	57.3	60.3	66.6
40	51.8	55.8	59.3	63.7	66.8	73.4
45	57.6	61.7	65.4	70.0	73.2	80.1
50	63.2	67.5	71.4	76.2	79.5	86.7
55	68.8	73.3	77.4	82.3	85.7	93.2
60	74.4	79.1	83.3	88.4	92.0	99.6
65	80.0	84.8	89.2	94.4	98.1	106.0
70	85.5	90.5	95.0	100.4	104.2	112.3
75	91.1	96.2	100.8	106.4	110.3	118.6
80	96.6	101.9	106.6	112.3	116.3	124.8
85	102.1	107.5	112.4	118.2	122.3	131.0
90	107.6	113.1	118.1	124.1	128.3	137.2
95	113.0	118.8	123.9	130.0	134.2	143.3
100	118.5	124.3	129.6	135.8	140.2	149.4

Table C

Values of mod t with a probability of being exceeded in a random sampling v : number of degree of freedom

v/p	0.500	0.10	0.05	0.02	0.01
1	1.000	6.34	12.71	31.82	63.66
2	0.816	2.92	4.30	6.96	9.92
3	0.765	2.35	3.18	4.54	5.84
4	0.741	2.13	2.78	3.75	4.60
5	0.727	2.02	2.57	3.36	4.03
6	0.718	1.94	2.45	3.14	3.71
7	0.711	1.90	2.36	3.00	3.50
8	0.706	1.86	2.31	2.90	3.36
9	0.703	1.83	2.26	2.82	3.25
10	0.700	1.81	2.23	2.76	3.17
11	0.697	1.80	2.20	2.72	3.11
12	0.695	1.78	2.18	2.68	3.06
13	0.694	1.77	2.16	2.65	3.01
14	0.692	1.76	2.14	2.62	2.98
15	0.691	1.75	2.13	2.60	2.95
16	0.690	1.75	2.12	2.58	2.92
17	0.689	1.74	2.11	2.57	2.90
18	0.688	1.73	2.10	2.55	2.88
19	0.688	1.73	2.09	2.54	2.86
20	0.687	1.72	2.09	2.53	2.84
21	0.686	1.72	2.08	2.52	2.83
22	0.688	1.72	2.07	2.51	2.82
23	0.685	1.71	2.07	2.50	2.81
24	0.685	1.71	2.06	2.49	2.80
25	0.684	1.71	2.06	2.48	2.79
26	0.684	1.71	2.06	2.48	2.78
27	0.684	1.70	2.05	2.47	2.77
28	0.683	1.70	2.05	2.47	2.76
29	0.683	1.70	2.04	2.46	2.76
30	0.683	1.70	2.04	2.46	2.75
35	0.682	1.69	2.03	2.44	2.72
40	0.681	1.68	2.02	2.42	2.71
45	0.68	1.68	2.02	2.41	2.69
50	0.679	1.68	2.01	2.40	2.68
60	0.678	1.69	2.00	2.39	2.66
α	0.674	1.64	1.96	2.33	2.58

REFERENCES

1. Bean, E. M. L., *Estimation and sampling variance in the health interview survey*. National Centre for Health Statistics, Washington, D. C., Series 2, 38; 1970.

2. Balloc, N. B., *Validation of morbidity survey data by comparison with hospital records*. Jour. Amer. stat. Assoc. 49, 832-846; 1954.

3. Cornfield, J, *The determination of sample size*. Amer. Jour. Pub. Health 41, 654-661; 1951.

4. Dalanius, T., *Sampling in Sweden. Contributions to the methods and theories of sample survey practice*. Almquist and Wicksell, Stockholm, 1957.

5. Deming, W. E., *Sample Design in Business Research*. John Wiley and Sons, New York, 1960.

6. Des Raj, *On sampling with probabilities proportional to size*. Ganita 5, 175-82; 1954.

7. Fisher, R. A., *Statistical Methods for Research Workers*. Oliver and Boyd. Edinburgh, 13th ed., Section 21, 4th ed., 1952.

8. Frankel, M. R., *Infcrcncc from survcy samplcs*. Institute for Social Research, Ann. Arbor, Mich. 1971.

9. Kish, L., *Survey sampling*. John Wilcy & Sons, Ncw York, 1965.

10. Murthy, M. N., *Sampling theory and methods*. Statistical Publishing Society, Calcutta, India, 1967.

11. National Bureau of Standards, *Tables of the Binomial Probability Distribution*, U. S. Government Printing Office, Washington, D. C., 1950.

12. Nordin, J. A., *Determining sample size*, Jour. Amer. Stat. Assoc., 39, 497-506, 1972.

13. Sen, A R., *Some theory of sampling on successive occasions*. Australian Jour. Stat. 15, 105-110, 1973 (b).

14. Sneddecor, G. W. and Cochran, W. G., *Statistical methods*. Iowa stale University Press, Ames, Iowa, 6th edition, 1967.

15. Sukhatme, P. V., *Sampling theory of surveys, with applications*. Food and Agriculture Organisation, Rome, 2nd ed. 1970.

16. Trueblood, R. M., and Cyrit, R. M., *Sampling techniques in accounting*,Prentice-Hall, Englewood Cliffs, N. J., 1957.

17. W. Edwards Demihg, *Some theory of Sampling*, John Wiley and Sons, New York, 1950.

18. R. A. Fisher, *Statistical Methods for Research Workers*, Oliver and Boyd, Edinburgh and London, 10th ed., 1948.

19. Paul G. Hoel, *Introduction to Mathematical Statistics*, John Wiley and Sons, New York, 1947.

20. H. F. Dodge and H. G. Romig, *Sampling Inspection Tables*, John Wiley and Sons, New York, 1944.

21. E.S.Pearson, *The applications of statistical methods to Industrial Standardization and Quality Control*, British Standards Institutions London, 1935.

22. Statistical Research Group, columbia University, *Sequential analysis of statistical data*, Columbia University Press, New York, 1945.

23. W. A. Shewhart, *Economic control of quality of manufactured product*, D. Van Nostrand Co., New York, 1931.

24. W. A. Shewhart, *Statistical methods from the viewpoint of quality control*, U. S. Dept. of Agriculture, Graduate School, 1939.

25. Abraham Wald, *Sequential Analysis*, John Wiley and Sons, New York, 1947.

26. C. I. Bliss, *The calculation of the dosage: Mortality Curve*, Ann. Applied Biol 22, 134-167, 1935.

27. J. H. Gaddurn, *Reports on biological standards,* Med. Research Council Brit, special rept. Ser. 183, 1933.

28. G. W. Snedecor, *Statistical Methods*, Iowa State College Press, Ames, Iowa, 4th ed., 1946

29. L. H. C. Tippett, *Biometrika* 17, 386, 1926.

30. R. A. Fisher, *Applications of «student's» Distribution,* Metron 5, 3-17, 1925.

31. R. A. Fisher, *The Design of Experiments*, Oliver and Boyd, Edinburgh and London, 4th ed., 1947.

32. R. A. Fisher, *The use of multiple measurements in Taxonomic problems*, Ann. Eugen 7, 179-188, 1936.

33. Tore Dalenius, *Bibliography on Sampling*, Swedish Employers' Confederation, Stockholm, 1950.

34. W. Edwards Deming, *Some theory of sampling,* chapter 1, John Wiley and Sons, New York, 1950.

35. W. A. Hendericks, *Mathematics of Sampling,* Va. Agr. Exp. Stat. Spec. Tech. Bull., Blacksburg, 1948.

36. Earl. E Houseman, *Design of samples for surveys*, Agr. Econ. Research, 1 3-10, 1949.

37. P. C. Mahalanobis, *On large scale sample survey,* Phil. Trans. Roy. Soc., series B, 231, 329-451,1946.

38. Philip J. McCarthy, *Sampling-Elementary Principles*, N. Y. Slate school Indus. Labor Relations Bull. 15, Cornell University Ithaca, N. Y., 1951.

39. F. Yates, *Sampling methods for censuses and surveys*, chapter 1 & 2, Charles Griffen & Company, London, 1949.

40. F. Yates, *A review of recent statistical developments in sampling and sampling surveys*, J. Roy. stat. soc., 109, 12-45, 1946.

41. W. G. Cochran, *The use of analysis of variance in enumeration by sampling*, J. Amer. stat. Assoc., 34, 492-510, 1939.

42. R. J. Jessen, *Statistical investigation of a sample survey for obtaining farm facts*, Iowa Agr. Exp. Stat. Res. Bull. 304, 1942.

43. M. H. Hansen and W. N. Hurwitz, *A new sample of the population*, Estadistica II, 483-497, 1940.

44. M. H. Hansen and W. N. Hurwitz, *On the theory of sampling from finite populations*, Annals Math. Stat., 14, 332-362, 1943.

45. L. H. Madow, *Systematic sampling and its relation to other sampling designs*, J. American. Stat. Asson., 41, 204-217, 1946.

46. W. G. Madow and L. H. Madow, *On the theory of Systematic sampling*, I, Annals Math. stat., 15, 1-24,1944.
47. W. R. Buckland, *A review of the literature of systematic sampling*, J. Roy. Stat. Soc., Series B 13, 208-215, 1951.
48. M. H. Hansen, W. N. Hurwitz and W. G. Madow, *Sample survey methods and theory: Methods and applications*, Vol. 1, John Wiley & sons, Inc., London, 1956.
49. Lwanga, S.K., and Lameshow, S., *Sample size determination in health studies, A practical manual*, World Health Organisation, Geneva, 1991.
50. Hill, A. Bradford, *Principles of medical statistics*, 8th edn., London: Lancet, 1996.
51. Wilts, L. J., *Medical survey and clinical trails*, London, New York, Oxford University Press, 1969.
52. Gene A, Mc Grady *et.al*, *An outbreak of necrotizing entrocolitis association with transfusion of packed red blood cells*, American Journal of Epidemiology, Vol. 126, 65-72, 1985.
53. Robert S. *et.al*, *Risk factors for urinary tract infection, American Journal of Epidemiology*, Vol. 126, No. 4, 685-694, 1987.
54. Toman K, *Sensitivity, specificity and predictive value of diagnostic tests*. Bull. Int. Union Tub., 56, 18,1981.
55. Walker, H. N., *Studies in the history of statistical method: Baltimore*: The Williams and Wilkins Company, 1929.
56. Westergoard, H., *Contributions to the history of statistics,* London: P. S. King & Son, 1932.
57. Kendall, M.G. and Plackett R. L. eds., *Studies in the history of statistics and probability*, Vol II, New York: Macmillan Publishing Co., Inc., 1977.
58. Pearson, E.S., and Kendall M. G., eds., *Studies in the history of statistics and probability*. Darien conn.: Hafner Publishing Co., Inc., 1970.
59. Porter, T. M., *The rise of statistical thinking, 1820-1900*. Princetoon: Princeton University Press, 1986.

60. Stigler, S. M., *The history of statistics*, Cambridge: Harvard University Press, 1986.

61. Feller, W., *An introduction to probability theory and its applications*, Vol. I, 3rd ed. New York: John Wiley & Sons, Inc. 1968.

62. Parzen , E., *Modern probability theory and its applications*, New York: John Wiley & Sons, Inc., 1960.

63. Hogg, R.V. and Craig, A.T., *Introduction to mathematical statistics*, 4th ed., New York; Mcmillan Publishing Co., Inc., 1978.

64. Kendall, M.G. and Stuart A, *The advanced theory of statistics*, Vol. I, 4th ed. New York: Mcmillan Publishing Co, Inc., 1950,

65. Yule, G.U., and Kendall, M. G., *An introduction to the theory of statitics*, 14 th ed., New York; Hafner Publishing Co., Inc., 1950.

66. Cramer, H., *Mathematical methods of statistics*, Princeton, N.J., Princeton University Press, 1950.

67. Row, C. R., *Advanced statistical methods in Biometric research*, New York, John Wiley & Sons, Inc., 1952.

68. Mood, A. M., Graybill, F. A. and Boes, D.C., *Introduction to the theory of statistics*, 3rd ed., New York: Mc-Graw Hill Book Company, 1974.

69. Lehmann, E. L., *Testing statistical hypothesis*, New York: John Wiley & Sons, Inc., 1950.

70. Hoel, P., *Introduction to mathematical Statistics*, 3rd ed., New York: John Wiley and Sons., Inc., 1962.

71. Anderson, V. L., and McLean, R. A., *Design of Experiments: A realistic approach*, New York: Marcel Dekker, Inc., 1974.

72. Cochran, W. G. and Cox, G.M., *Experimental design*, 2nd ed., New York: John Wiley and Sons, Inc., 1957.

73. Snedoor, G. W. and Cochran W. G., *Statistical methods*, 8th ed., Ames, IOWA, Iowa University Press, 1989.

74. Siegel, S., *Non-parametric statistics for the behavioural sciences*, New York; Mc Graw Hill Book Company, 1956.

75. Freund J.E., *Introduction to probability*, Encino, Calif: Dickenson Publishing Co., Inc., 1973.

76. Goldberg,S. *Probability–An introduction*, Mineola, N.Y.:Dover Publications.Inc. (republication of 1960 edition).

77. Fraser, D.A.S., *Probability and statistics: Theory and applications*, North Scituate, Mass: Dwcbury Press, 1976.

78. Acheson, E. D., *Medical record linkage*, London, Oxford University Press, 1967.

79. P. Armitage, *Statistical methods in medical research*, Blackwell Scientific Publications, Oxford and Edinburgh, 1971.

80. Bailey, N.T.J., A *classification of methods of ascertainment and analysis in estimating the frequencies of recessive in man,* Ann. Eugen. 16, 223-225, 1951.

81. Bartelett, M.S., *Properties of sufficiency and statistical tests*. Proc. R. Soc., A 160, 268-282, 1937.

82. Benjamin B., *Health and Vital Statistics*, London: Allen and Unwin.

83. Cochran W. G., *Sampling Techniques,* 2nd ed., New York; Wiley, 1963.

84. Cox, D. R., *Planning of Experiments*, New York: Wiley, 1958.

85. Cox, D. R., *Demography*, 4th ed., Cambridge University Press, 1970.

86. Draper, N.R. and Smith H., *Applied Regression Analysis*, New York, Wiley, 1966.

87. Finney, D. J., Latscha R., Bennett, B.M. and H S U P, *Tables for testing significance at a 2X2 contingency Table,* Cambridge: University Press, 1963.

88. Fisher, R. A., *The Significance of deviations from expectation in a Poisson series*. Biometrics, 6, 17-24: reprinted in 20, 265-272, 1964.

89. Fisher R, A. and Yates F., *Statistical tables for biological, agricultural and medical research*, 6th ed., Edinburgh: Oliver and Boyd, 1963.

90. Greenhouse, S.W. and Mantel, N., *The evaluation of diagnostic tests,* Biometrics 6, 399-412, 1950.

91. Hill, A. Bradford, *Statistical methods in clinical and preventive medicine*, Edinburgh: Livingstone, 1962.

92. Hill A. Bradford, *Principles of Medical statistics*, 8th edn., London: Lancet, 1966.

93. Kendall, M.G., *A course in Multivariate analysis*, London :Griffin, 1957.

94. King, .E. P., *A statistical design for drug screening*, Biometrics, 19, 429-440, 1963.

95. Kramer, M. and Greenhouse, S. W., *Determination of sample size and Selection of cases in psychopharmacology: Problems in Evaluation*, ed. J.O. Cole and R.W. Geerard, 356-371, Washington National Academy of Sciences, National Research Council, 1959.

96. Moser, C.A., *Survey methods in social investigations*, London: Heinemann, 1958.

97. Seal A. L., *Multivariate statistical analysis for biologists*, London: Methuen, 1964.

98. Yates F., *Contingency Tables involving small numbers and Chi-square test*, J. R. Satist.Soc., Supple l, 217-235, 1934 (a).

99. Biemer P. and L.Lyberg, *Introduction to Survey Quality*, Wiley, 2003.

100. Lehtonen R., and E. Pahkinen, *Practical Methods for Design and Analysis of Complex Surveys*, Wiley, 2003.

101. Casella G., and R. Berger, *Statistical Inference*, Wadsworth Pub. Co., 2001.

102. Lehmann E. and G. Casella, *Theory of Point Estimation*, Springer Verlag, NewYork, 1998.

103. Levy P. and S. Lemeshow, *Sampling of Populations: Methods and Applications*, Wiley, 1999.

INDEX